Advanced ERCP for Complicated and Refractory Biliary and Pancreatic Diseases

Dong Ki Lee
Editor

Advanced ERCP for Complicated and Refractory Biliary and Pancreatic Diseases

Springer

Editor
Dong Ki Lee
Department of Internal Medicine
Gangnam Severance Hospital
Yonsei University College of Medicine
Seoul
South Korea

ISBN 978-981-13-0607-5 ISBN 978-981-13-0608-2 (eBook)
https://doi.org/10.1007/978-981-13-0608-2

This Springer imprint is published by the registered company Springer Nature Singapore Pte Ltd.
The registered company address is: 152 Beach Road, #21-01/04 Gateway East, Singapore 189721, Singapore

It is with great admiration, respect, and love that I dedicate this book to a courageous, intelligent, and wonderful woman, my wife, Kyung Won, who is truly the "wind beneath my wings."

Contents

1 High-Level Biliary Strictures After Living-Donor Liver Transplantation

Young Min Kim, Tae Ryong Chung, and Dong Ki Lee

Introduction

Biliary complications after surgery, such as liver transplantation (LT) and cholecystectomy, include biliary stricture and leakage and formation of a biliary cast, sludge, and/or stone. The incidence of biliary complications after LT is 10–35% [1, 2]. Despite advances in surgical techniques and the development of immunosuppressants, biliary complications after LT remain a major cause of morbidity and, in severe cases, mortality.

Biliary stricture is the most common complication after LT, accounting for ~40% of all biliary complications [3–8]. The symptoms of biliary stricture range from none to pruritus and abdominal pain. If biliary stricture is overlooked, severe complications such as ascending cholangitis, liver abscess, and secondary biliary cirrhosis can result. Therefore, high-risk patients should be monitored closely. Moreover, in patients with high-level biliary stricture, the intrahepatic duct is narrow, and the distal part of the stent has a high rate of migration over the stricture.

In this chapter, we focus on the definition, incidence, etiology, pathophysiology, risk factors, and management of high-level biliary stricture after living-donor LT (LDLT).

Definition

Biliary strictures after LT are classified as anastomotic (AS) or non-anastomotic (NAS) strictures according to location. AS occurs at the site of anastomosis between the choledochal duct of the donor and the choledochal duct of the jejunal Roux limb of the recipient. NAS also occurs in other parts of the biliary system [9, 10] and patients with both types of strictures have been reported. In this chapter, we will discuss high-level biliary strictures, which occur at or around the bifurcation of the left and right hepatic ducts [11]. Endoscopic retrograde cholangiopancreatography (ERCP) images of high- and low-level biliary strictures are shown in Fig. 1.1.

Incidence

Benign biliary stricture (BBS) is a common complication after LT. The incidence of biliary stricture after LDLT is 25–32% [3, 12–15] compared with <15% after deceased-donor LT (DDLT) [14, 16, 17]. In LDLT, anastomosis between the right hepatic duct of the donor and the bile duct of the recipient is highly complex. The right hepatic duct has many anatomic variations, including multiple bile ducts, poor blood supply, and a

Y. M. Kim · T. R. Chung · D. K. Lee (✉)
Department of Internal Medicine, Gangnam Severance Hospital, Yonsei University College of Medicine, Seoul, South Korea
e-mail: dklee@yuhs.ac

D. K. Lee (ed.), *Advanced ERCP for Complicated and Refractory Biliary and Pancreatic Diseases*,
https://doi.org/10.1007/978-981-13-0608-2_1

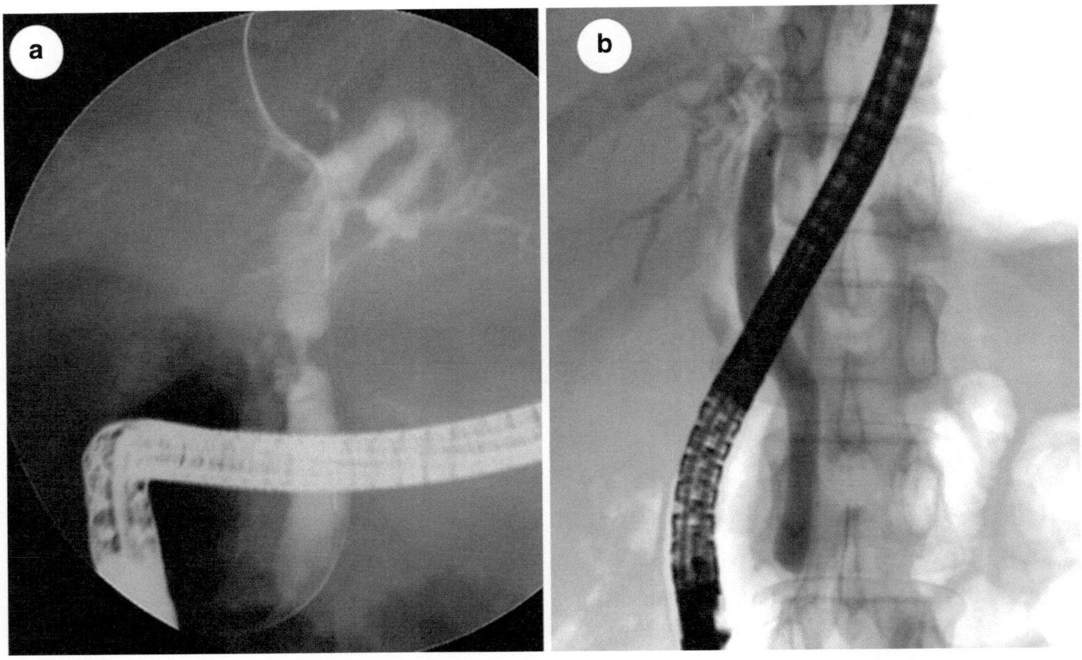

Fig. 1.1 Two types of benign biliary stricture (BBS) according to the location of stricture. (**a**) Shows low-level BBS and is mainly observed in patients who have undergone a deceased donor liver transplantation. On the other hand, (**b**) shows high-level BBS and is observed mainly in patients who have undergone living donor liver transplantation

short stump [6, 14, 15, 18]. Also, hypertrophy of the received liver aggravates ASs. Biliary stricture is more common after LDLT (33.3%) than after DDLT (9.6%) [7, 19–22]. LDLT is the treatment of choice for end-stage liver disease, particularly in East Asia, including South Korea, because it is more difficult to obtain organs from deceased donors than is the case in Western nations. In Asia, the incidence of biliary stricture has decreased from 30% to 15–25% due to accumulation of experience with LDLT [6, 23–27].

In a prospective study of 531 patients who underwent LT from 1979 to 2003, AS occurred in 47 (42 duct-to-duct anastomosis and 5 hepaticojejunal Roux-en-Y anastomosis) patients, and the cumulative risks of AS at 1, 5, and 10 years were 6.6%, 10.6%, and 12.3%, respectively [1].

Etiology

The causes of biliary strictures include LT, postoperative injury after cholecystectomy, pancreatitis, primary sclerosing cholangitis, and stone disease. A 68-year-old female underwent laparoscopic cholecystectomy 25 years prior and had BBS due to recurrent common hepatic duct (CHD) and common bile duct stones. An ERCP cholangiogram showed a stricture of, and a stone in, the left intrahepatic duct (Fig. 1.2). A 44-year-old female underwent left hemihepatectomy for intrahepatic cholangiocarcinoma. An ERCP cholangiogram showed a stricture of the CHD, and abdominal computed tomography (CT) showed bile leakage due to postoperative injury (Fig. 1.3).

We will focus on the etiology of biliary strictures after LDLT (Table 1.1). AS can be caused by the surgical technique and local ischemia, whereas NAS can be caused by, for example, hepatic artery thrombosis or immunological factors, prolonged cold ischemia, and vascular insufficiency [10, 28–30]. Biliary strictures early after LT are caused by technical factors. In contrast, those occurring late after LT are typically caused by hepatic artery thrombosis, preservation-induced injury, prolonged cold and warm ischemia, altered bile composition, and immunological injury.

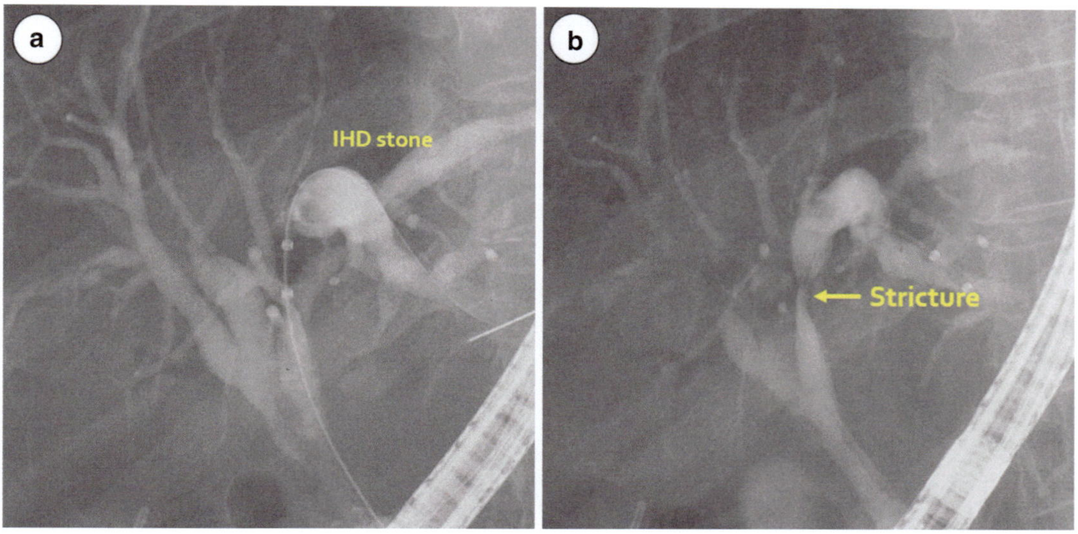

Fig. 1.2 Benign biliary stricture due to intrahepatic bile duct stone. An ERCP cholangiogram shows a stone (**a**) and stricture (**b**) in the left hepatic duct

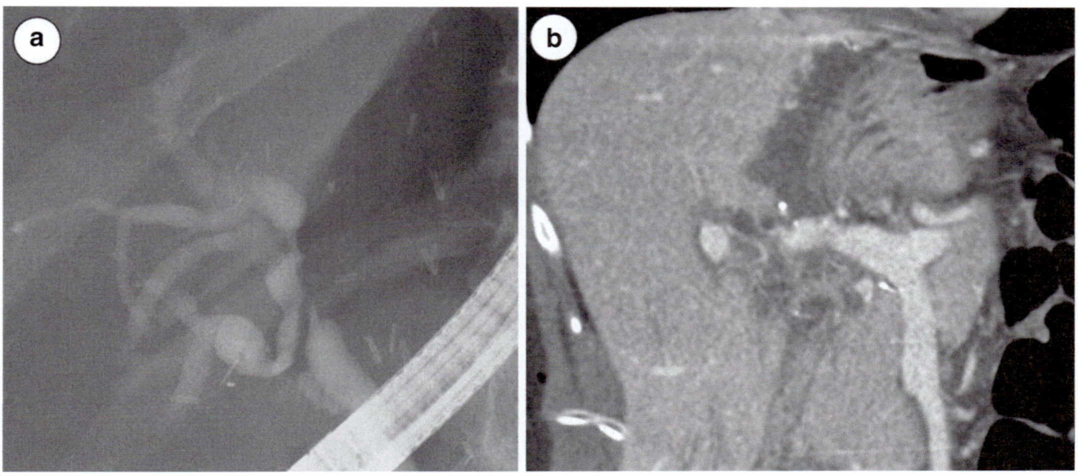

Fig. 1.3 Benign biliary stricture due to postoperative injury after hemihepatectomy. An ERCP cholangiogram shows stricture of the common hepatic duct (**a**), and abdominal CT shows bile leakage (**b**)

Pathophysiology

Biliary tract injury such as surgery induces an inflammatory response, resulting in fibrosis and narrowing of the lumen of the bile duct.

Cytokines and chemokines are key mediators of hepatobiliary inflammation [31]. Pro-inflammatory cytokines such as interleukin-6, tumor necrosis factor-alpha, and interferon-gamma induce a cell-mediated immune response and promote hepatobiliary injury. Also, chemokine ligand (CCL) 2, CCL5, and fractalkine (CX3CL1) induce transendothelial migration of leukocytes, resulting in induction of an inflammatory cascade [32]. Genetic polymorphisms in the chemokine receptors (CCRs) that mediate leukocyte trafficking alter their expression and function, affecting hepatobiliary inflammation after LT [33, 34]. The association between a loss-of-function mutation in CC chemokine receptor 5 delta 32 and occurrence of ischemic-type biliary lesions has been

Table 1.1 Etiology for biliary stricture after liver transplantation

Anastomotic stricture
Surgical technique
Local ischemia
Non-anastomotic stricture
Hepatic artery thrombosis
Immunological factors
Prolonged cold ischemia times
Vascular insufficiency
Early stage after transplantation
Technical reasons
Later stage after transplantation
Hepatic artery thrombosis
Preservation-induced injury
Prolonged cold and warm ischemia times
Altered bile composition
Immunological injury

Table 1.2 Risk factors for biliary stricture after liver transplantation

Verdonk et al. [1]
Postoperative bile leakage
Female donor/male recipient combination
Labob et al. [38]
CX3CR1-249II allele
Liver transplantation for acute liver failure
ABO-compatible non-identical liver transplantation
Forrest et al. [39]
Hepatic artery thrombosis
Primary sclerosing cholangitis
Postoperative day 7 total bilirubin >55 μmol/L
Jeong et al. [40]
Short duct diameter
Ductoplasty
Cytomegalovirus infection

investigated [30, 34], and the effects of human leucocyte antigen (HLA) mismatch and anti-HLA antibodies on liver allograft survival are controversial [30, 34–38].

Chronic stricture results in atrophy of the hepatic segment of the lobe that drains into the involved bile duct and hypertrophy of the unaffected segments, leading eventually to secondary biliary cirrhosis and portal hypertension.

Risk Factor

Among 531 patients who underwent LT, postoperative bile leakage, female donor/male recipient combination, and a short stay in the intensive care unit were associated with AS in univariate analyses. Of these, postoperative bile leakage and female donor/male recipient combination were independent risk factors for AS [1].

In a cross-sectional study of 162 patients who underwent LT from 2009 to 2010 [38], LT for acute liver failure, ABO-compatible non-identical LT, and donor-specific anti-HLA class II AB were associated with AS in univariate analyses. Of these, LT for acute liver failure and ABO-compatible non-identical LT were independent risk factors for AS. Also, specific chemokine receptor polymorphisms and altered cytokine profiles in the recipient promoted fibrotic tissue remodeling leading to biliary stricture. Screening for anti-HLA antibodies enables early detection of biliary stricture in high-risk patients.

Hepatic artery thrombosis and primary sclerosing cholangitis are independent risk factors for biliary stricture after LT [39]. Interestingly, a total bilirubin level >55 μmol/L on postoperative day 7 was also an independent risk factor and may be a clinical indicator of biliary stricture. In another study, hepatic artery thrombosis, a small-diameter duct, ductoplasty, and cytomegalovirus infection were independent risk factors for biliary complications after LT [40]. The risk factors for high-level biliary stricture after LT are listed in Table 1.2.

Endoscopic Management

Difficulty in Endoscopic Treatment of BBS

Endoscopic treatment in recipients of LDLT with complex BBS with multiple ductal anastomoses and a bizarre configuration can be difficult [41]. The success rate of endoscopic treatment of AS is lower in LDLT patients (58–76%) than in DDLT patients (80–90%) [6, 17, 42]. In particular, endoscopic treatment of BBS in LDLT patients characterized by high-level biliary stricture is more difficult than DDLT because of its anatomical nature (Fig. 1.1). In particular, endoscopic treatment of BBS is more difficult in LDLT patients with high-level biliary strictures than in DDLT patients (Fig. 1.1). The reconstructed bile ducts in LDLT patients are characterized by twisted biliary strictures or small-caliber, multiple, complex anastomotic bile ducts caused by anastomotic fibrosis and hypertrophy of the donor liver [43]. Endoscopic treatment is problematic because manipulation of the device (including the guidewire) is difficult, multiple plastic stent insertion is hampered by a lack of space in the intrahepatic bile duct (IHD), a long stent is required, and only the proximal part of the stent passes the stricture site. Consequently, there is a high probability of stent migration and dysfunction. Transient narrowing of the biliary anastomosis that occurs 1–2 months after LT is predominantly due to postoperative edema and inflammation, endoscopic treatment of which is highly likely to be successful. However, if late-onset biliary stricture after LDLT occurs or diagnosis is delayed, the probability of failure of primary endoscopic therapy is relatively high [44].

Balloon Dilatation and/or Plastic Stent Insertion

Endoscopic management, consisting of biliary sphincterotomy, balloon dilatation, and stent replacement, is generally the first-line treatment for biliary stricture after LDLT [45]. Extant reports on endoscopic management of BBS after LDLT are listed in Table 1.3. Repeated ERCPs at 2–3 month intervals are preferred and require upsizing of the plastic stent (8.0–11.5 Fr) or maintenance of six to eight stents for at least 1 year (Figs. 1.4 and 1.5) [46]. There has been much debate as to whether balloon dilatation alone is superior to balloon dilatation with stent placement for treating biliary stricture. Although stent placement is associated with a higher incidence of complications, balloon dilatation with stent placement is superior to balloon dilatation alone [47–49]. Balloon dilation (BD) with multiple plastic stent (MPS) results in a clinical success rate 50–75% higher than that of BD alone [48]. In addition, insertion of multiple stents is more effective for stricture dilatation than is insertion of a single stent [49, 50]. Endoscopic sphincterotomy is often used to relieve AS, but some clinicians prefer to insert multiple large internal stents into the narrowing bile duct, which prevents ERCP-induced pancreatitis or enterobiliary reflux due to compression of the pancreatic orifice. Moreover, patients receiving LT should be given immunosuppressive agents, and the risk of infection must be considered. Patients with biliary stricture after LDLT in whom an internal endoscopic stent was placed above the intact

Table 1.3 Treatment outcomes of endoscopic management of anastomotic biliary stricture in living-donor liver transplantation

Author (year)	No. of patients (*n*)	Technique	No. of procedures per patients (mean)	Technical success rate (%)	Clinical success rate (%)	Recurrence rate (%)	Complication rate (%)	Recurrence treatment
Lee et al. (2011) [78]	137	BD + stent	4.8	46.7	–	–	–	–
Kim et al. (2011) [79]	147	BD + stent	6.3	55.8	36.9	11.5	7.2	ERCP
Kurita et al. (2011) [51]	94	BD + stent	1.4	79.7	90.1	9.9	22.3	ERCP, PTBD, re-LT
Hsieh et al. (2013) [80]	41	BD + stent	4.0	84.2	100.0	21.0	17.1	ERCP
Chok et al. (2014) [81]	56	BD ± stent	3.0	–	73.2	–	40.0	–

BD biliary drainage, *ERCP* endoscopic retrograde cholangiopancreatography, *PTBD* percutaneous transhepatic biliary drainage, *LT* liver transplantation

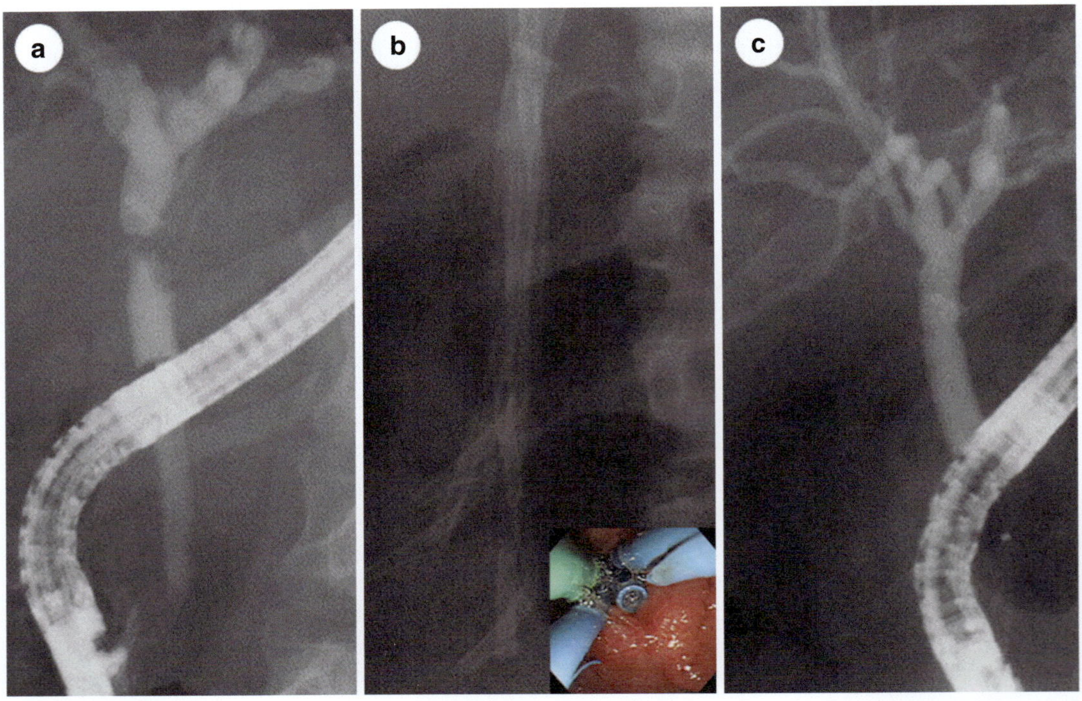

Fig. 1.4 High-level benign biliary stricture treated with multiple plastic stents (MPSs). An ERCP cholangiogram shows a high-level biliary stricture (**a**). After 3 months, five MPSs were inserted at the stricture site (**b**), and the stricture was resolved (**c**)

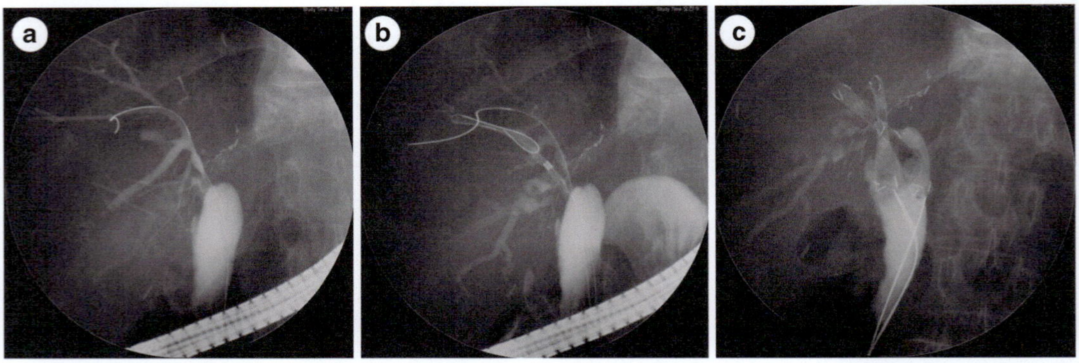

Fig. 1.5 Limitation in plastic stent insertion due to pouched-type benign biliary stricture. An ERCP cholangiogram shows a pouched-type biliary anastomosis (**a**). The ability to position MPS was limited. Instead, after difficult passage of a guidewire through the orifice at the site of the pouched-type stricture (**b**), two FCSEMSs were inserted at the stricture site (**c**)

sphincter of Oddi achieved long-term stent patency and a high remission rate [51]. However, because endoscopic sphincterotomy facilitates dilatation of the stricture, placement of stents, and removal of stones during repeated ERCP procedures, additional studies are needed.

Self-Expanding Metal Stents

Self-expanding metal stents (SEMSs) can also be used to treat biliary strictures. Early anastomotic biliary stricture (ABS) (<6 months post-LT) generally shows a good therapeutic response to single endoscopic therapy, but treatment is prolonged by a stricture at the site of anastomosis, likely due to ischemic injury [1]. In addition, post-LDLT ABS occurs at a high level and involves acute angulated bile duct anastomosis and a narrow luminal space in the upper intrahepatic bile duct above the ABS. These features hamper the treatment of high-level biliary strictures. SEMS are of large diameter (30 Fr), which reduces the number of ERCP attempts and accelerates stricture resolution. The main reasons of stent occlusion are stent ingrowth and overgrowth and biliary stone and sludge formation in the stent [52–55]. Fully covered SEMS (FCSEMSs) overcome most of the disadvantages of uncovered SEMS and can be removed endoscopically, facilitating treatment of BBS. Various types of FCSEMS are available (Table 1.4 and Fig. 1.6).

Table 1.4 Biliary fully covered self-expanding metal stents (FCSEMs) commercially available

Manufacturer	Model	Material	Diameter (mm)	Length (cm)
Boston Scientific	The WallFlex Biliary RX stent	Platinol covered with permalume	8, 10	4, 6, 8
Taewoong Medical	Niti-S Biliary stent	Nitinol covered with silicone	6, 8, 10	4, 5, 6, 7, 8, 9, 10, 12
M.I. Tech	Flap with Lasso	Nitinol covered with silicone	8, 10	4, 12
Standard SciTech	Bonastent	Nitinol covered with silicone	10	4, 5, 6, 7, 8, 9, 10

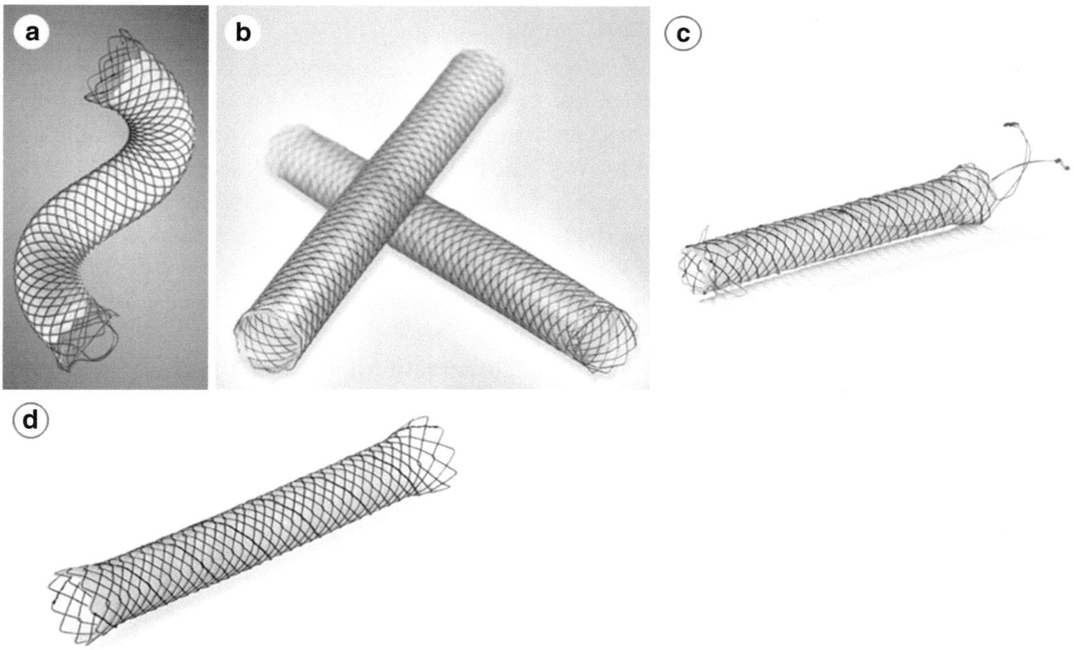

Fig. 1.6 Commercially available fully covered self-expanding metal stents (FCSEMSs). WallFlex Biliary RX stent by Boston Scientific, MA (**a**). Niti-S Biliary stent by Taewoong Medical, South Korea (**b**). Flap with Lasso stent by M.I. Tech, South Korea (**c**). Bonastent by Standard SciTech, South Korea (**d**). (Adapted from (**a**) http://www.bostonscientific.com/en-US/products/stents%2D%2Dgastrointestinal/wallflex-biliary-rx-stents.html. (**b**) http://www.stent.net/products/gastroenterology/niti-s-self-expandable-metal-stent/niti-s-biliary-stent/s-biliary-stent-covered-2/. (**c**) http://www.mitech.co.kr/custom/prCustomView.do?disp_idx=DPIDX00010&menu_nix=FS9X8VzA. (**d**) https://www.mediteksystems.com/bonastent-standard-sci-tech/bonastent-biliary/#.XGecpegzaUk)

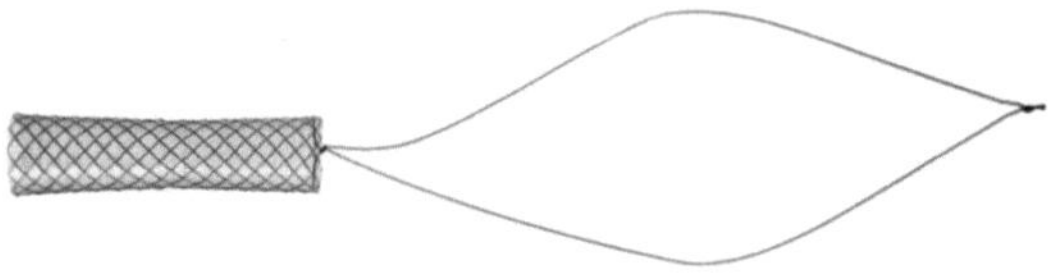

Fig. 1.7 Modified fully covered self-expanding metal stents (FCSEMSs) named Kaffes. The central waist is located at the center of the stricture site and is shorter than those of other stents. The string facilitates stent removal. (Adapted from http://www.stent.net/products/gastroenterology/niti-s-self-expandable-metal-stent/niti-s-biliary-stent/kaffes-biliary-stent-2/)

Compared with plastic stents, FCSEMSs have better durability and patency and require fewer ERCP procedures [56, 57]. The recurrence and complication rates of FCSEMSs are comparable with those of plastic stents [56]. In randomized controlled trials of DDLT patients, a SEMS and the use of multiple plastic stents were similar in terms of the rate of stricture resolution, but the SEMS required fewer total interventions [56, 58]. Stent migration is a major disadvantage of FCSEMSs. According to a recent meta-analysis of SEMSs for AS, the overall SEMS migration rate was ~16% [59]. In addition, sludge or stones may form in the stent cavity, and FCSEMS can be indwelling for no more than 3–4 months. We evaluated the efficacy of a short FCSEMS with a string and central waist (Fig. 1.7) (Kaffes stent; Taewoong Medical, Seoul, South Korea) [60] in 35 LDLT patients with refractory stricture. The stricture resolution rate was 83% and the stent migration rate 6%, and the Kaffes stent did not migrate. Several cases of treatment with FCSEMS insertion are shown in Figs. 1.8, 1.9, and 1.10.

Percutaneous Treatment

In general, percutaneous treatment can be applied in patients with Roux-en-Y reconstruction surgery or a severely stenotic or disconnected bile duct that cannot be passed by an endoscopic retrograde approach [61] (Fig. 1.11). Percutaneous therapy is often considered a second-line alternative treatment, despite its high success rate, because the procedure is invasive and may cause post-procedural discomfort. Percutaneous therapy also has risks of bleeding, pseudoaneurysm, bile leakage, and infection [62]. However, percutaneous transhepatic drainage (PTBD) can be successful in cases of ERCP failure, especially in patients with hilar-level BBS. Endoscopic therapy in patients with a pouched bile-duct anastomosis has the lowest success rate. In our previous study [63], 15 of 22 patients (68%) with post-LDLT biliary strictures in whom endoscopic therapy failed were treated successfully by PTBD. This is also true for patients with malignant hilar lesions [64].

Rendezvous Technique

An endoscopic technique and percutaneous transhepatic cholangiography can be combined to facilitate bile duct cannulation, known as the rendezvous method. In addition, replacing the PTBD catheter with an internal-drainage stent via ERCP is difficult if passage of the guidewire is obstructed by angulated or twisted biliary strictures. The rendezvous technique can overcome this difficulty (Fig. 1.12). In the classic rendezvous technique, the guidewire is passed through the PTBD tract for an endoscopic approach to the bile duct. However, because it is not easy to manipulate, the rendezvous technique using the Kumpe (KMP) catheter (5 Fr, 40 cm; Cook, Bloomington, IN) was used to treat biliary strictures after LDLT [65] In that study, the KMP catheter resulted in a significantly shorter procedure time than that using a guidewire. End-to-end contact between an ERCP cannula and the end of a KMP catheter can be achieved because the tip of the KMP catheter is short, angled, and easy to rotate. Thus, KMP catheter rendezvous techniques may be recommended for recipients of LDLT who have angulated or twisted anastomotic biliary strictures.

Surgery

Endoscopic management is the most important treatment for BBS but is unsuitable for recurrent or refractory BBS. Therefore, surgical

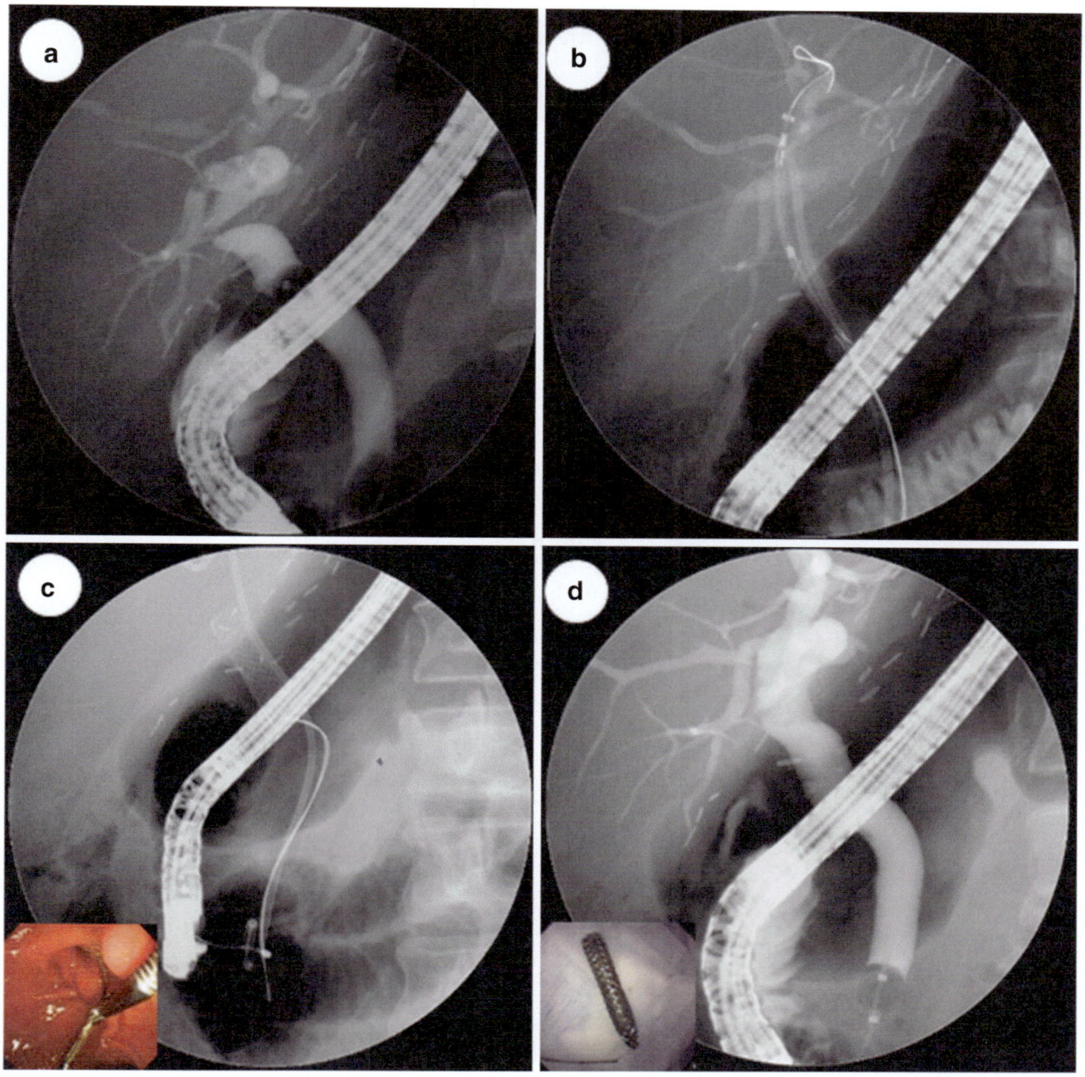

Fig. 1.8 First case of hilar BBS after LDLT treated with the Kaffes FCSEMS. An ERCP cholangiogram shows the shape and length of the stricture site (**a**). The guidewire was passed through the stricture site (**b**), and the Kaffes stent was located and deployed. A plastic stent was co inserted to prevent IHD occlusion draining into the CHD. After ~3 months, the Kaffes stent was removed by grasping the long string using alligator forceps (**c**), and the stricture had resolved (**d**)

treatment may be considered to prevent sepsis and graft failure when refractory biliary strictures recur despite endoscopic or percutaneous treatment [66]. Surgical treatment includes repair of the biliary anastomosis, conversion from duct-to-duct anastomosis to hepaticojejunostomy (HJ), and retransplantation. HJ anastomosis comprises end-to-side and side-to-side HJ. Side-to-side HJ has several theoretical advantages over end-to-side HJ. First, there is no need to dissect the posterior aspect of the bile duct, thus avoiding injury to the hepatic artery due to post-LT adhesion. Second, side-to-side HJ can be used for endoscopic treatment at the time of stricture relapse. However, side-to-side HJ is only possible when the native common bile duct is of sufficient length. Therefore, side-to-side HJ may be suitable for

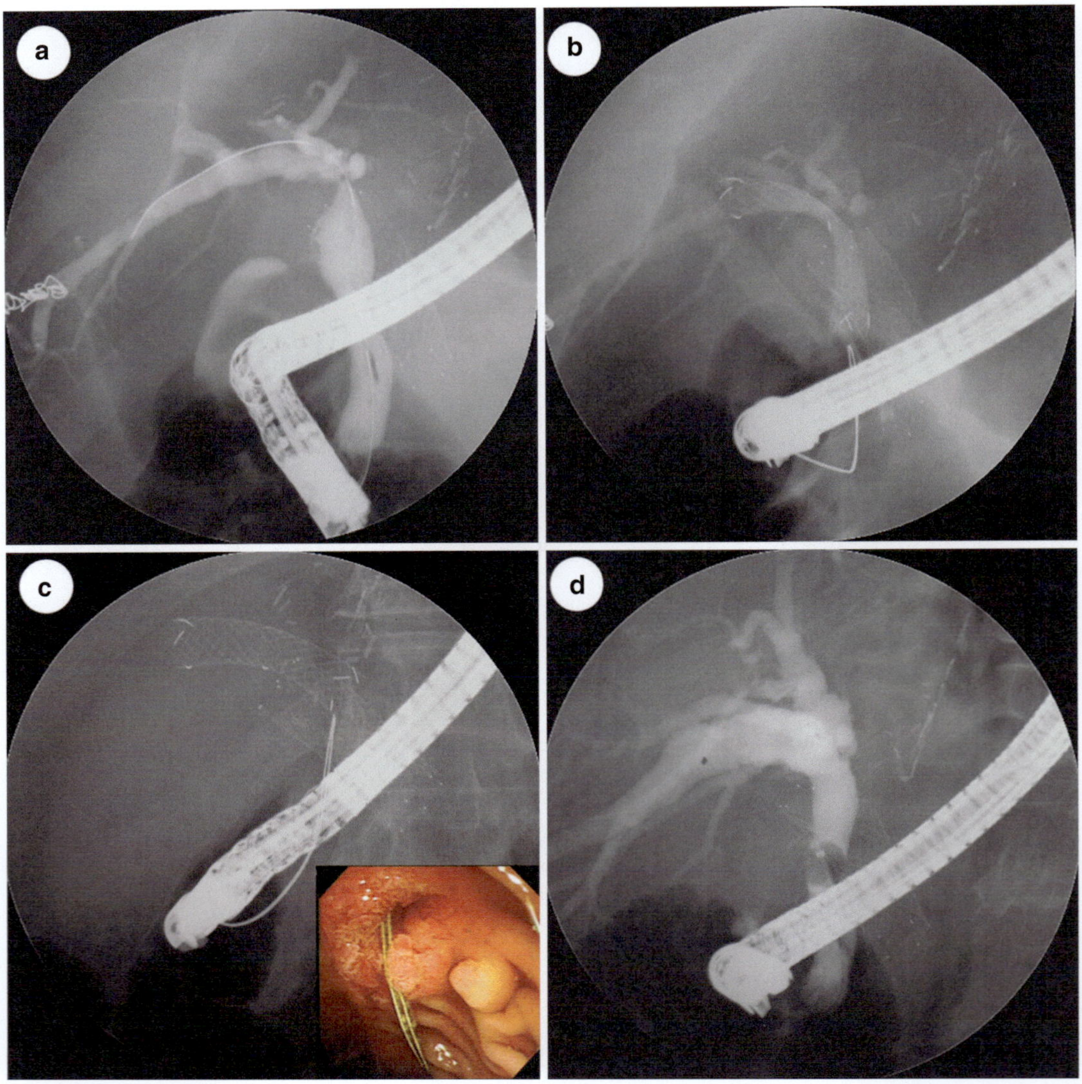

Fig. 1.9 Second case of hilar BBS after LDLT treated with the Kaffes FCSEMS. (**a**) An ERCP cholangiogram shows the shape and length of the stricture site. The guidewire was passed through the stricture site (**b**), and the Kaffes stent was deployed. After ~3 months, the Kaffes stent was removed by grasping the string using alligator forceps (**c**), and the stricture had resolved (**d**)

reconstruction of the bile duct after failed endoscopic treatment [67].

New Attempts

New types of balloons and stents can be used for the management of biliary strictures. The balloon dilatation method has a relatively high failure rate for severely fibrotic anastomotic bile ducts. In that case, percutaneous cutting balloon incision and dilation may be used to treat biliary AS after LT [68]. During balloon inflation, a 1-cm-long microsurgical blade is exposed to incise the stenotic segment. There are no major or minor procedure-related complications related to the procedure, and failure was reported in only one case.

In a 2012 study, among 13 patients with symptomatic AS after LT paclitaxel-eluting balloon dilation, 12 had no recurrence for 24 months, and the long-term clinical success rate was 92.3% [69].

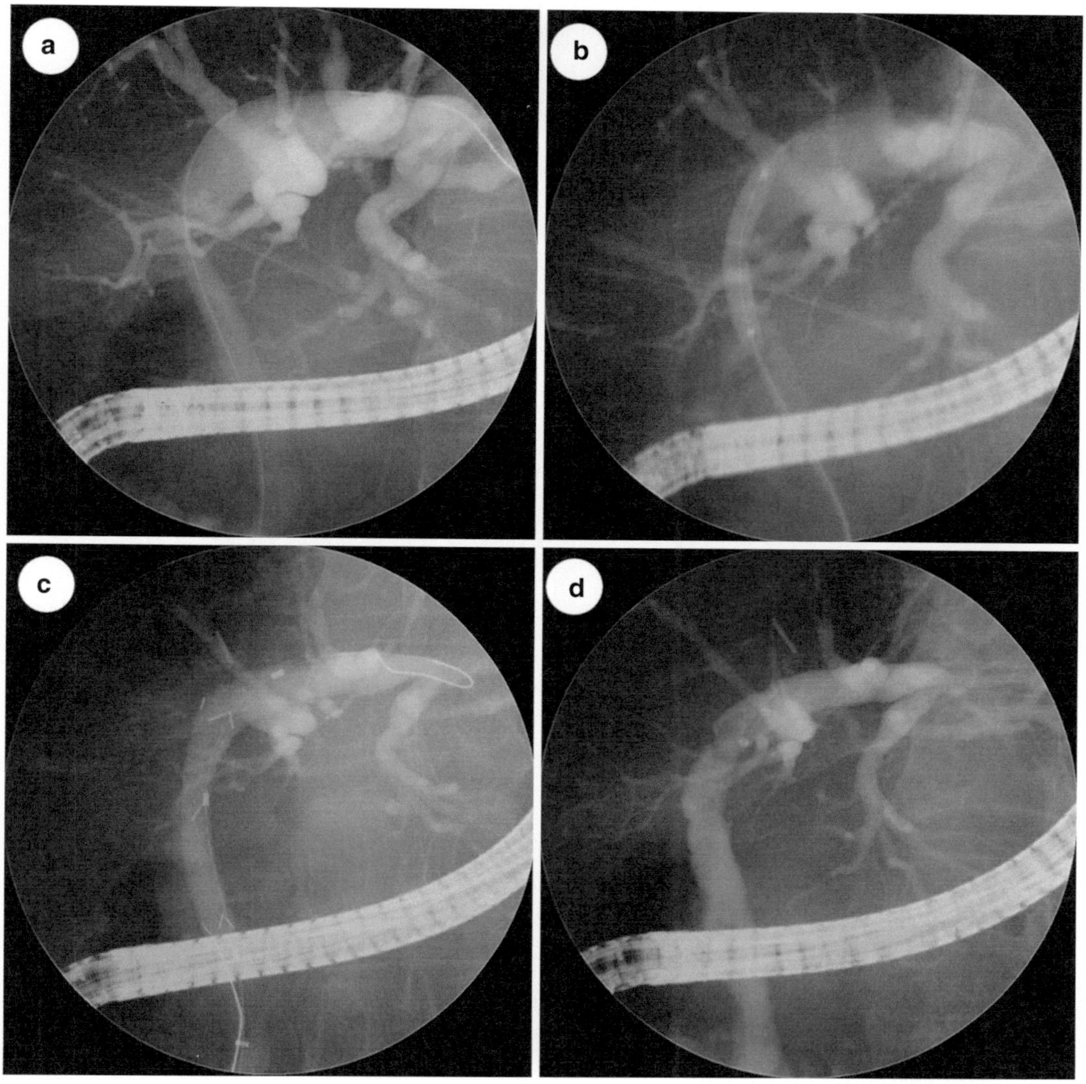

Fig. 1.10 Third case of hilar BBS after LDLT treated with the Kaffes FCSEMS. A 49-year-old male was referred to our hospital for anastomotic BBS 10 years after a right lobectomy for hepatocellular cancer and was successfully treated with an FCSEMS. BBS at the hilar level (**a**). The guidewire was passed through the stricture site, balloon dilatation was performed (**b**), and a Kaffes stent was deployed (**c**). After ~3 months, the Kaffes stent was removed, and the stricture had resolved (**d**)

Direct cholangioscopy (SpyGlass; Boston Scientific Inc., Natick, MA) enables direct visualization of the inner wall of the bile duct and is in use in selected medical centers. The SpyGlass per oral cholangioscopy system is designed to be used by a single operator, as opposed to the two operators required for the mother–baby scope technique. The SpyGlass system comprises the SpyGlass fiber optic probe (reusable) and the SpyScope access and delivery catheter, a single-use disposable delivery system. This method not only enables clear visualization of the opening of the stricture but also simultaneously facilitates rapid cannulation, obviating the need for a repeat ERCP/percutaneous approach or for revision surgery [70].

Self-expanding stents made of bioabsorbable material are also treatment options for BBS [71]. The material most commonly used in self-expanding biodegradable biliary stents is the

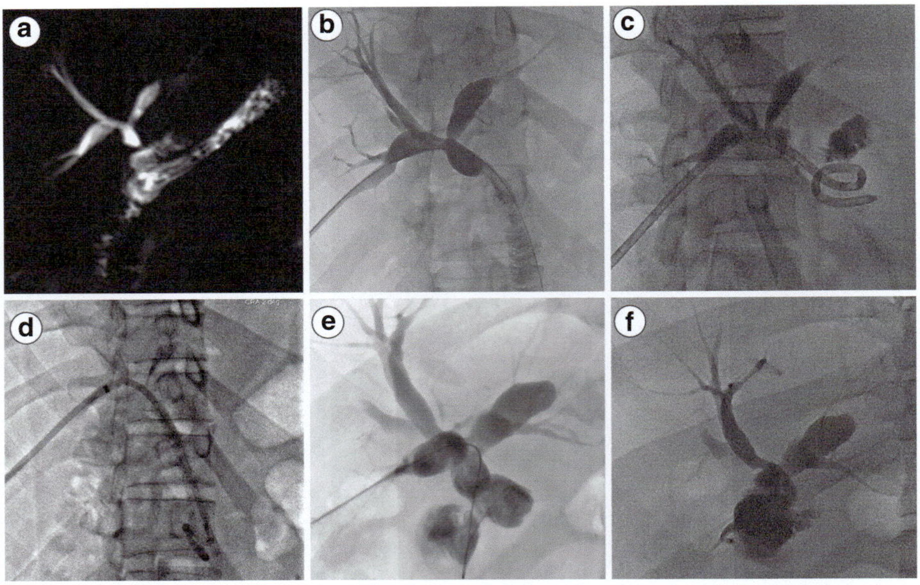

Fig. 1.11 High-level biliary stricture treated with percutaneous treatment. A 53-year-old female presented with high-level biliary stricture after Roux-en-Y choledochojujenostomy due to a choledochal cyst. An MRCP image (**a**) shows a biliary stricture at the choledochojujenostomy site. Because of the biliary reconstruction, the stricture was impossible to approach via ERCP, so we passed the guidewire via a percutaneous approach (**b**). The PTBD was passed through the stricture site, and the tip was located in the jejunum (**c**). A fully covered retrievable biliary stent was placed along the PTBD tract (**d**). PTBD exchange was performed every 2 months, and the stricture was resolved 6 months later (**e**). Finally, both stents and the PTBD were removed (**f**)

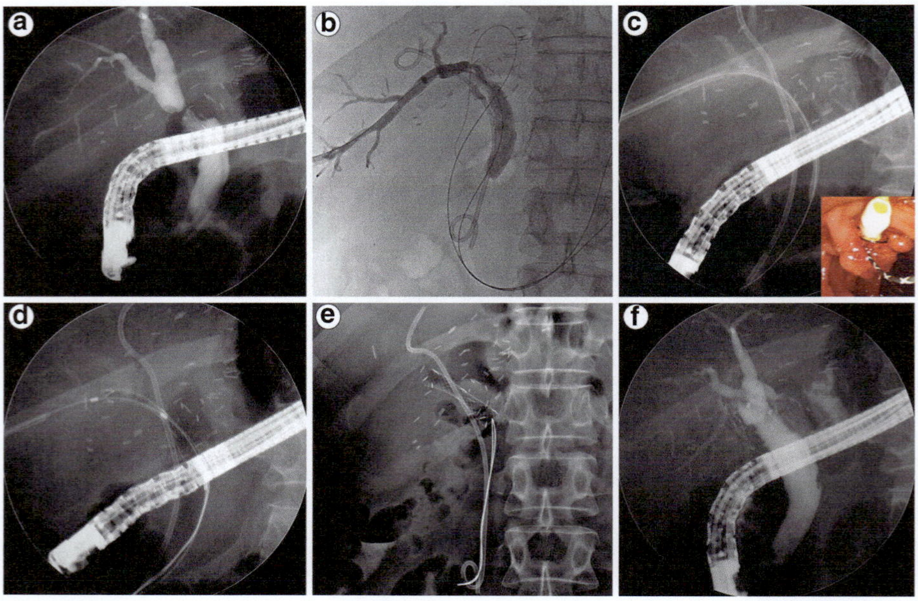

Fig. 1.12 High-level biliary stricture treated with rendezvous technique. A 54-year-old male with a hilar stricture due to non-B, non-C hepatocellular cancer after LDLT successfully treated with the rendezvous technique. An ERCP cholangiogram shows that the contrast dye extended to the distal IHD, but guidewire passage failed (**a**). The guidewire was passed through the stricture site using a percutaneous approach via the B6 bile duct (**b**). The guidewire was lowered through the PTBD tract to the duodenum by the anterograde method (**c**), and a Kaffes stent was inserted through the guidewire by the retrograde method (**d**, **e**). After 3 months, the stricture was resolved (**f**)

synthetic polymer poly-dioxanone. Biodegradable biliary stents did not result in unexpected adverse events after 2 years of follow-up, and the long-term success rate was >80% [72, 73].

In 2005, magnetic compression anastomosis was introduced as an interventional treatment to create an anastomosis between the enlarged bile duct and the small intestine. This method involves opening the bile duct causing ischemic necrosis of the stenotic biliary duct by gradually compressing two strong magnets between the two narrowed bile ducts. It enables a new tract to be formed between two completely blocked or disconnected biliary tracts [74–77]. This method is described in Chaps. 3 and 4.

Conclusion

In conclusion, high-level biliary strictures, which occur at or around the bifurcation of the left and right hepatic ducts, are common complications after LDLT. The causes of high-level strictures are diverse, and their pathophysiology is associated with the inflammatory response. Clinicians should take into account the risk factors for high-level strictures and closely monitor patients with these factors. Endoscopic management is typically the first-line treatment for biliary strictures after LDLT. The FCSEMS is superior to use of multiple plastic stents in terms of treatment outcomes, and specially designed types of FCSEMSs are available commercially.

References

1. Verdonk RC, Buis CI, Porte RJ, van der Jagt EJ, Limburg AJ, van den Berg AP, et al. Anastomotic biliary strictures after liver transplantation: causes and consequences. Liver Transpl. 2006;12(5):726–35.
2. Verdonk RC, Buis CI, van der Jagt EJ, Gouw AS, Limburg AJ, Slooff MJ, et al. Nonanastomotic biliary strictures after liver transplantation, part 2: management, outcome, and risk factors for disease progression. Liver Transpl. 2007;13(5):725–32.
3. Gondolesi GE, Varotti G, Florman SS, Munoz L, Fishbein TM, Emre SH, et al. Biliary complications in 96 consecutive right lobe living donor transplant recipients. Transplantation. 2004;77(12):1842–8.
4. Hwang S, Lee SG, Sung KB, Park KM, Kim KH, Ahn CS, et al. Long-term incidence, risk factors, and management of biliary complications after adult living donor liver transplantation. Liver Transpl. 2006;12(5):831–8.
5. Morioka D, Egawa H, Kasahara M, Ito T, Haga H, Takada Y, et al. Outcomes of adult-to-adult living donor liver transplantation: a single institution's experience with 335 consecutive cases. Ann Surg. 2007;245(2):315–25.
6. Shah SA, Grant DR, McGilvray ID, Greig PD, Selzner M, Lilly LB, et al. Biliary strictures in 130 consecutive right lobe living donor liver transplant recipients: results of a Western center. Am J Transplant. 2007;7(1):161–7.
7. Chang JH, Lee IS, Choi JY, Yoon SK, Kim DG, You YK, et al. Biliary stricture after adult right-lobe living-donor liver transplantation with duct-to-duct anastomosis: long-term outcome and its related factors after endoscopic treatment. Gut Liver. 2010;4(2):226–33.
8. Zimmerman MA, Baker T, Goodrich NP, Freise C, Hong JC, Kumer S, et al. Development, management, and resolution of biliary complications after living and deceased donor liver transplantation: a report from the adult-to-adult living donor liver transplantation cohort study consortium. Liver Transpl. 2013;19(3):259–67.
9. Jagannath S, Kalloo AN. Biliary complications after liver transplantation. Curr Treat Options Gastroenterol. 2002;5(2):101–12.
10. Guichelaar MM, Benson JT, Malinchoc M, Krom RA, Wiesner RH, Charlton MR. Risk factors for and clinical course of non-anastomotic biliary strictures after liver transplantation. Am J Transplant. 2003;3(7):885–90.
11. Larghi A, Tringali A, Lecca PG, Giordano M, Costamagna G. Management of hilar biliary strictures. Am J Gastroenterol. 2008;103(2):458–73.
12. Kasahara M, Egawa H, Takada Y, Oike F, Sakamoto S, Kiuchi T, et al. Biliary reconstruction in right lobe living-donor liver transplantation: comparison of different techniques in 321 recipients. Ann Surg. 2006;243(4):559–66.
13. Tsujino T, Isayama H, Sugawara Y, Sasaki T, Kogure H, Nakai Y, et al. Endoscopic management of biliary complications after adult living donor liver transplantation. Am J Gastroenterol. 2006;101(10):2230–6.
14. Yazumi S, Yoshimoto T, Hisatsune H, Hasegawa K, Kida M, Tada S, et al. Endoscopic treatment of biliary complications after right-lobe living-donor liver transplantation with duct-to-duct biliary anastomosis. J Hepatobiliary Pancreat Surg. 2006;13(6):502–10.
15. Tashiro H, Itamoto T, Sasaki T, Ohdan H, Fudaba Y, Amano H, et al. Biliary complications after duct-to-duct biliary reconstruction in living-donor liver transplantation: causes and treatment. World J Surg. 2007;31(11):2222–9.
16. Londono MC, Balderramo D, Cardenas A. Management of biliary complications after orthotopic liver transplantation: the role of endoscopy. World J Gastroenterol. 2008;14(4):493–7.

17. Sharma S, Gurakar A, Jabbour N. Biliary strictures following liver transplantation: past, present and preventive strategies. Liver Transpl. 2008;14(6):759–69.
18. Ohkubo M, Nagino M, Kamiya J, Yuasa N, Oda K, Arai T, et al. Surgical anatomy of the bile ducts at the hepatic hilum as applied to living donor liver transplantation. Ann Surg. 2004;239(1):82–6.
19. Kato H, Kawamoto H, Tsutsumi K, Harada R, Fujii M, Hirao K, et al. Long-term outcomes of endoscopic management for biliary strictures after living donor liver transplantation with duct-to-duct reconstruction. Transpl Int. 2009;22(9):914–21.
20. Duffy JP, Kao K, Ko CY, Farmer DG, McDiarmid SV, Hong JC, et al. Long-term patient outcome and quality of life after liver transplantation: analysis of 20-year survivors. Ann Surg. 2010;252(4):652–61.
21. Melcher ML, Pomposelli JJ, Verbesey JE, McTaggart RA, Freise CE, Ascher NL, et al. Comparison of biliary complications in adult living-donor liver transplants performed at two busy transplant centers. Clin Transpl. 2010;24(5):E137–44.
22. Kim PT, Marquez M, Jung J, Cavallucci D, Renner EL, Cattral M, et al. Long-term follow-up of biliary complications after adult right-lobe living donor liver transplantation. Clin Transpl. 2015;29(5):465–74.
23. Sugawara Y, Makuuchi M. Advances in adult living donor liver transplantation: a review based on reports from the 10th anniversary of the adult-to-adult living donor liver transplantation meeting in Tokyo. Liver Transpl. 2004;10(6):715–20.
24. Liu CL, Fan ST, Lo CM, Wei WI, Chan SC, Yong BH, et al. Operative outcomes of adult-to-adult right lobe live donor liver transplantation: a comparative study with cadaveric whole-graft liver transplantation in a single center. Ann Surg. 2006;243(3):404–10.
25. Soejima Y, Taketomi A, Yoshizumi T, Uchiyama H, Harada N, Ijichi H, et al. Biliary strictures in living donor liver transplantation: incidence, management, and technical evolution. Liver Transpl. 2006;12(6):979–86.
26. Wadhawan M, Kumar A. Management issues in post living donor liver transplant biliary strictures. World J Hepatol. 2016;8(10):461–70.
27. Rao HB, Ahamed H, Panicker S, Sudhindran S, Venu RP. Endoscopic therapy for biliary strictures complicating living donor liver transplantation: Factors predicting better outcome. World J Gastrointest Pathophysiol. 2017;8(2):77–86.
28. Pfau PR, Kochman ML, Lewis JD, Long WB, Lucey MR, Olthoff K, et al. Endoscopic management of postoperative biliary complications in orthotopic liver transplantation. Gastrointest Endosc. 2000;52(1):55–63.
29. Moser MA, Wall WJ. Management of biliary problems after liver transplantation. Liver Transpl. 2001;7(11 Suppl 1):S46–52.
30. Moench C, Uhrig A, Lohse AW, Otto G. CC chemokine receptor 5delta32 polymorphism-a risk factor for ischemic-type biliary lesions following orthotopic liver transplantation. Liver Transpl. 2004;10(3):434–9.
31. Strazzabosco M, Fabris L, Spirli C. Pathophysiology of cholangiopathies. J Clin Gastroenterol. 2005;39(4 Suppl 2):S90–s102.
32. Isse K, Harada K, Zen Y, Kamihira T, Shimoda S, Harada M, et al. Fractalkine and CX3CR1 are involved in the recruitment of intraepithelial lymphocytes of intrahepatic bile ducts. Hepatology. 2005;41(3):506–16.
33. Kruger B, Schroppel B, Murphy BT. Genetic polymorphisms and the fate of the transplanted organ. Transplant Rev (Orlando). 2008;22(2):131–40.
34. op den Dries S, Buis CI, Adelmeijer J, Van der Jagt EJ, Haagsma EB, Lisman T, et al. The combination of primary sclerosing cholangitis and CCR5-Delta32 in recipients is strongly associated with the development of nonanastomotic biliary strictures after liver transplantation. Liver Int. 2011;31(8):1102–9.
35. Neumann UP, Guckelberger O, Langrehr JM, Lang M, Schmitz V, Theruvath T, et al. Impact of human leukocyte antigen matching in liver transplantation. Transplantation. 2003;75(1):132–7.
36. Muro M, Marin L, Miras M, Moya-Quiles R, Minguela A, Sanchez-Bueno F, et al. Liver recipients harbouring anti-donor preformed lymphocytotoxic antibodies exhibit a poor allograft survival at the first year after transplantation: experience of one centre. Transpl Immunol. 2005;14(2):91–7.
37. Castillo-Rama M, Castro MJ, Bernardo I, Meneu-Diaz JC, Elola-Olaso AM, Calleja-Antolin SM, et al. Preformed antibodies detected by cytotoxic assay or multibead array decrease liver allograft survival: role of human leukocyte antigen compatibility. Liver Transpl. 2008;14(4):554–62.
38. Iacob S, Cicinnati VR, Dechene A, Lindemann M, Heinemann FM, Rebmann V, et al. Genetic, immunological and clinical risk factors for biliary strictures following liver transplantation. Liver Int. 2012;32(8):1253–61.
39. Forrest EA, Reiling J, Lipka G, Fawcett J. Risk factors and clinical indicators for the development of biliary strictures post liver transplant: Significance of bilirubin. World J Transplant. 2017;7(6):349–58.
40. Jeong S, Wang X, Wan P, Sha M, Zhang J, Xia L, et al. Risk factors and survival outcomes of biliary complications after adult-to-adult living donor liver transplantation. United European Gastroenterol J. 2017;5(7):997–1006.
41. Koneru B, Sterling MJ, Bahramipour PF. Bile duct strictures after liver transplantation: a changing landscape of the Achilles' heel. Liver Transpl. 2006;12(5):702–4.
42. Azzam AZ, Tanaka K. Biliary complications after living donor liver transplantation: a retrospective analysis of the Kyoto experience 1999–2004. Indian J Gastroenterol. 2017;36(4):296–304.
43. Wang SF, Huang ZY, Chen XP. Biliary complications after living donor liver transplantation. Liver Transpl. 2011;17(10):1127–36.

44. Seo JK, Ryu JK, Lee SH, Park JK, Yang KY, Kim YT, et al. Endoscopic treatment for biliary stricture after adult living donor liver transplantation. Liver Transpl. 2009;15(4):369–80.
45. Gomez CM, Dumonceau JM, Marcolongo M, de Santibanes E, Ciardullo M, Pekolj J, et al. Endoscopic management of biliary complications after adult living-donor versus deceased-donor liver transplantation. Transplantation. 2009;88(11):1280–5.
46. Tsujino T, Isayama H, Kogure H, Sato T, Nakai Y, Koike K. Endoscopic management of biliary strictures after living donor liver transplantation. Clin J Gastroenterol. 2017;10(4):297–311.
47. Kulaksiz H, Weiss KH, Gotthardt D, Adler G, Stremmel W, Schaible A, et al. Is stenting necessary after balloon dilation of post-transplantation biliary strictures? Results of a prospective comparative study. Endoscopy. 2008;40(9):746–51.
48. Schwartz DA, Petersen BT, Poterucha JJ, Gostout CJ. Endoscopic therapy of anastomotic bile duct strictures occurring after liver transplantation. Gastrointest Endosc. 2000;51(2):169–74.
49. Zoepf T, Maldonado-Lopez EJ, Hilgard P, Malago M, Broelsch CE, Treichel U, et al. Balloon dilatation vs. balloon dilatation plus bile duct endoprostheses for treatment of anastomotic biliary strictures after liver transplantation. Liver Transpl. 2006;12(1):88–94.
50. Morelli J, Mulcahy HE, Willner IR, Cunningham JT, Draganov P. Long-term outcomes for patients with post-liver transplant anastomotic biliary strictures treated by endoscopic stent placement. Gastrointest Endosc. 2003;58(3):374–9.
51. Kurita A, Kodama Y, Minami R, Sakuma Y, Kuriyama K, Tanabe W, et al. Endoscopic stent placement above the intact sphincter of Oddi for biliary strictures after living donor liver transplantation. J Gastroenterol. 2013;48(9):1097–104.
52. Culp WC, McCowan TC, Lieberman RP, Goertzen TC, LeVeen RF, Heffron TG. Biliary strictures in liver transplant recipients: treatment with metal stents. Radiology. 1996;199(2):339–46.
53. Harada N, Shirabe K, Soejima Y, Taketomi A, Yoshizumi T, Asonuma K, et al. Intrahepatic artery pseudoaneurysm associated with a metallic biliary stent after living donor liver transplantation: report of a case. Surg Today. 2013;43(6):678–81.
54. Dumonceau JM, Deviere J, Delhaye M, Baize M, Cremer M. Plastic and metal stents for postoperative benign bile duct strictures: the best and the worst. Gastrointest Endosc. 1998;47(1):8–17.
55. Siriwardana HP, Siriwardena AK. Systematic appraisal of the role of metallic endobiliary stents in the treatment of benign bile duct stricture. Ann Surg. 2005;242(1):10–9.
56. Tal AO, Finkelmeier F, Filmann N, Kylanpaa L, Udd M, Parzanese I, et al. Multiple plastic stents versus covered metal stent for treatment of anastomotic biliary strictures after liver transplantation: a prospective, randomized, multicenter trial. Gastrointest Endosc. 2017;86(6):1038–45.
57. Kaffes A, Griffin S, Vaughan R, James M, Chua T, Tee H, et al. A randomized trial of a fully covered self-expandable metallic stent versus plastic stents in anastomotic biliary strictures after liver transplantation. Therap Adv Gastroenterol. 2014;7(2):64–71.
58. Martins FP, De Paulo GA, Contini MLC, Ferrari AP. Metal versus plastic stents for anastomotic biliary strictures after liver transplantation: a randomized controlled trial. Gastrointest Endosc. 2018;87(1):131.e1–e13.
59. Kao D, Zepeda-Gomez S, Tandon P, Bain VG. Managing the post-liver transplantation anastomotic biliary stricture: multiple plastic versus metal stents: a systematic review. Gastrointest Endosc. 2013;77(5):679–91.
60. Jang SI, Sung SY, Park H, Lee KH, Joo SM, Lee DK. Salvage therapy using self-expandable metal stents for recalcitrant anastomotic strictures after living-donor liver transplantation. Therap Adv Gastroenterol. 2017;10(3):297–309.
61. Mita A, Hashikura Y, Masuda Y, Ohno Y, Urata K, Nakazawa Y, et al. Nonsurgical policy for treatment of bilioenteric anastomotic stricture after living donor liver transplantation. Transpl Int. 2008;21(4):320–7.
62. Sung RS, Campbell DA Jr, Rudich SM, Punch JD, Shieck VL, Armstrong JM, et al. Long-term follow-up of percutaneous transhepatic balloon cholangioplasty in the management of biliary strictures after liver transplantation. Transplantation. 2004;77(1):110–5.
63. Kim ES, Lee BJ, Won JY, Choi JY, Lee DK. Percutaneous transhepatic biliary drainage may serve as a successful rescue procedure in failed cases of endoscopic therapy for a post-living donor liver transplantation biliary stricture. Gastrointest Endosc. 2009;69(1):38–46.
64. Jang SI, Hwang JH, Lee KH, Yu JS, Kim HW, Yoon CJ, et al. Percutaneous biliary approach as a successful rescue procedure after failed endoscopic therapy for drainage in advanced hilar tumors. J Gastroenterol Hepatol. 2017;32(4):932–8.
65. Chang JH, Lee IS, Chun HJ, Choi JY, Yoon SK, Kim DG, et al. Comparative study of rendezvous techniques in post-liver transplant biliary stricture. World J Gastroenterol. 2012;18(41):5957–64.
66. Chok KS, Lo CM. Prevention and management of biliary anastomotic stricture in right-lobe living-donor liver transplantation. J Gastroenterol Hepatol. 2014;29(10):1756–63.
67. Chok KS, Chan SC, Cheung TT, Chan AC, Sharr WW, Fan ST, et al. Outcomes of side-to-side conversion hepaticojejunostomy for biliary anastomotic stricture after right-liver living donor liver transplantation. HBPD Int. 2013;12(1):42–6.
68. Atar E, Bachar GN, Bartal G, Mor E, Neyman H, Graif F, et al. Use of peripheral cutting balloon in the management of resistant benign ureteral and biliary strictures. J Vasc Interv Radiol. 2005;16(2 Pt 1):241–5.
69. Husing A, Reinecke H, Cicinnati VR, Beckebaum S, Wilms C, Schmidt HH, et al. Paclitaxel-eluting

balloon dilation of biliary anastomotic stricture after liver transplantation. World J Gastroenterol. 2015;21(3):977–81.
70. Wright H, Sharma S, Gurakar A, Sebastian A, Kohli V, Jabbour N. Management of biliary stricture guided by the spyglass direct visualization system in a liver transplant recipient: an innovative approach. Gastrointest Endosc. 2008;67(7):1201–3.
71. Siiki A, Rinta-Kiikka I, Sand J, Laukkarinen J. A pilot study of endoscopically inserted biodegradable biliary stents in the treatment of benign biliary strictures and cystic duct leaks. Gastrointest Endosc. 2018;87(4):1132–7.
72. Mauri G, Michelozzi C, Melchiorre F, Poretti D, Pedicini V, Salvetti M, et al. Benign biliary strictures refractory to standard bilioplasty treated using polydoxanone biodegradable biliary stents: retrospective multicentric data analysis on 107 patients. Eur Radiol. 2016;26(11):4057–63.
73. Lorenzo-Zuniga V, Moreno-de-Vega V, Marin I, Boix J. Biodegradable stents in gastrointestinal endoscopy. World J Gastroenterol. 2014;20(9):2212–7.
74. Okajima H, Kotera A, Takeichi T, Ueno M, Ishiko T, Hirota M, et al. Magnet compression anastomosis for bile duct stenosis after duct-to-duct biliary reconstruction in living donor liver transplantation. Liver Transpl. 2005;11(4):473–5.
75. Jang SI, Choi J, Lee DK. Magnetic compression anastomosis for treatment of benign biliary stricture. Dig Endosc. 2015;27(2):239–49.
76. Parlak E, Koksal AS, Kucukay F, Eminler AT, Toka B, Uslan MI. A novel technique for the endoscopic treatment of complete biliary anastomosis obstructions after liver transplantation: through-the-scope magnetic compression anastomosis. Gastrointest Endosc. 2017;85(4):841–7.
77. Muraoka N, Uematsu H, Yamanouchi E, Kinoshita K, Takeda T, Ihara N, et al. Yamanouchi magnetic compression anastomosis for bilioenteric anastomotic stricture after living-donor liver transplantation. J Vasc Interv Radiol. 2005;16(9):1263–7.
78. Lee YY, Gwak GY, Lee KH, Lee JK, Lee KT, Kwon CH, et al. Predictors of the feasibility of primary endoscopic management of biliary strictures after adult living donor liver transplantation. Liver Transpl. 2011;17(12):1467–73.
79. Kim TH, Lee SK, Han JH, Park DH, Lee SS, Seo DW, et al. The role of endoscopic retrograde cholangiography for biliary stricture after adult living donor liver transplantation: technical aspect and outcome. Scand J Gastroenterol. 2011;46(2):188–96.
80. Hsieh TH, Mekeel KL, Crowell MD, Nguyen CC, Das A, Aqel BA, et al. Endoscopic treatment of anastomotic biliary strictures after living donor liver transplantation: outcomes after maximal stent therapy. Gastrointest Endosc. 2013;77(1):47–54.
81. Chok KS, Chan SC, Cheung TT, Sharr WW, Chan AC, Fan ST, et al. A retrospective study on risk factors associated with failed endoscopic treatment of biliary anastomotic stricture after right-lobe living donor liver transplantation with duct-to-duct anastomosis. Ann Surg. 2014;259(4):767–72.

Totally Obstructed Biliary Stricture I: Concept and Methods of Magnetic Compression Anastomosis

2

Yool Lae Kim, Sung Ill Jang, and Dong Ki Lee

History

The concept of compression articulation was originally proposed in 1826 by Denan, who described a newly formed anastomotic fistula caused by ischemic compression of tissue [1]. Denan's spring-loaded device was further developed by Murphy in 1892 and became known as the Murphy button [2–5]. This technique allows for the formation of a circular anastomosis of the intestinal tract by ischemic compression of the tissues between the two buttons and is used to prepare a sutureless connection through end-to-end or side-to-side ischemic compression. It was the first surgical device made for such a purpose [6]. In 1991, an attempt was made to compress an anastomosis using a compression button and an improved Murphy button in an animal study [7]. This device was used to create a compression anastomosis by contacting two screws. The physical contact can be replaced by a magnetic force mediated by a magnetic field. The effects of magnetic force in the intestinal tract were analyzed after swallowing a magnet in some children who had natural perforation or fistulas [8–11]. In 1980, Jansen et al. [12] conducted the first human experiment to achieve tissue compression with magnetic force compression. Magnetic compression-induced mucosal anastomosis was successfully performed in five patients undergoing colonic resection. In 1993, Saveliev et al. [13] conducted clinical and laboratory studies on mongrel dogs, and cholecystoenteric, enteroenteric, and magnetic cholecystogastric anastomoses were successful. In addition, data from four patients who underwent cholecystogastric anastomosis and one patient who underwent cholecystoduodenal anastomosis indicated the possibility of endoscopic magnetic cholecystoenteric anastomosis [14]. Attempts have been made to evaluate the concept and clinical utility of magnetic resonance [15]. In 1998, Yamanouchi et al. [16] introduced the magnetic compression anastomosis (MCA) method and successfully established a bile duct-small intestinal fistula. Other clinical results have also been reported [17–32].

Magnets

Magnetic force is very important for the success of MCA. Rare earth magnets are classified as neodymium-iron-boron magnets and samarium-cobalt (Sm-Co) magnets. Both types are suitable for MCA because of their high flux density and retention. However, the retention of Sm-Co magnets is stronger than that of neodymium-iron-boron

Y. L. Kim · S. I. Jang · D. K. Lee (✉)
Department of Internal Medicine, Gangnam Severance Hospital, Yonsei University College of Medicine, Seoul, South Korea
e-mail: aerojsi@yuhs.ac; dklee@yuhs.ac

D. K. Lee (ed.), *Advanced ERCP for Complicated and Refractory Biliary and Pancreatic Diseases*,
https://doi.org/10.1007/978-981-13-0608-2_2

magnets, and they are used more frequently [17–20, 26, 33]. A magnetic force determination algorithm (MAGDA) is used to calculate the magnetic force of a magnet [14, 33]. It has been assumed that calculating magnetic forces will help predict the success of MCA. Several variables, such as the shape of the magnet, diameter, nature of the material, magnetic grades, strength, and experimentally estimated or derived strength between in vivo magnets, are inputted into the MAGDA.

Animal Studies

In the 1990s, efforts were made to induce compression anastomosis through magnetic attraction between strong rare earth magnets. In 1995, Cope et al. [34, 35] demonstrated the feasibility and safety of MCA by creating bilioenteric and enteroenteric anastomoses in pigs. Cope used neodymium-iron fluoride or rare earth Sm-Co magnets to perform cholecystogastric and cholecystojejunal anastomoses in pigs, and a bilioenteric anastomosis formed as a result of MCA after 9–16 weeks [34]. Preliminary studies have shown that magnets can be used to make enteroenteric anastomoses without a short-term leak in pigs [35]. The shape of the magnet used in subsequent MCA studies was modified to amplify the magnetic effect, and further animal studies were performed. Jamshidi et al. [21] performed MCA using a uniform and tapered suture method compared with an additional hand-stapled anastomosis. In addition, gross appearance, histology, and mechanical stability were evaluated, and functional radiological evaluation was performed. No severe complications or stenoses were observed. The rupture pressures of the anastomosis formed by MCA and the anastomosis formed by surgery did not differ. On pathological examination, the anastomosis formed by MCA demonstrated continuity of serous, submucosal, and mucosal layers, and no ischemia or necrosis was observed. Thus, the MCA was safe and similar, or even superior, to anastomosis made with conventional sutures or a stapler [21]. In addition, the same team showed that MCA-assisted enteroenterostomy is feasible using modified magnets in the form of convex-concave radial symmetry [36]. Achieving a reliable enteric anastomosis requires the design and development of a controlled MCA system (magnamosis) that optimizes magnetic coupling, distance between magnets, and surface matching [37]. A magnamosis device has three main features: (1) two convex-concave radial symmetrical rings that self-align magnetically, (2) ring-shaped magnets allowing immediate opening, and (3) radial terrain specially designed to facilitate necrosis at the center and to heal nearby. This ensures that the anastomosis will not be punctured.

In addition to modifications to the magnets, animal studies were performed to optimize the endoscopic magnet supply [38]. A modular soft magnetic anastomosis device was developed without leakage. One study used a partially covered stent to improve the modular shape of the magnet and the opening of the MCA fistula [39]. Inserting a partially covered stent into the gastroenteric anastomosis formed by the MCA maintained the opening for more than 7 weeks. A compression anastomosis using magnets has been experimentally tested in blood vessels and the biliary and gastrointestinal tracts [40].

Human Studies

In 1998, Yamanouchi et al. [16] successfully introduced the MCA method and successfully established a bile duct-small intestinal fistula. Other clinical results have also been reported [17–32]. Thereafter, MCA has been successfully used for biliobiliary anastomoses and bilioenteric anastomoses. Long-term follow-up data on side effects and restenosis after the procedure are still lacking. However, some results have demonstrated the stability and effectiveness of the method. Jang et al. studied 39 patients who underwent MCA, and recanalization was successful in 35 patients [41]. One patient had mild cholangitis, and none died. The average follow-up period was 41.9 months, and restenosis was confirmed in one patient.

Indication of MCA

The development of nonsurgical treatments, including endoscopic and percutaneous approaches, enables reperfusion of benign or malignant postoperative severe biliary strictures [25, 42–45]. However, non-operative treatment has limited effectiveness for severe biliary strictures or complete occlusion, and inserting and maintaining a drain catheter is necessary in patients who fail to respond to stricture treatment using conventional methods. Therefore, the indications of MCA are severe biliary stricture or a complete obstruction that cannot be treated using endoscopic or percutaneous treatment (Fig. 2.1) [17–24].

Methods

Outline of the Procedure

The magnets used in MCA are cylindrical Sm-Co rare earth magnets that can be delivered in a variety of ways [33]. The most common delivery pathways are percutaneous and peroral. The MCA procedure is divided into four steps: (1) delineating the track to deliver the magnet, (2) magnet approximation, (3) magnet removal, and (4) maintenance and removal of the internal catheter.

Step 1: Track Formation for Magnet Delivery

The percutaneous transhepatic biliary drainage (PTBD) route is formed using a PTBD catheter to deliver the magnet. The PTBD catheter is exchanged with an 18-Fr sheath prior to MCA approximation, allowing for convenient insertion of the magnet through the PTBD catheter, which reduces intrahepatic duct damage. After a full endoscopic sphincterotomy (EST) and balloon dilatation or retrieval, a fully covered self-expandable metal stent (FCSEMS) is temporarily inserted into the common bile duct (CBD) to facilitate delivery of the magnet via the oral route (Fig. 2.2).

Step 2: Magnet Approximation

A screw attached to one magnet is fixed to a polypectomy snare and the magnet is moved to the anastomosis site via the 18-Fr PTBD

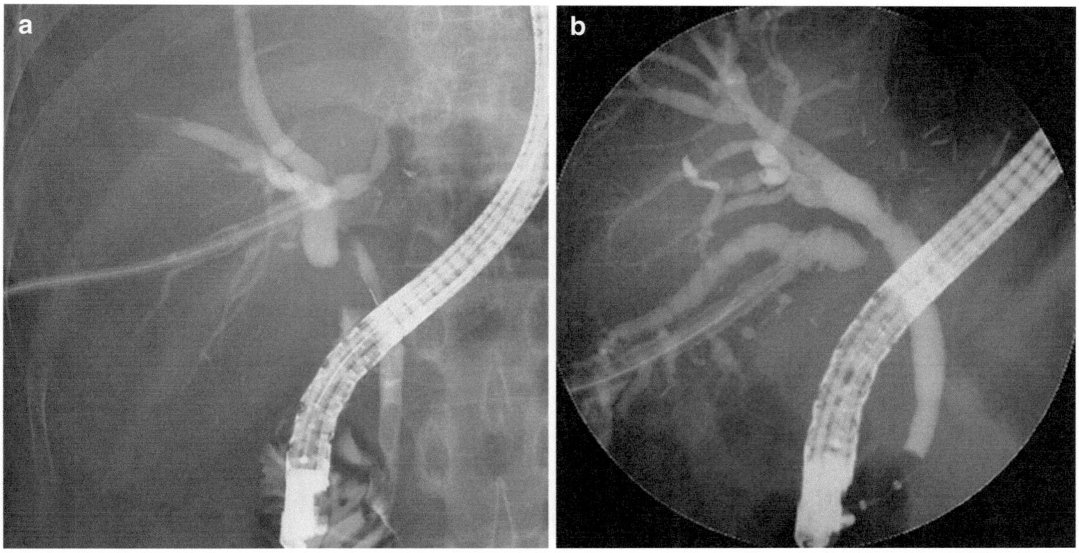

Fig. 2.1 Indications for magnetic compression anastomosis (MCA). MCA was performed for a refractory benign biliary stricture that could not be treated using conventional endoscopic and/or percutaneous methods because of a complete obstruction through which the (**a**) guide wire or (**b**) dye was unable to pass

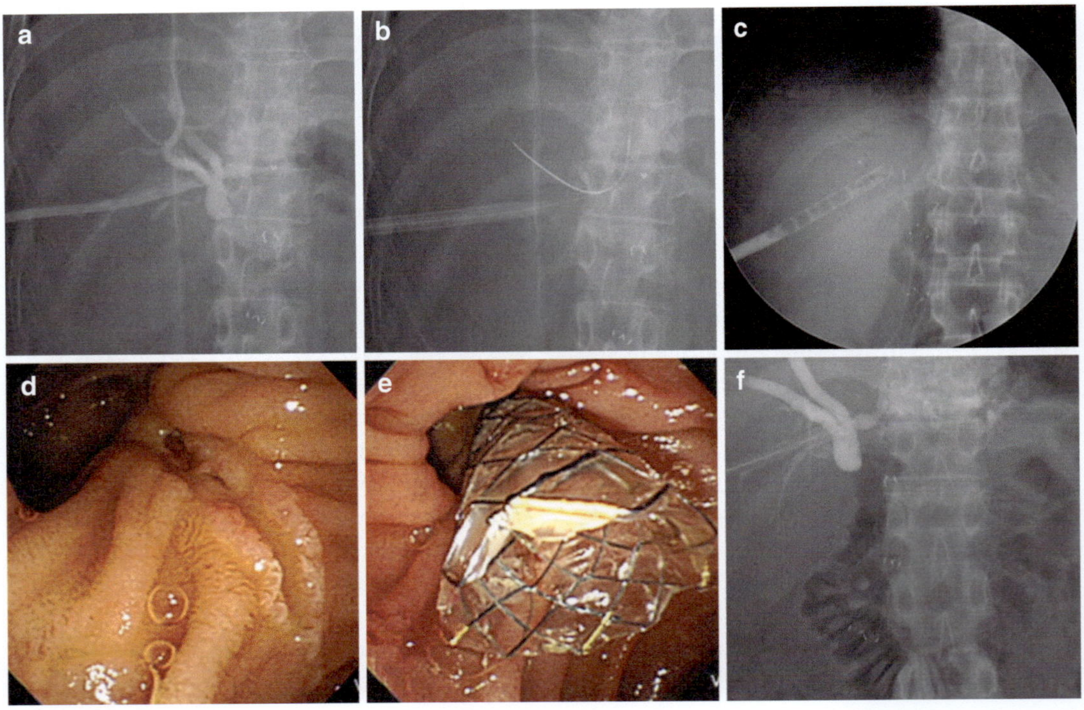

Fig. 2.2 Magnet delivery routes. (**a**) A percutaneous transhepatic biliary drainage (PTBD) tract was formed and dilated to 16-Fr size. (**b**) The PTBD catheter was changed to an 18-Fr sheath to deliver the magnet without injuring the duct. (**c**) The location of the 18-Fr sheath was confirmed using contrast dye under fluoroscopy. (**d**) The orifice of the ampulla was opened after endoscopic sphincterotomy using endoscopic retrograde cholangiopancreatography (ERCP). (**e**) A retrievable fully converted self-expandable metal stent (FCSEMS) was inserted into the common bile duct to facilitate delivery of the magnet. (**f**) The location of FCSEMS was confirmed using contrast dye under fluoroscopy

sheath. The polypectomy snare passes through the channel of an endoscopic retrograde cholangiopancreatography (ERCP) scope, and the other magnet is fixed in front of the scope. The magnets are moved to the anastomosis site via FCSEMS, and MCA approximation is possible owing to the attraction between the two magnets. The magnet is advanced through the PTBD and ERCP tracks using a balloon catheter to better approximate the magnet. The approximation of the two magnets is confirmed by radiography. Next, the long sheath tube is removed, and an indwelling PTBD catheter is inserted. The FCSEMS inserted in the CBD is removed immediately after the magnets are approximated (Fig. 2.3).

Step 3: Magnet Removal

When a fistula is formed due to ischemic necrosis caused by an approximated magnet, the magnet is moved naturally to the duodenum (Fig. 2.4). However, if spontaneous movement does not occur after 8–10 weeks, the magnet can be pushed out using a guidewire or catheter. Percutaneous transhepatic cholangioscopy (PTCS) can also be used to remove the magnet through the PTBD tube (Fig. 2.5).

Magnet Preparation

As the silk thread and magnet are separate and the magnet is difficult to manipulate during the procedure, we developed our own rare-earth magnets. We connected the silk thread by making a hole in the opposite side of the magnet. In addition, we made the magnets 4 mm in diameter, resulting in a 50% stronger magnetic force than the previously used magnets (Fig. 2.6) [17].

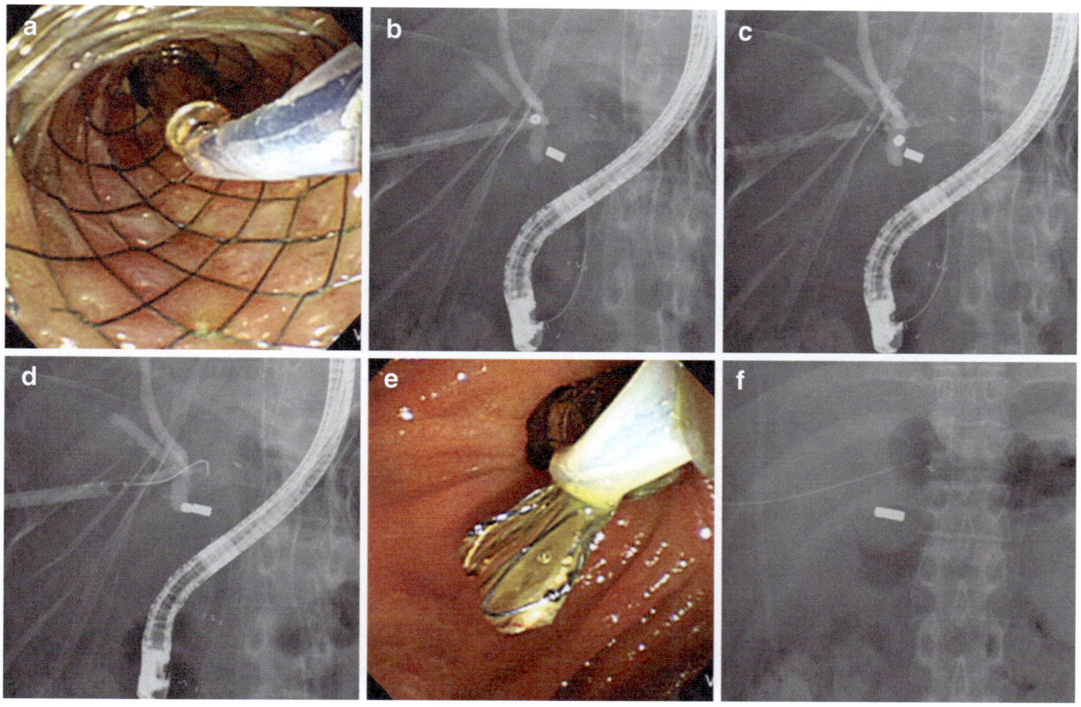

Fig. 2.3 The process of magnet approximation. (**a**) A magnet attached to a polypectomy snare is delivered via fully converted self-expandable metal stent (FCSEMS) using an endoscopic retrograde cholangiopancreatography (ERCP) scope through the CBD. (**b**) Another magnet is delivered via an 18-Fr percutaneous transhepatic biliary drainage (PTBD) sheath. (**c**) Two magnets draw close together due to the magnetic attraction between them. (**d**) The approximation of magnets is confirmed by fluoroscopy. (**e**) The FCSEMS in the common bile duct (CBD) was removed using a polypectomy snare. (**f**) The PTBD catheter (16 Fr) was inserted after magnet approximation was established

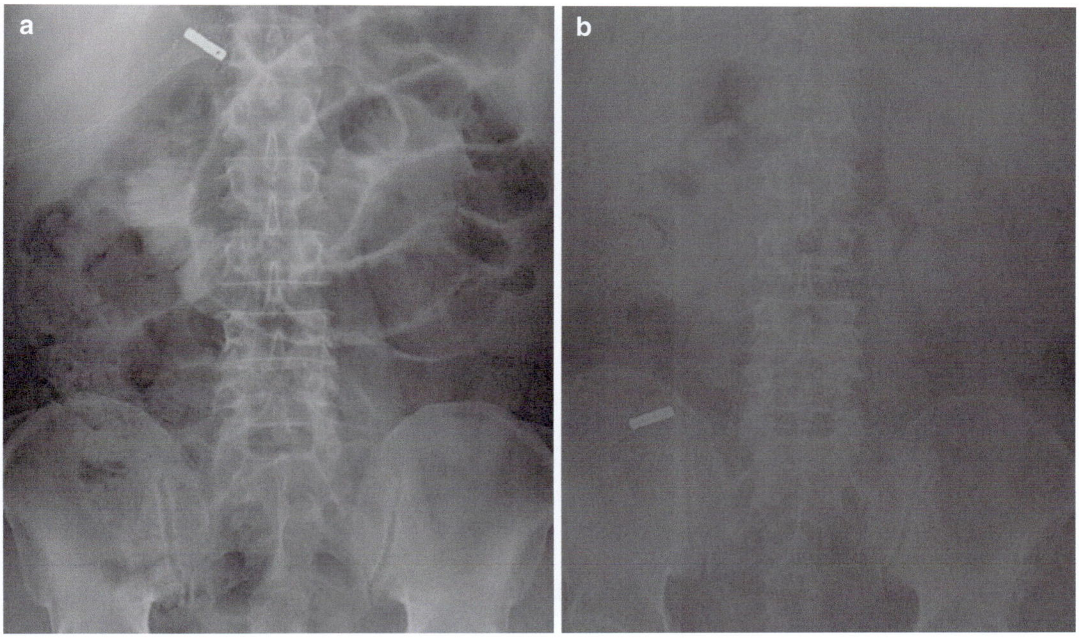

Fig. 2.4 A simple abdominal image showing a spontaneously removed magnet. The approximated magnets may move to the bowel within 4–6 weeks after approximation. (**a**) The approximated magnets were located at the stricture site. (**b**) Magnets that were removed spontaneously are present in the intestinal tract after 3 weeks

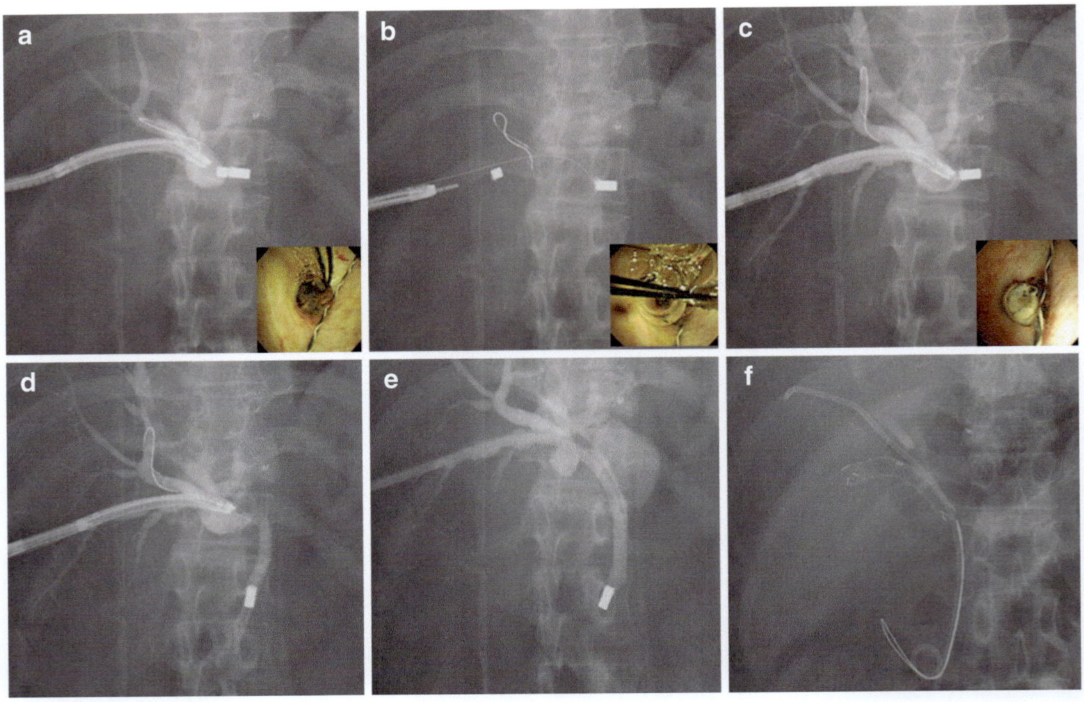

Fig. 2.5 The process of magnet removal using percutaneous transhepatic cholangioscopy (PTCS). If the approximated magnets do not move spontaneously to the bowel within 8–10 weeks, they can be removed using a PTCS scope. (**a**) The approximated magnets are visualized using a PTCS scope. (**b**) The silk thread attached to the magnet was used to ease detachment from the approximated magnets. (**c**, **d**) The other magnet is removed by contrast injection or pushing with a catheter. (**e**) A 16-Fr percutaneous transhepatic biliary drainage (PTBD) catheter is inserted through the newly formed fistula after the detached magnet is moved to the common bile duct (CBD). (**f**) A fully converted self-expandable metal stent (FCSEMS) is inserted at the newly formed fistula, and the previous PTBD catheter is removed

Pre-evaluation for MCA

The pre-MCA evaluation is limited to planning outcomes and treatment methods. This problem should be improved. The success of MCA is determined by several factors, such as length of the stenosis, shape of the bile duct, orientation of the magnet, and the biliary axis. The main causes of MCA failure are a long stenosis, tapered or twisted bile duct, or misalignment [17, 18]. The longer the stenosis, the weaker the magnetic force. In this situation, necrosis due to compression does not occur, and no fistula forms. Therefore, an accurate assessment of the length of the stenosis is important before MCA. However, current noninvasive imaging studies, such as computed tomography (CT), ultrasound, and magnetic resonance cholangiopancreatography, cannot be used to accurately assess the length of a stenosis. The evaluation of cholangiogram-based biliary ducts is fairly accurate, but it has the disadvantage of requiring invasive procedures, such as ERCP and PTBD. In addition to stenosis length, the axis and shape of the bile duct are important parts of the MCA pre-evaluation. If the bile duct is tapered and twisted, even if the stenosis is short, the magnet cannot reach the stenosis and the actual distance between the two magnets will be longer than the length measured before MCA, eventually leading to MCA failure (Fig. 2.7) [17]. The axis of the bile duct also determines the alignment direction of the magnet. Even if the distance between the magnets is short and MCA is successful, if the magnets align in parallel, the weak magnetic force eventually causes the procedure to fail [17, 18]. Noninvasive examinations are limited for finding suitable MCA candidates because factors such as

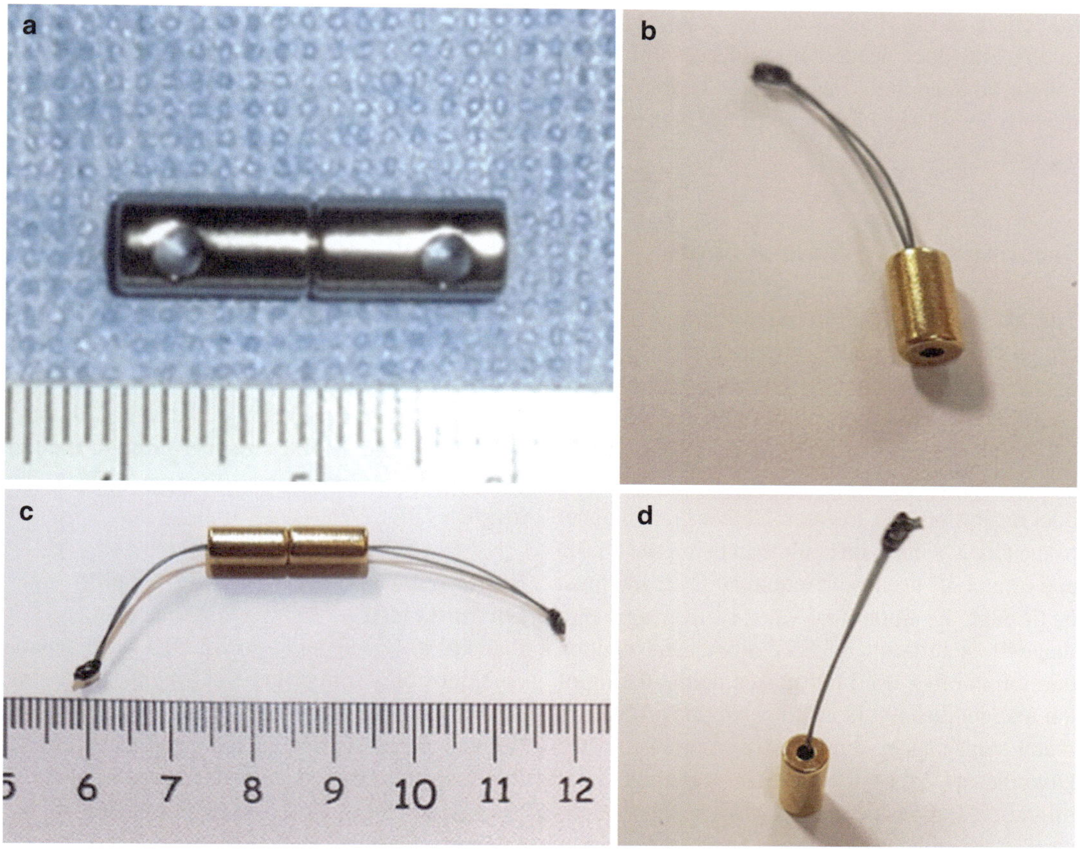

Fig. 2.6 Magnet preparation. (**a**) The originally used magnet had a side hole. (**b–d**) A hole was drilled in the new magnet on the side opposite the alignment side. A silk thread was passed through the hole and attached with strong adhesive. This magnet was smaller but stronger than the first

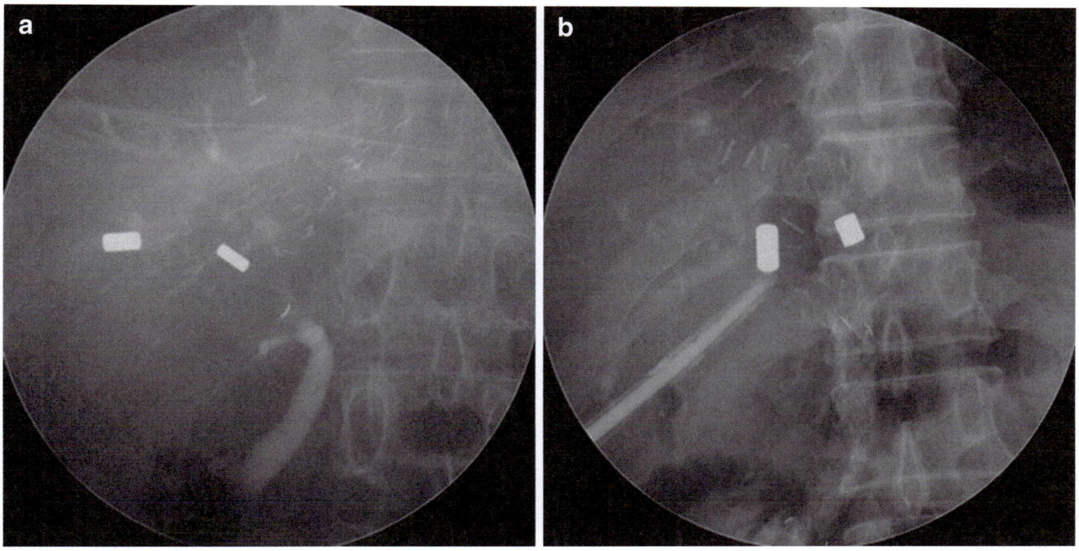

Fig. 2.7 Cholangiogram showing failed magnetic compression anastomosis (MCA). The main causes of unsuccessful MCA are long length of the stricture (**a**), tapered or tortuous duct, and/or parallel axis of alignment (**b**)

the length of the stenosis and the shape and axis of the bile duct needed for a successful MCA cannot be accurately determined. Therefore, the results can only be known when MCA is actually applied.

Securing the Two-Magnet Route

The choice of magnet delivery method depends on the type of anesthesia required, history of the operation, and patient characteristics. Biliobiliary anastomosis delivers magnets through PTBD and ERCP. It is better to use 16- or 18-Fr sheaths through the PTBD tract to prevent damage to the duct during magnet transfer. Delivering a magnet to the CBD is more difficult than using the PTBD and often fails because it requires ERCP and must be through the ampulla of Vater. Delivering 5-mm magnets is difficult by EST alone, and balloon dilation is often used but makes manipulation of the magnet difficult [17]. To solve this problem, a metal stent can be temporarily inserted into the ampulla of Vater [17, 29]. To minimize stent migration and pancreatitis, it is advisable to minimize stent indwelling time, so that the stent is inserted 1 day before administration of MCA. In general, transferring magnets through ERCP in a Roux-en-Y bilioenteric anastomosis is difficult due to the long length of the E-loop and A-limbs and the risk of perforation. In this case, a colonoscopic scope with a transparent cap and a balloon endoscope may be helpful [18]. In all cases, however, there is no guarantee of success, and there is risk of intestinal perforation. A method to deliver a magnet through the skin/intestinal fistula operatively has been reported as an alternative [18, 46]. The magnet delivery method should be selected by considering patient characteristics, surgical history, and required anastomosis, but further development of safe and effective delivery methods is needed.

Route 1: PTBD Track and Endoscopic Approach

An endoscopic approach is the most commonly used MCA method for biliary stenosis after living-donor liver transplantation (LDLT). It is a method of transferring magnets by securing a percutaneous pathway and carrying other magnets through an oral approach to achieve magnetic alignment (Fig. 2.8).

Route 2: PTBD Tract and PTBD Tract

Both the left intrahepatic duct (IHD) and right IHD are anastomosed to the jejunum, and the right IHD is occluded. Two percutaneous transhepatic cholangioscopy scopes are used to deliver the magnet using percutaneous transhepatic biliary drainage through the right IHD tube (one scope) and another magnet through the left IHD tube (second scope) to approximate the magnets (Fig. 2.9).

Route 3: PTBD Tract and a Surgically Formed Fistula

Patients who have undergone LDLT with hepaticojejunostomy often have difficulty accessing peroral endoscopy to the afferent loop. The procedures are described in more detail below. In this case, the magnet can be effectively delivered by passing the endoscope after incision in the afferent loop by performing a surgical intervention (Fig. 2.10).

Removing the Magnets and Maintaining the Re-canalized Fistulous Tract

Removal of the Magnets

As a result of magnet approximation, the stricture tissue becomes sandwiched between the two magnets, and resulting compression causes ischemic necrosis to occur. As the magnets gradually approach each other, the attraction between them strengthens, and ischemic necrosis is accelerated, causing the formation of a new fistula. The approximated magnets may undergo spontaneous migration into the bile duct or bowel through this newly formed fistula (Fig. 2.4). To confirm whether the magnets pass through the anastomosis site, plain abdominal radiographs are taken at 2-week intervals for 6–8 weeks after successful

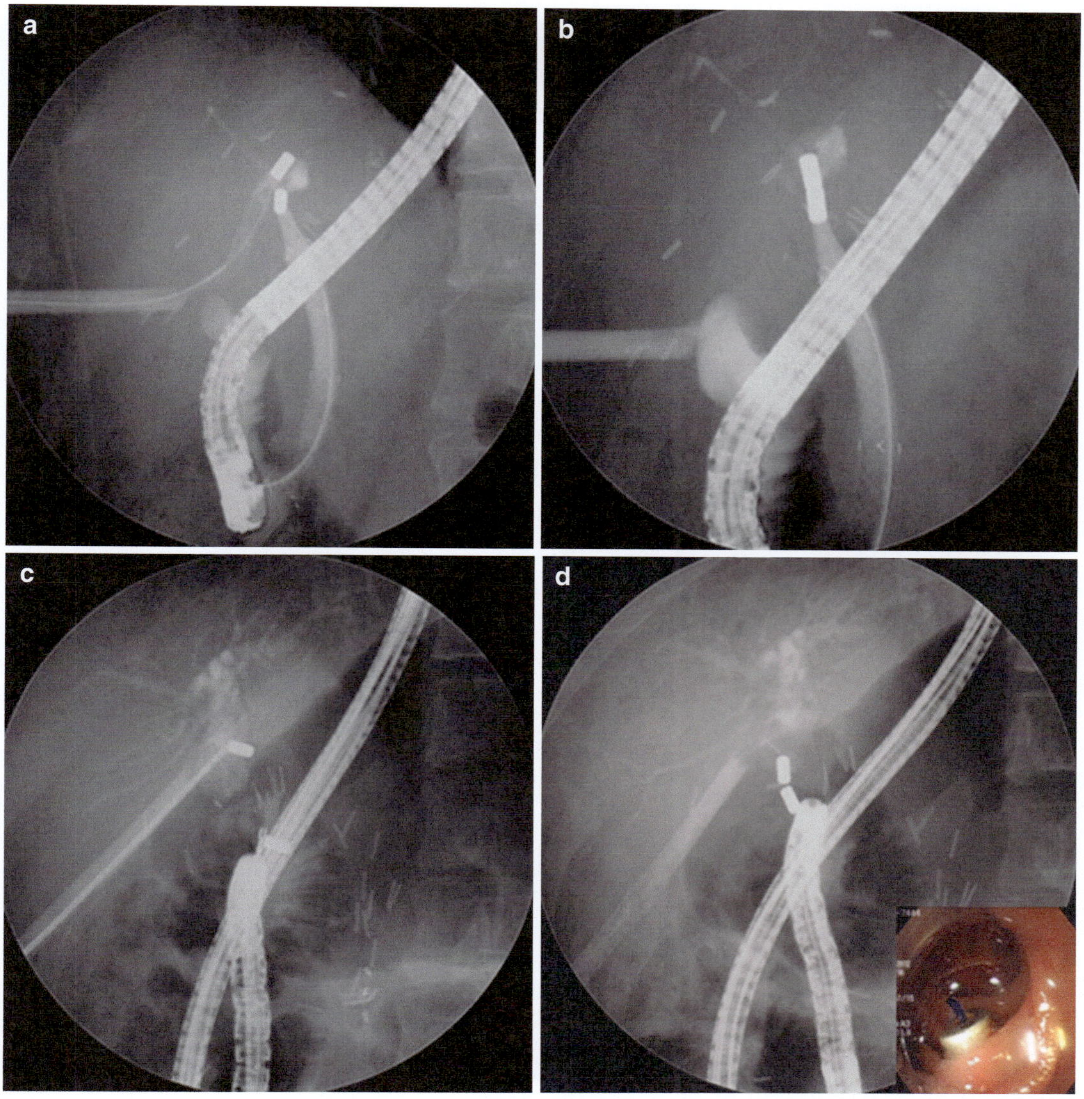

Fig. 2.8 Magnet delivery method: percutaneous transhepatic biliary drainage (PTBD) tract and peroral tract. (**a**, **b**) One magnet is delivered via the PTBD tract and another magnet is delivered via the common bile duct (CBD) in a patient with biliobiliary stricture after living-donor liver transplantation. (**c**, **d**) One magnet is delivered via the PTBD tract and another magnet is delivered via the jejunum using cap-assisted colonoscopy in a patient with bilioenteric stricture after Whipple's operation

magnet approximation. If the magnets maintain a close approximation without spontaneously moving after 10 weeks, they are removed through the PTBD tract using a PTCS scope (Fig. 2.5).

In a previous study, the mean time for successful magnet removal after magnet array was 53.3 days (range, 9–181 days) for a biliobiliary anastomosis and 7–40 days for a bilioenteric anastomosis [31]. The time to successful removal of the magnet array is determined by the distance between the two magnets, the strength of the magnetic field, and the histological differences at the occlusion site. The distance between the two magnets (2–7 mm) is shorter for a bilioenteric anastomosis than for a biliobiliary anastomosis (2–15 mm). In general, partial reperfusion requires a minimum of 10 days for a short occlusion and up to 1 month for long lesions [31].

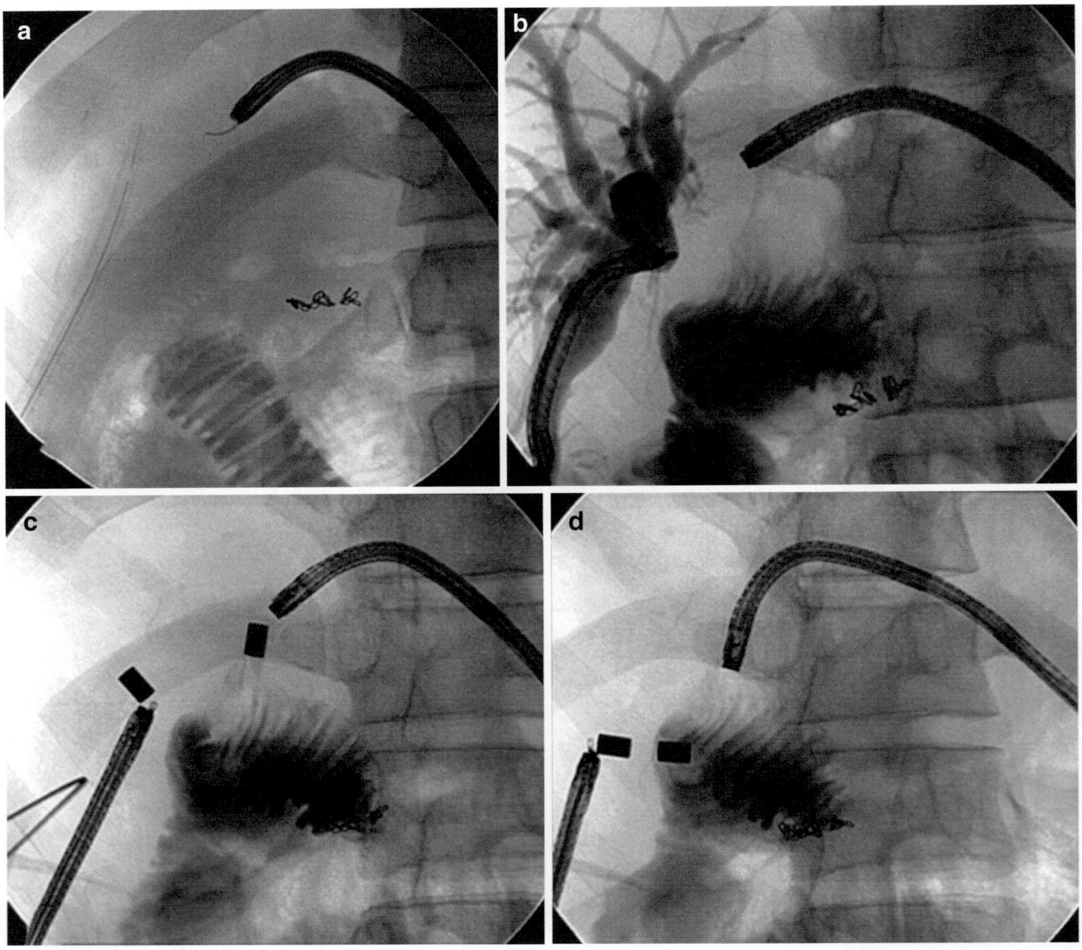

Fig. 2.9 Magnetic compression anastomosis (MCA) using different delivery pathways to form bilioenteric anastomosis. (**a**) A catheter is inserted into the right intrahepatic duct (IHD) and percutaneous transhepatic cholangioscope (PTCS) enters the left IHD. (**b**) PTCS enters the ight IHD and total obstruction of the IHD and jejunum is confirmed. (**c**) Magnet delivery using both PTCS. (**d**) The magnet is delivered to the left IHD through the jejunum using the PTCS. Magnet approximation is achieved through magnetic force

Recanalized Fistulous Tract

After the magnets have been removed, and the recanalized fistula has been confirmed endoscopically or fluoroscopically, a PTCS catheter or FCSEMS is temporarily inserted to maintain the tract after removing the magnets 4–6 months later (Fig. 2.11). Research on these two methods has been carried out. A total of 49 patients were enrolled in the study. The comparison between PTCS ($n = 16$) and FCSEMS ($n = 33$) showed that both methods were equivalent in terms of safety and efficacy. However, as PTCS has a long indwelling duration and has the disadvantage of being replaced, it is more convenient for patients to use FCSEMS [47].

Recoiling

Current long-term clinical follow-up data after MCA treatment are insufficient. However, because MCA forms a fistula as a result of tissue necrosis without enlargement of fibrous tissue, the risk of restenosis due to reorganization of the fibrous tissue is low. Restenosis was not reported for 3 years in one patient who underwent a bilio-biliary anastomosis [30]. Twenty-one patients with biliary stenosis after LDLT were followed up for 331 days, and one patient underwent reperfusion using PTBD [17]. In one study, no restenosis was observed for 50 months [18]. No recurrence was observed 30 days after MCA in

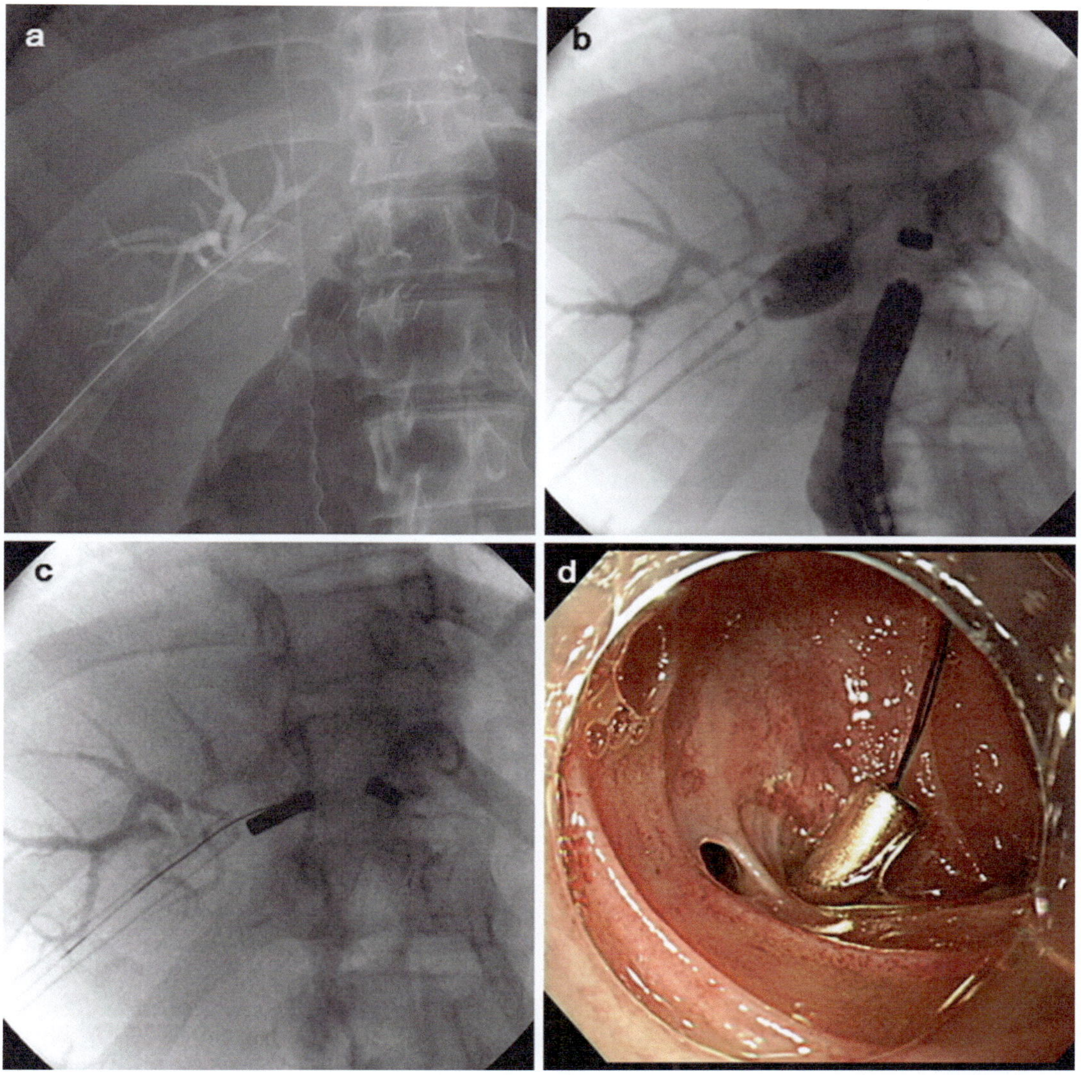

Fig. 2.10 Magnet delivery using the percutaneous transhepatic biliary drainage (PTBD) tract and a surgical fistula. (**a**) A stricture occurred after living-donor liver transplantation with hepaticojejunostomy, and the contrast agent did not move to the jejunum. (**b**) Magnet delivery via percutaneous transhepatic cholangioscopy and intraoperative endoscopy to the incision in the afferent loop are performed. (**c**) Magnet approximation was successful by increasing magnetic power after increasing the number of magnets in the PTBD side. (**d**) The magnet in the jejunum was seen at the endoscopic view after approximation

patients with malignant tumors [22]. The low recurrence rate after MCA has been confirmed in a large, long-term follow-up study.

Safety and Feasibility

The validity and safety of biliobiliary and bilioenteric anastomoses made using MCA has been demonstrated in both human and animal studies. In addition, Avaliani et al. [22] used MCA to form anastomoses between the bile duct and the duodenum or jejunum in 34 patients with malignant strictures, but MCA was not used to recanalize a malignant obstruction. A re-procedure was required in six subjects. However, MCA is not routinely performed to treat malignant biliary obstructions that can often be treated using conventional peroral or percutaneous methods.

Doppler ultrasonography and follow-up may be performed because of the possibility of rupture

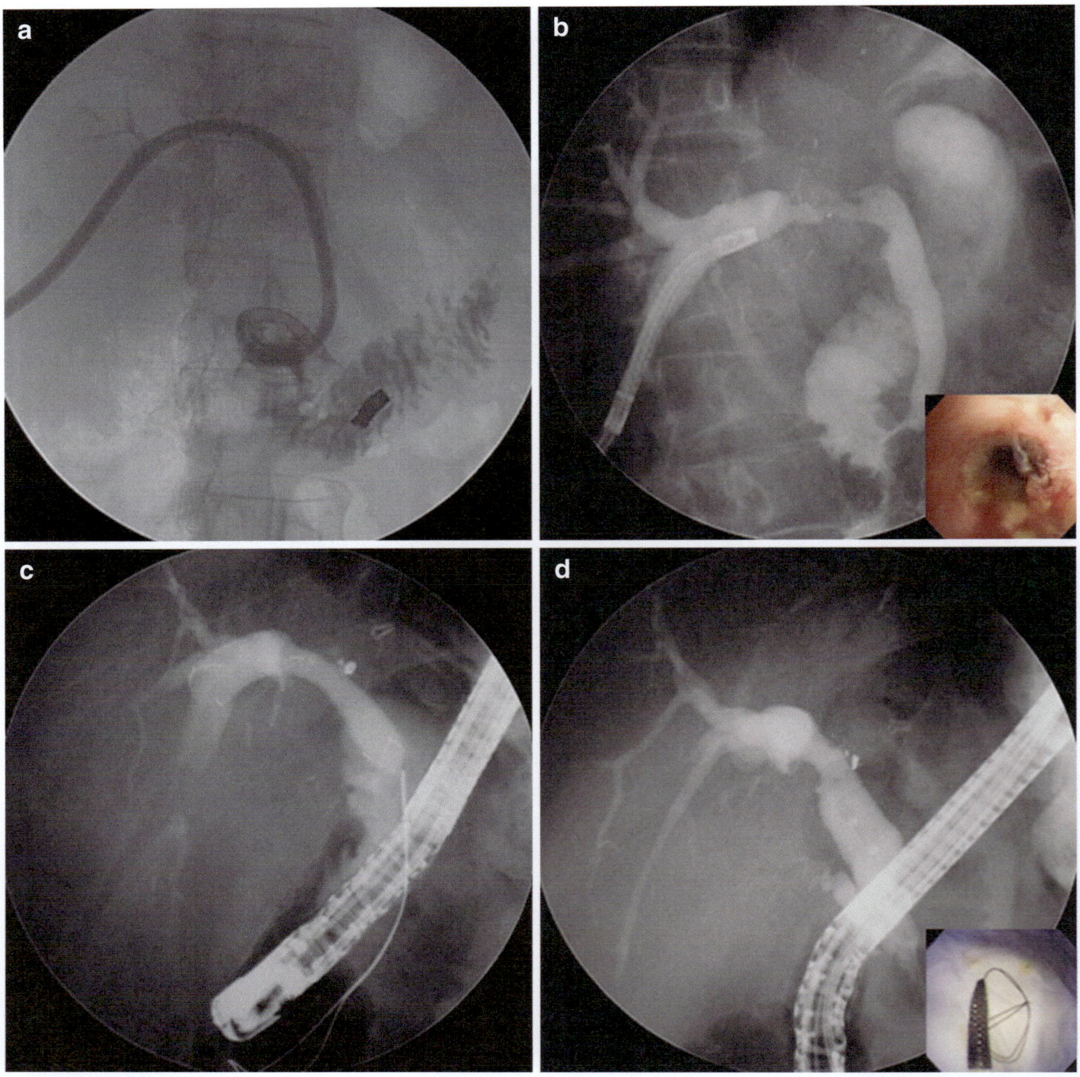

Fig. 2.11 Two methods for maintaining a new fistula created by magnetic compression anastomosis (MCA). (**a**) Magnets were approximated via two delivery tracts in patients with post-living-donor liver transplantation (LDLT) stenosis. (**b**) A percutaneous transhepatic cholangioscopy (PTCS) catheter was inserted through the new fistula after removing the magnets. The PTCS catheter was maintained for 6 months by exchanging every 3 months and removed thereafter. A well-established fistula was seen on PTCS. (**c**) The magnets were approximated via two delivery tracts in patients with post-LDLT stenosis. (**d**) A fully covered self-expandable metal stent (FCSEMS) was inserted endoscopically through the new fistula after removing the magnets. The FCSEMS was removed after 3 months. The FCSEMS removed is shown at the bottom right of the photograph

during MCA treatment if there are blood vessels between the two magnets [26, 46]. However, no vascular tears or other complications have been reported in clinical trials. This is thought to be due to the relatively long time required to form the channel after MCA. Using two magnets makes them closer to each other. Therefore, compression or rupture is not anticipated even if there are blood vessels between them.

Summary

MCA is a feasible and safe non-surgical treatment for occluded benign biliary strictures that are difficult to resolve using conventional endoscopic or percutaneous methods. MCA assessment methods, small and powerful magnets, and effective magnet delivery systems must be developed to predict outcomes for effective MCA and successful re-opening. In addition, endoscopists should fully understand the mechanism and principles of MCA and expand the clinical indications of MCA to apply and develop technologies in various fields. Although the number of cases reported to date is small, MCA is effective and safe, with a lower recurrence rate and less invasiveness than other treatments for benign biliary stenosis.

References

1. Kaidar-Person O, et al. Compression anastomosis: history and clinical considerations. Am J Surg. 2008;195(6):818–26.
2. Jamshidi R, et al. Magnamosis: magnetic compression anastomosis with comparison to suture and staple techniques. J Pediatr Surg. 2009;44(1):222–8.
3. Aggarwal R, Darzi A. Compression anastomoses revisited. J Am Coll Surg. 2005;201(6):965–71.
4. Kopelman D, et al. Compression gastrointestinal anastomosis. Expert Rev Med Devices. 2007;4(6):821–8.
5. Hardy KJ. Non-suture anastomosis: the historical development. Aust N Z J Surg. 1990;60(8):625–33.
6. Murphy JB. Cholecysto-intestinal, gastro-intestinal, entero-intestinal anastomosis, and approximation without sutures. Med Rec N Y. 1892;42:665–76.
7. Swain CP, Mills TN. Anastomosis at flexible endoscopy: an experimental study of compression button gastrojejunostomy. Gastrointest Endosc. 1991;37(6):628–31.
8. Pryor HI 2nd, et al. Multiple magnetic foreign body ingestion: a surgical problem. J Am Coll Surg. 2007;205(1):182–6.
9. Centers for Disease, C and Prevention. Gastrointestinal injuries from magnet ingestion in children--United States, 2003–2006. MMWR Morb Mortal Wkly Rep. 2006;55(48):1296–300.
10. Cauchi JA, Shawis RN. Multiple magnet ingestion and gastrointestinal morbidity. Arch Dis Child. 2002;87(6):539–40.
11. Honzumi M, et al. An intestinal fistula in a 3-year-old child caused by the ingestion of magnets: report of a case. Surg Today. 1995;25(6):552–3.
12. Jansen A, et al. Early experiences with magnetic rings in resection of the distal colon. Neth J Surg. 1980;32(1):20–7.
13. Saveliev VS, Avaliani MV, Bashirov AD. Endoscopic magnetic cholecystodigestive anastomoses: personal technique for palliative treatment of distal bile duct obstruction. J Laparoendosc Surg. 1993;3(2):99–112.
14. Lambe T1, Ríordáin MG, Cahill RA, Cantillon-Murphy P. Magnetic compression in gastrointestinal and bilioenteric anastomosis: how much force? Surg Innov. 2014;21(1):65–73.
15. Savelev VS, et al. Endoscopic biliodigestive anastomosis with the use of magnets (experimental and clinical study). Khirurgiia (Mosk). 1993;3:10–8.
16. Yamanouchi E, et al. A new interventional method: magnetic compression anastomosis with rare-earth magnets. Cardiovasc Intervent Radiol. 1998;22(Suppl 1):S155.
17. Jang SI, et al. Magnetic compression anastomosis is useful in biliary anastomotic strictures after living donor liver transplantation. Gastrointest Endosc. 2011;74(5):1040–8.
18. Jang SI, et al. Recanalization of refractory benign biliary stricture using magnetic compression anastomosis. Endoscopy. 2014;46(1):70–4.
19. Takao S, et al. Magnetic compression anastomosis for benign obstruction of the common bile duct. Endoscopy. 2001;33(11):988–90.
20. Itoi T, et al. Magnetic compression anastomosis: a novel technique for canalization of severe hilar bile duct strictures. Endoscopy. 2005;37(12):1248–51.
21. Okajima H, et al. Magnet compression anastomosis for bile duct stenosis after duct-to-duct biliary reconstruction in living donor liver transplantation. Liver Transpl. 2005;11(4):473–5.
22. Avaliani M, et al. Magnetic compression biliary-enteric anastomosis for palliation of obstructive jaundice: initial clinical results. J Vasc Interv Radiol. 2009;20(5):614–23.
23. Oya H, et al. Magnetic compression anastomosis for bile duct stenosis after donor left hepatectomy: a case report. Transplant Proc. 2012;44(3):806–9.
24. Suyama K, et al. Recanalization of obstructed choledochojejunostomy using the magnet compression anastomosis technique. Am J Gastroenterol. 2010;105(1):230–1.
25. Mita A, et al. Nonsurgical policy for treatment of bilioenteric anastomotic stricture after living donor liver transplantation. Transpl Int. 2008;21(4):320–7.
26. Mimuro A, et al. A novel technique of magnetic compression anastomosis for severe biliary stenosis. Gastrointest Endosc. 2003;58(2):283–7.
27. Lim HC, et al. Magnet compression anastomosis for bilioenteric anastomotic stricture after removal of a choledochal cyst: a case report. Korean J Gastrointest Endosc. 2010;41:180–4.
28. Akita H, et al. Use of a metallic-wall stent in the magnet compression anastomosis technique for bile duct obstruction after liver transplantation. Liver Transpl. 2008;14(1):118–20.
29. Yukawa N, et al. A case of magnetic compression anastomosis between the common bile duct and the duodenum after distal gastrectomy with Roux-Y reconstruction and cholecystectomy. Nihon Shokakibyo Gakkai Zasshi. 2008;105(10):1523–8.
30. Matsuno N, et al. A nonsuture anastomosis using magnetic compression for biliary stricture after living donor liver transplantation. Hepato-Gastroenterology. 2009;56(89):47–9.
31. Itoi T, et al. Magnetic compression duct-to-duct anastomosis for biliary obstruction in a patient with living donor liver transplantation. Gut Liver. 2010;4(Suppl 1):S96–8.
32. Itoi T, et al. Magnetic compression anastomosis for biliary obstruction: review and experience at Tokyo

Medical University Hospital. J Hepatobiliary Pancreat Sci. 2011;18(3):357–65.
33. Lambe T, et al. Magnetic compression in gastrointestinal and bilioenteric anastomosis: how much force? Surg Innov. 2014;21(1):65–73.
34. Cope C. Evaluation of compression cholecystogastric and cholecystojejunal anastomoses in swine after peroral and surgical introduction of magnets. J Vasc Interv Radiol. 1995;6(4):546–52.
35. Cope C. Creation of compression gastroenterostomy by means of the oral, percutaneous, or surgical introduction of magnets: feasibility study in swine. J Vasc Interv Radiol. 1995;6(4):539–45.
36. Pichakron KO, et al. Magnamosis II: magnetic compression anastomosis for minimally invasive gastrojejunostomy and jejunojejunostomy. J Am Coll Surg. 2011;212(1):42–9.
37. Wall J, et al. MAGNAMOSIS IV: magnetic compression anastomosis for minimally invasive colorectal surgery. Endoscopy. 2013;45(8):643–8.
38. Gonzales KD, et al. Magnamosis III: delivery of a magnetic compression anastomosis device using minimally invasive endoscopic techniques. J Pediatr Surg. 2012;47(6):1291–5.
39. Cope C, et al. Stent placement of gastroenteric anastomoses formed by magnetic compression. J Vasc Interv Radiol. 1999;10(10):1379–86.
40. Yan X, et al. Portacaval shunt established in six dogs using magnetic compression technique. PLoS One. 2013;8(9):e76873.
41. Jang SI, et al. Treatment of completely obstructed benign biliary strictures with magnetic compression anastomosis: follow-up results after recanalization. Gastrointest Endosc. 2017;85(5):1057–66.
42. Dumonceau JM, et al. Plastic and metal stents for postoperative benign bile duct strictures: the best and the worst. Gastrointest Endosc. 1998;47(1):8–17.
43. Bonnel DH, et al. Placement of metallic stents for treatment of postoperative biliary strictures: long-term outcome in 25 patients. AJR Am J Roentgenol. 1997;169(6):1517–22.
44. Ernst O, et al. Biliary leaks: treatment by means of percutaneous transhepatic biliary drainage. Radiology. 1999;211(2):345–8.
45. Vogel SB, et al. Evaluation of percutaneous transhepatic balloon dilatation of benign biliary strictures in high-risk patients. Am J Surg. 1985;149(1):73–9.
46. Muraoka N, et al. Yamanouchi magnetic compression anastomosis for bilioenteric anastomotic stricture after living-donor liver transplantation. J Vasc Interv Radiol. 2005;16(9):1263–7.
47. Jang SI, et al. Maintenance of the fistulous tract after recanalization via magnetic compression anastomosis in completely obstructed benign biliary stricture. Scand J Gastroenterol. 2018;53:1393–8.

3 Totally Obstructed Biliary Stricture II: Clinical Applications and Results of Magnetic Compression Anastomosis

Sung Ill Jang, Mo Jin Won, and Dong Ki Lee

Introduction

Potentially fatal complications commonly develop in the biliary system after biliary surgery, including liver transplantation, despite continuous advancement of surgical techniques. An anastomotic stricture may develop due to hypertrophic changes and ischemic injury caused by extensive stripping of the blood vessels of the bile duct of the donor liver during surgery. The development of acute angulation and torsion between the recipient and donor bile ducts renders management more difficult [1–4]. Although anastomotic stricture is the most common surgical complication in living-donor liver transplantation (LDLT), no standardized treatment protocol for such strictures has been established [5–8].

In the early period of LDLT, most bile duct complications were treated surgically. However, surgical treatment is associated with high rates of morbidity and mortality and may not be recommended for patients with serious complications, such as bile duct inflammation [9]. When an interventional radiology technique is used after percutaneous transhepatic biliary drainage (PTBD), bile ducts occluded by stenosis may be recanalized with a guidewire and balloon dilator. Balloon dilation or the placement of plastic or metal stents, guided by endoscopic retrograde cholangiopancreatography (ERCP), may also yield favorable results [3]. Advances in non-surgical methods, including endoscopic and percutaneous techniques, have enabled recanalization of biliary strictures. Overall, non-surgical treatment of anastomotic stenosis and obstruction after biliary operation is more effective than surgical treatment [7, 10].

Unfortunately, balloon dilation or stent insertion cannot be performed when the guidewire does not pass through the duct-to-duct anastomotic obstruction percutaneously or endoscopically because of complete obstruction, severe stenosis, or deviation of the duct. In such patients, an external PTBD catheter must be maintained to support life, which burdens the responsible physician and the patient.

In 1998, Yamanouchi et al. [11] introduced magnetic compression anastomosis (MCA), which is now an accepted non-surgical technique for the reconstruction of anastomotic sites in the digestive system [12–22]. In this chapter, we classify biliary strictures that develop after biliary surgery as biliobiliary and bilioenteric and discuss the clinical results of MCA for each stricture type.

S. I. Jang · M. J. Won · D. K. Lee (✉)
Department of Internal Medicine, Gangnam Severance Hospital, Yonsei University College of Medicine, Seoul, South Korea
e-mail: aerojsi@yuhs.ac; dklee@yuhs.ac

D. K. Lee (ed.), *Advanced ERCP for Complicated and Refractory Biliary and Pancreatic Diseases*,
https://doi.org/10.1007/978-981-13-0608-2_3

MCA for Biliobiliary Stricture

MCA for Treatment of Post-LDLT Stricture

Despite advances in surgical techniques, fatal complications frequently arise after liver transplantation. Anastomotic strictures develop in 5–15% of deceased-donor liver transplant (DDLT) recipients and 28–32% of LDLT recipients [23]. The ischemic injury [2] and the hypertrophic change [1] caused by extensive detachment of the blood vessels during surgery induce duct-to-duct anastomotic stenosis [3]. In addition, torsion and sharp angles between the donor and recipient bile ducts hamper the management of stenosis [4]. Bile duct anastomosis is the most common surgical complication of LDLT, but no protocol for its treatment has been established [5–8, 24].

The magnets used in MCA are cylindrical Sm-Co rare-earth magnets of various powers that can be delivered by a variety of methods; the most common methods are percutaneously and per oral. MCA can be divided into the following four steps (Fig. 3.1): (1) tract formation for magnet delivery, (2) magnet approximation, (3) magnet removal, and (4) maintenance and removal of the internal catheter.

1. Tract formation for magnet delivery. A PTBD tract for magnet delivery is formed using a 16-Fr PTBD catheter. The PTBD catheter is exchanged for an 18-Fr sheath prior to MCA

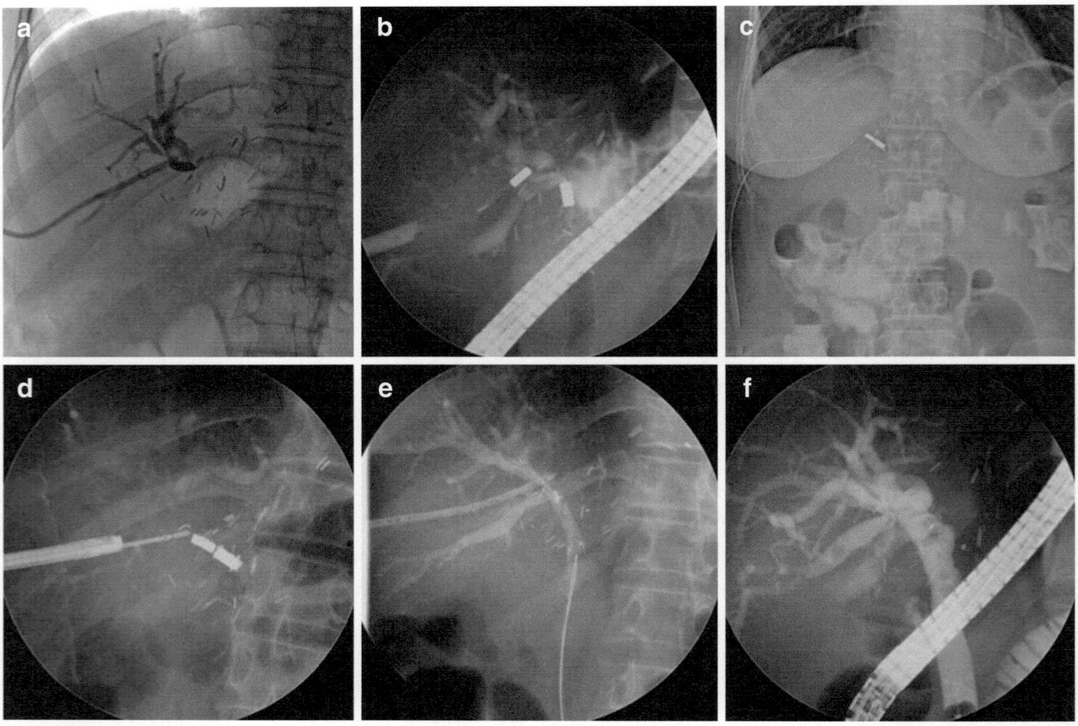

Fig. 3.1 Cholangiograms showing magnetic compression anastomosis for a biliobiliary stricture developing after living-donor liver transplantation. (**a**) After insertion of a percutaneous transhepatic biliary drainage (PTBD) catheter, the tract was dilated to 16 Fr. (**b**) After insertion of a covered self-expandable metal stent into the common bile duct (CBD), a magnet attached to a polypectomy snare was delivered using an endoscopic retrograde cholangiopancreatography scope through the CBD. A second magnet was fixed to alligator forceps and moved toward the anastomosis site through the PTBD tract after insertion of an 18-Fr sheath. (**c**) The magnets were approximated, and the PTBD catheter was inserted. (**d**) After 6 weeks, the approximated magnets were removed by percutaneous transhepatic cholangioscopy through the PTBD tract. (**e**) A retrievable, fully covered self-expandable metal stent (FCSEMS) was inserted for 6 months. (**f**) Finally, the FCSEMS was removed and a new fistula was formed

approximation to facilitate magnet insertion via the PTBD tract and to reduce duct injury. In the common bile duct (CBD) tract, full endoscopic sphincterotomy and balloon dilation or transient insertion of a retrievable, fully covered self-expandable metal stent (FCSEMS) are used to facilitate magnet delivery.

2. Magnet approximation. A thread attached to a magnet is fixed to a polypectomy snare, and the magnet is moved to the anastomosis site via the PTBD tract. The polypectomy snare is passed through the channel of an ERCP scope, and a second magnet is fixed in front of the scope. The magnet is moved to the anastomosis site through the FCSEMS, and MCA approximation occurs as a result of attraction between the two magnets. To better approximate the magnets, a balloon catheter may be used to advance the magnets through the PTBD and ERCP tracts. Approximation of the two magnets is confirmed radiographically. Next, the long sheath tube is removed and an indwelling PTBD catheter is inserted. The FCSEMS in the CBD is removed immediately after magnet approximation.
3. Magnet removal. When a fistula forms because of ischemic necrosis caused by the approximated magnets, the magnets spontaneously migrate to the duodenum. However, if spontaneous migration does not occur after 8–10 weeks, the magnets can be pushed out using a guidewire or catheter. The magnets can also be removed through the PTBD tract via percutaneous transhepatic cholangioscopy (PTCS).
4. Maintenance and removal of the internal catheter. After magnet removal, a 14–16-Fr internal catheter is inserted into the fistula and maintained in situ for 4–6 months to reduce the probability of re-stenosis of the fistulous tract. An FCSEMS is more useful than an internal catheter because the FCSEMS allows formation of a larger fistula. However, an FCSEMS is more likely to migrate than is an indwelling catheter. Further work is necessary to confirm the efficacy of FCSEMS use.

The results of MCA for biliobiliary strictures (BBSs) are summarized in Table 3.1. MCA showed a higher clinical success rate (87.5%) and lower recurrence rate (7.1%) than did other conventional endoscopic and percutaneous methods. In the treatment of BBSs, the clinical success rate differs depending on the etiology and the treatment method used. Postoperative and stone-related strictures respond well to endoscopic management, but idiopathic and chronic pancreatitis-related strictures have low response rates [25]. The clinical success rate of endoscopic BBS treatment is 90% for postoperative strictures, but 65% for chronic pancreatitis-related strictures; in comparison, the success rate of percutaneous treatment is 61.4–90.9% [26–29]. Although improvements in conventional methods have increased their technical success rates, these procedures are not successful in cases of stenosis through which the guidewire cannot be passed; thus, they cannot be used to resolve all cases of BBS. In addition, the clinical success rates of these procedures are lower than the technical success rates because of restenosis. Forceful disruption of the stricture scar caused by repeated pneumatic dilation causes traumatic damage to the tissue and ultimately provokes a new fibrotic reaction, which can lead to restenosis [30]. A recent trial conducted with patients with complete CBD interruption showed the feasibility of the intraperitoneal rendezvous method for biliary reconstruction, but further research is needed [31].

The only early adverse event was mild cholangitis in one patient. No late adverse event was noted during follow-up. Early adverse events after MCA have not been reported in other studies, including in those involving LDLT recipients. The only reported adverse event is cholangitis, which can be resolved by conservative management [20, 21]. Hence, the MCA procedure is safe in post-LDLT and other immunocompromised patients. Doppler ultrasound-based screening and follow-up are performed because of the risk of vessel rupture during the early stages of MCA, when blood vessels are present between the two magnets [15, 17]. However, no clinical report has described blood vessel rupture or any related adverse event. Thus, compression or rupture of the intervening vessels does not occur, possibly because the

Table 3.1 Outcomes of recanalization using magnetic compression anastomosis in patients with biliobiliary strictures

Year	Author	Type of report	Age/sex	Reason for operation	Previous operation	Distance between magnets (mm)	Anastomosis
2003	Mimuro et al.	Case	76/F	Pancreatic cancer	DP	12	Partial
2005	Itoi et al.	Case	76/F	Hilar bile duct cancer	None	8	Partial
2005	Okajima et al.	Case	44/F	Fulminant hepatitis	LDLT	2	Complete
2008	Akita et al.	Case	34/F	NA	LDLT	2	Complete
2009	Matsuno et al.	Case	53/M	NA	LDLT	2	Complete
2010	Itoi et al.	Case	60/M	NA	LDLT	NA	Complete
2011	Itoi et al.	Case	40/F	Metastasis live tumor derived from colon cancer	Right three segmental + S3 partial hepatectomy	15	Complete
2011	Jang et al.	Original	Mean 53.8 M:F = 9:3	LC (3), HCC (7), HF (2)	LDLT	NA	Complete
2012	Oya et al.	Case	24/M	NA	LDLT	NA	Partial
2014	Jang et al.	Case	45/M	Abdominal trauma	Embolization	4	Complete
			38/F	Cholecystitis	Cholecystitis	6	Complete
2017	Jang et al.	Original	39 patients	LC, HCC, HF	LDLT	NA	Complete
2018	Jiang et al.	Case	64/F	Metastatic liver tumor from rectal cancer	Right partial hepatectomy	NA	Complete

DP dorsal pancreatectomy, *HCC* hepatocellular carcinoma, *HF* hepatic failure, *LC* liver cirrhosis, *LDLT* living-donor liver transplantation, *NA* not available

magnets gradually move closer to each other over a prolonged period after approximation (biliobiliary anastomosis, mean 53.3 days; bilioenteric anastomosis, range 7–40 days) [21]. In a previous study, the only MCA-related adverse event occurring between magnet approximation and the removal of the indwelling catheter was slight fever, and in the present study, the only adverse event was mild cholangitis [32]. No procedure-related mortality has been reported. Moreover, no adverse event resulting from the procedure or the devices used in the procedure has been reported, as it is carried out using the conventional ERCP method and the PTBD tract. Magnet-related adverse events are thought to not occur because the magnet is an aseptic device that does not introduce foreign material into the body or induce inflammation or an immune reaction in the bile duct.

In the above study, reperfusion of the stenosis was observed in all ten patients in whom treatment was successful. The average time from disposition to magnet removal was 74.2 days; in two patients, the magnets could not be removed within 3 months due to the presence of dense fibrous tissue. In nine patients, the internal catheter was removed completely, and the mean indwelling duration was 183 days. One patient had cholecystitis and one had recurrent stenosis after MCA.

MCA is a safe and effective treatment for anastomotic stenosis after LDLT. It is associated with some complications, but it is less invasive than surgery and can be performed even in patients who have present contraindications for surgery. Stenosis length is an important factor in the success of MCA. Stenoses are usually longer and more distorted in LDLT than in DDLT recipients. The technical limitations of MCA include the length of the stenosis, the period after LDLT, the structure of the CBD, and the strength of the magnet. The maximal anastomotic stenosis length for which MCA is feasible is difficult to assess accurately and should be clarified in further studies. In addition, reperfusion after MCA may take about 2 months. However, if the magnet is not passed, intervention using a guidewire or balloon through the percutaneous tube may be performed. After removal of the magnet, a catheter should be inserted to prevent restenosis of the new track.

When MCA creates new tracks instead of resolving a previous stenosis, the recurrence rate of stenosis is likely lower than those obtained with conventional methods. In addition, the maintenance of an external PTBD catheter is not required, and the risk of complications, including infection, is low. However, confirmatory studies involving small populations and long-term follow up are needed. MCA may be effective in cases that cannot be treated by conventional methods, in addition to cases of stenosis caused by LDLT.

MCA for Treatment of Post-DDLT Stricture

Benign biliary stricture is a common complication after liver transplantation. LDLT is the treatment of choice for end-stage liver disease, especially in Asia, where organs from deceased donors are more difficult to obtain than in western nations. As experience of LDLT in Asia has increased, the incidence of biliary stricture has decreased from 30% to 15–25% [7, 33–37].

The incidence of biliary stricture is 25–32% after LDLT [38–42] and <15% after DDLT [23, 41, 43]. Furthermore, biliary stricture is more common after LDLT (33.3%) than after DDLT (9.6%) [44–48]. In LDLT, anastomosis between the right hepatic duct of the donor and the recipient bile duct is complex. In addition, the right hepatic duct has many variants, including multiple bile ducts, poor blood supply, and a short stump for anastomosis [7, 41, 42, 49].

MCA for the treatment of biliary stricture after DDLT is similar to that for the treatment of post-LDLT stricture (Fig. 3.2). The sites of stricture after LDLT are more distal than those developing after DDLT. Post-LDLT and post-DDLT strictures tend to be high and mid-level, respectively. Moreover, proximal duct dilatation is more severe in post-DDLT than in post-LDLT strictures, but the dilated ducts are less angulated and tortuous. Therefore, the magnet approximation and success rates are higher for post-DDLT than for post-LDLT strictures (Fig. 3.3).

MCA for Treatment of Post-cholecystectomy Stricture

The incidence of bile duct injury during laparoscopic cholecystectomy is 0.3–0.6%, higher than that achieved in the era of open cholecystectomy, despite advances in laparoscopic surgery and increasing surgical experience [50, 51]. Bile duct injury is the most serious complication of gastrointestinal surgery and has significant impacts on patients' quality of life.

Biliary injuries can be classified using the Bismuth [52], Strasberg [53], and Stewart–Way classification [54]. The Stewart–Way classification divides biliary injuries into four classes based on the mechanism and anatomy (Fig. 3.4) [54]. Stewart–Way class I injuries, which are by definition recognized intraoperatively, can be repaired immediately using fine monofilament absorbable sutures [55]. Stewart–Way class II injuries with stricture can be treated with multiple plastic stents and self-expanding covered metallic stents. The treatment of Stewart–Way classes III and IV injuries requires a multidisciplinary approach. Fiocca et al. [56] proposed a combined endoscopic–radiological rendezvous technique for the treatment of complete transection of the main bile duct, a Stewart–Way class III injury. This modality avoids the need for surgical reintervention, which is associated with morbidity and mortality risks. Class IV injuries, which involve non-transected sectorial bile ducts, can often be managed non-surgically with drainage and stenting via ERCP or

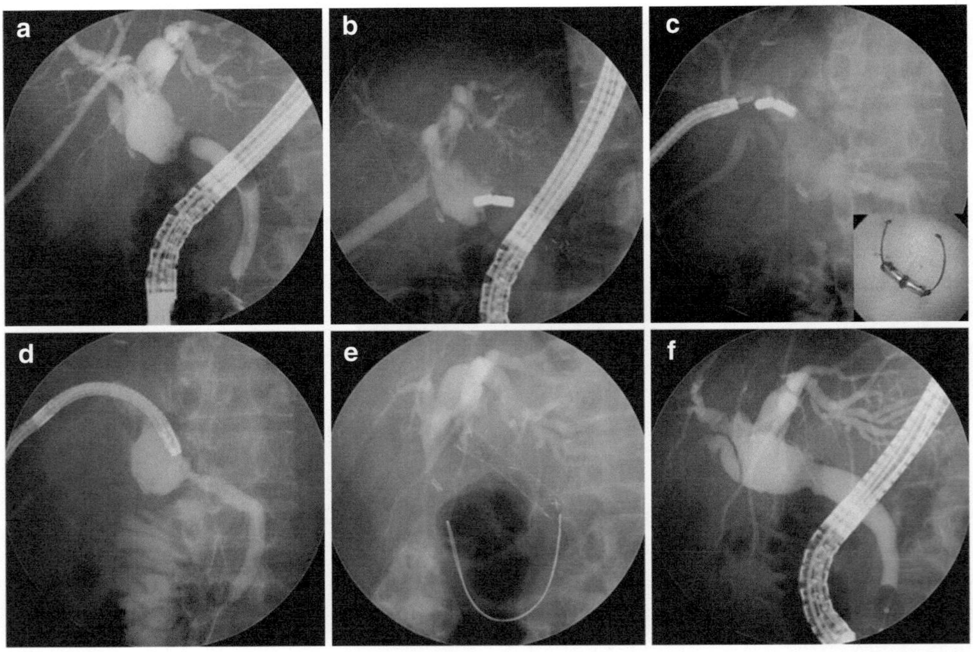

Fig. 3.2 Cholangiograms showing magnetic compression anastomosis for a biliobiliary stricture that developed after deceased-donor liver transplantation. (**a**) After insertion of a percutaneous transhepatic biliary drainage (PTBD) catheter, the tract was dilated to 16 Fr. (**b**) After insertion of a covered self-expandable metal stent into the common bile duct (CBD), a magnet attached to a polypectomy snare was delivered using an endoscopic retrograde cholangiopancreatography scope through the CBD. Another magnet was fixed to alligator forceps and moved toward the anastomosis site through the PTBD tract after insertion of an 18-Fr sheath. (**c**) The magnets were approximated, and the PTBD catheter was inserted. After 6 weeks, the approximated magnets were removed by percutaneous transhepatic cholangioscopy through the PTBD tract. Bottom-right color photograph shows the removed magnets. (**d**) Cholangiogram showing the newly formed fistula. (**e**) A retrievable, fully covered self-expandable metal stent (FCSEMS) was inserted for 6 months. (**f**) Finally, the FCSEMS was removed and a new fistula was formed (compare with [**d**])

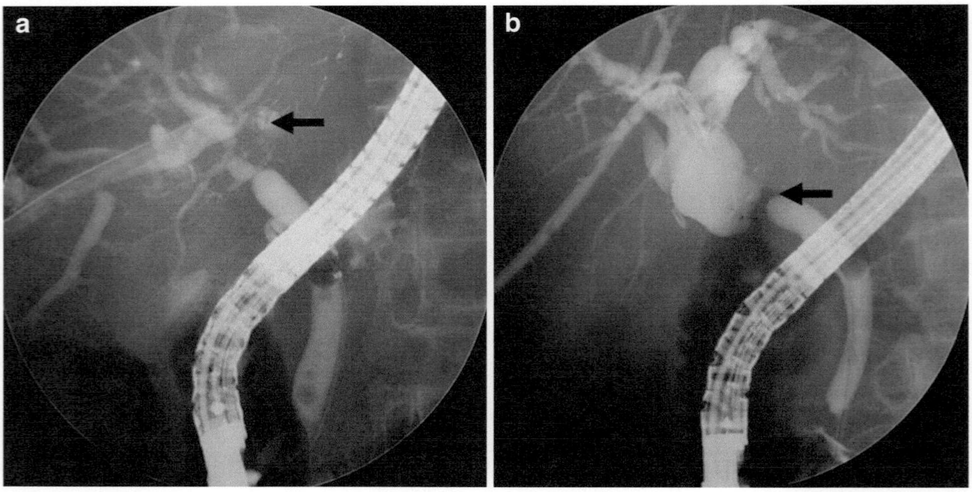

Fig. 3.3 Cholangiograms showing the levels and shapes of strictures after liver transplantation. (**a**) Cholangiogram showing an anastomotic stricture after living-donor liver transplantation (LDLT). (**b**) Cholangiogram showing an anastomotic stricture after deceased-donor liver transplantation (DDLT). The post-LDLT stricture is a high-level stricture, and the proximal duct dilatation in the post-DDLT stricture is more severe than in the post-LDLT stricture, but the dilated duct is less angulated and tortuous

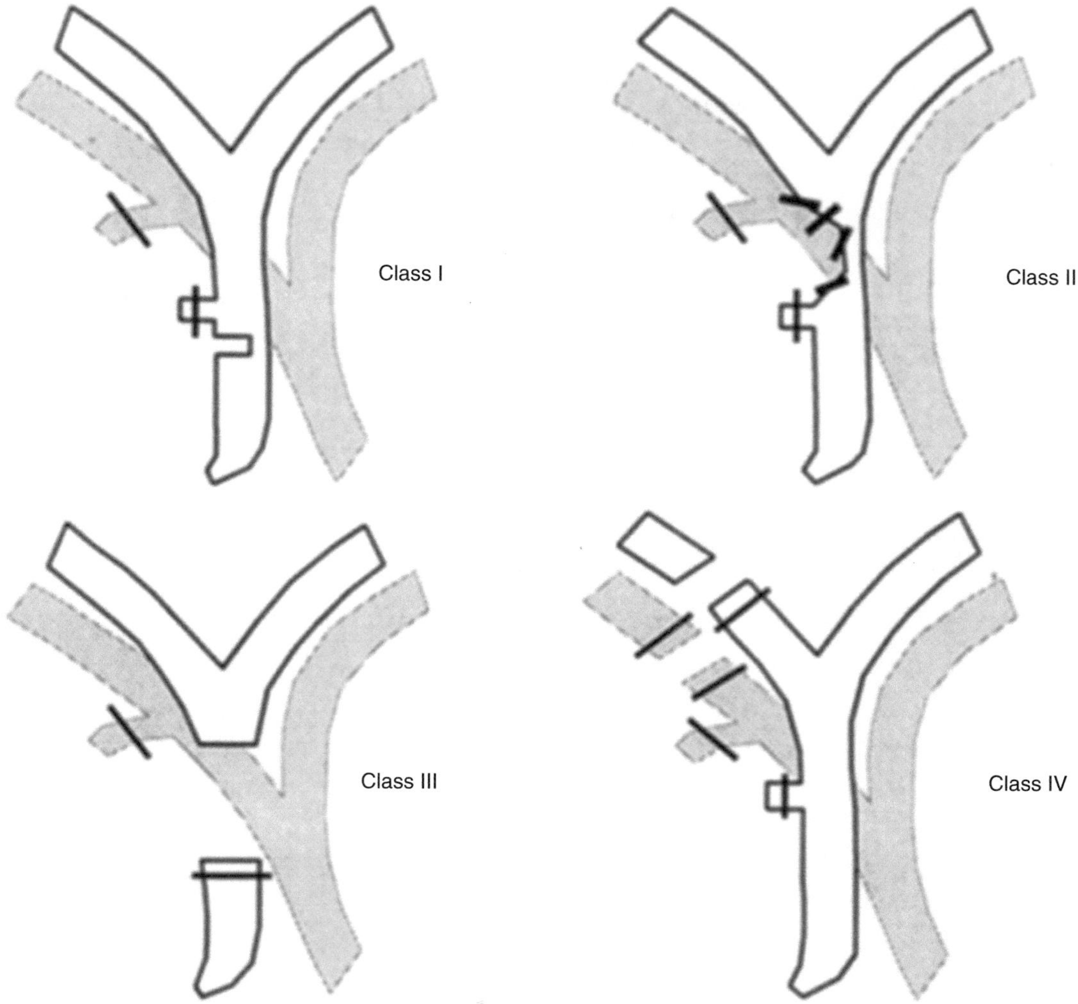

Fig. 3.4 Stewart–Way classification of bile duct injuries. (Adapted from [54])

PTCS. These endoscopic–radiological rendezvous techniques for the treatment of bile duct stricture or obstruction are feasible if the guidewire can be passed through the stricture lesion. MCA represents an alternative method in patients with Stewart–Way classes III and IV bile duct injuries (Figs. 3.5 and 3.6). The process of MCA in these patients is similar to that in those with post-LDLT strictures.

MCA for Treatment of Other Post-biliary Operation Stricture

Although most bile duct injuries occur after cholecystectomy, other hepatic surgeries, such as hepatectomy, may also cause major damage to the bile duct. Early-stage injuries result from complex dissection, poorly defined anatomy, or management of preoperative bleeding by clipping or diathermy [57]. Late-stage injuries can be caused by ischemia of the bile ducts, and stenoses may develop clinically decades after the original insult. Endoscopic treatment with plastic or metal stents is essential for stenosis after biliary surgery, including hepatectomy, and typically requires the expertise of multidisciplinary teams of endoscopists, radiologists, and surgeons. In these patients, endoscopic or percutaneous treatment can be effective if the guidewire can pass through the stricture. MCA is an alternative when conventional methods cannot be used to resolve

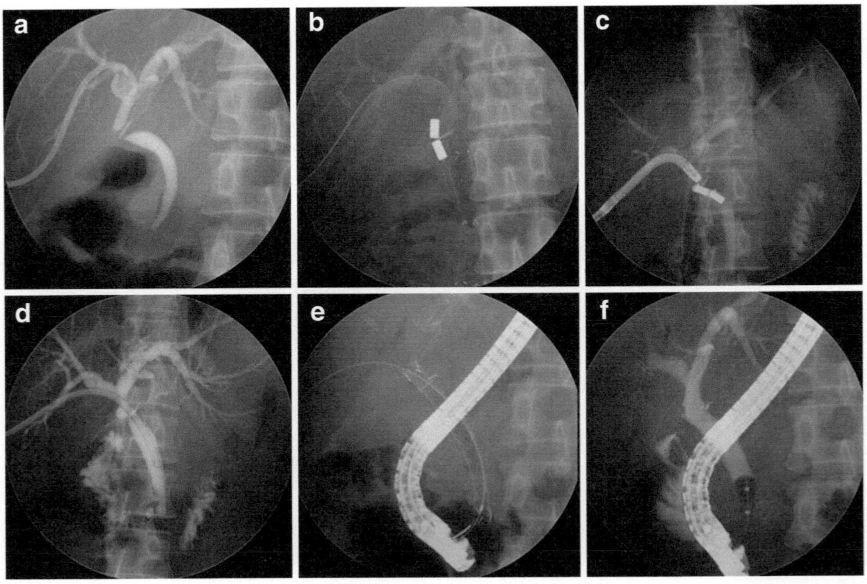

Fig. 3.5 Cholangiograms showing magnetic compression anastomosis (MCA) for a Stewart–Way class III biliobiliary stricture that developed after cholecystectomy. (**a**) Common bile duct stricture after cholecystectomy. (**b**) One magnet was delivered through the percutaneous transhepatic biliary drainage (PTBD) tract, and a second was approximated using a duodenoscope to form an MCA, leading to successful recanalization. (**c**) After 6 weeks, the approximated magnets were removed by percutaneous transhepatic cholangioscopy (PTCS) through the PTBD tract. (**d**) A PTCS catheter was placed through the right hepatic duct and common bile duct, with the distal tip in the jejunum. (**e**) A retrievable, fully covered self-expandable metal stent (FCSEMS) was inserted for 6 months. (**f**) Finally, the FCSEMS was removed and a new fistula formed

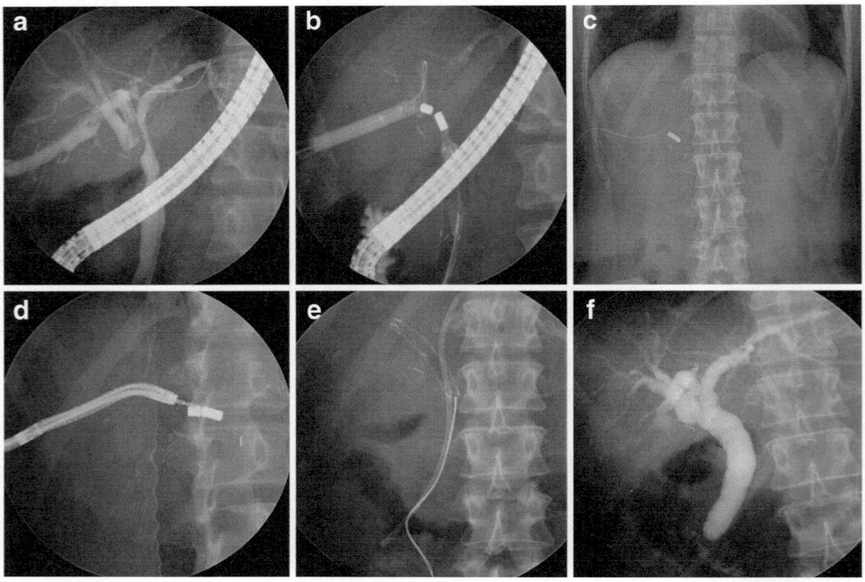

Fig. 3.6 Cholangiograms showing magnetic compression anastomosis (MCA) for a Stewart–Way class IV biliobiliary stricture that developed after cholecystectomy. (**a**) Right intrahepatic duct stricture after cholecystectomy. (**b**) One magnet was delivered through the percutaneous transhepatic biliary drainage (PTBD) tract, and a second was approximated using a duodenoscope to form an MCA, leading to successful recanalization. (**c**) The magnets were approximated, and the PTBD catheter was inserted. (**d**) After 6 weeks, the approximated magnets were removed by percutaneous transhepatic cholangioscopy through the PTBD tract. (**e**) A retrievable, fully covered self-expandable metal stent (FCSEMS) and a plastic stent were inserted for 6 months. (**f**) Finally, the FCSEMS was removed and a new fistula formed

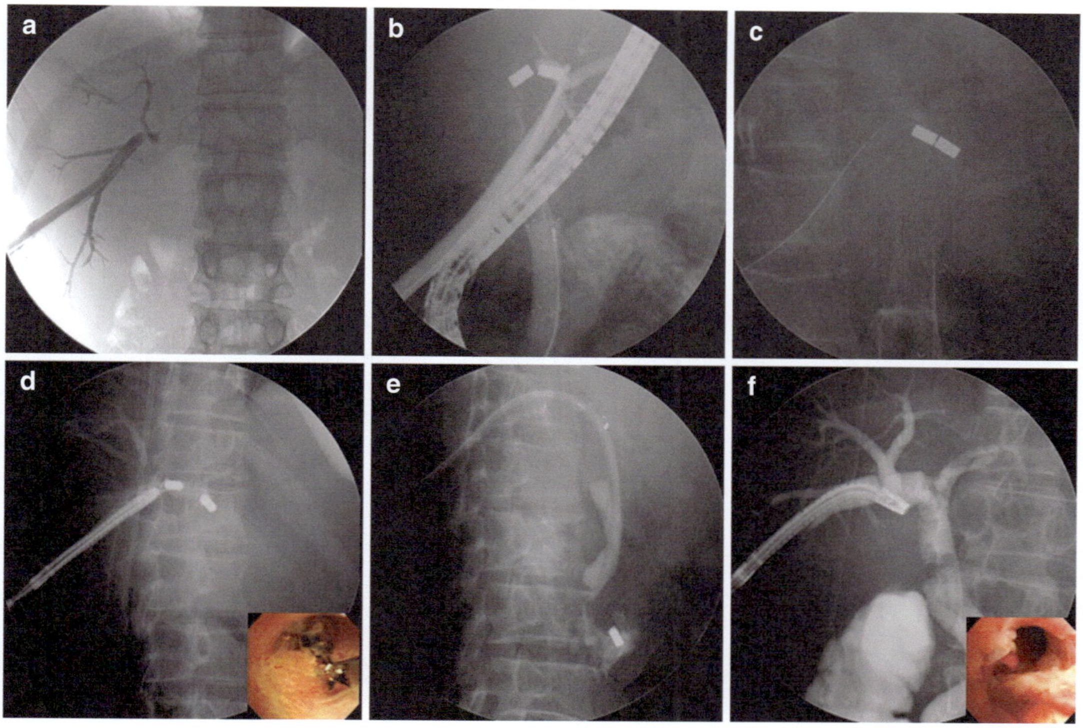

Fig. 3.7 Cholangiograms showing magnetic compression anastomosis (MCA) for a biliary stricture developing after surgery for a hepatic injury caused by a traffic accident. (**a**) Right intrahepatic duct stricture after hepatic surgery. (**b**) One magnet was delivered through the percutaneous transhepatic biliary drainage (PTBD) tract, and a second was approximated using a duodenoscope to form an MCA, leading to successful recanalization. (**c**) The magnets were approximated, and the PTBD catheter was inserted. (**d**) After 6 weeks, the approximated magnets were removed by percutaneous transhepatic cholangioscopy (PTCS) through the PTBD tract. (**e**) A PTCS catheter was inserted for 6 months. (**f**) Finally, the catheter was removed and a new fistula formed

post-biliary surgery strictures. The process of MCA in these patients is similar to that for post-LDLT strictures (Fig. 3.7).

MCA for Bilioenteric Stricture

MCA for Hepaticojejunostomy Site Stricture

The results of MCA for BBSs are summarized in Table 3.2. Benign biliary strictures are typically caused by postoperative complications, and the principal anastomosis method used is Roux-en-Y reconstruction (Fig. 3.8). In general, the MCA method used for bilioenteric anastomosis is similar to that used for biliobiliary anastomosis. However, the magnets can be delivered by a percutaneous–peroral tract (most frequent; Fig. 3.9), a surgically formed percutaneous–jejunum tract (Fig. 3.10), or a percutaneous–percutaneous tract (Fig. 3.11).

The method of magnet delivery to the percutaneous tract is identical to that described above, but a forward-viewing endoscope is used for the per oral approach. However, an endoscopic approach is difficult in patients with long afferent loops. In such cases, magnets may be delivered through a surgically created skin/intestinal fistula; single-balloon enteroscopy is reportedly useful in such situations. Rarely, the left and right intrahepatic ducts (IHDs) may be anastomosed separately to the jejunum, with the stricture evident on the right side. Two PTCS scopes are used in this context: one to deliver a magnet through the right IHD via the PTBD tract and the other to approximate the second magnet at the stricture site via the left IHD tract.

The above cases highlight the various delivery methods that may be used. The mean distance

Table 3.2 Outcomes of recanalization by magnetic compression anastomosis in patients with bilioenteric strictures

Year	Author	Type of report	Age/sex	Reason for operation	Previous operation	Distance between magnets (mm)	Anastomosis
2001	Takao et al.	Case	70/M	Gastric cancer	Subtotal gastrectomy (B-II)	2	Complete
2005	Muraoka et al.	Case	1/F	Fulminant hepatitis	LDLT (left lobe) with R-Y	2	Complete
			57/M	LC + HCC	LDLT (right lobe) with R-Y	5	Complete
2008	Yukawa et al.	Case	83/M	Gastric and gallbladder cancer	Distal gastrectomy with R-Y and cholecystectomy	NA	Complete
2009	Avaliani et al.	Original article	Mean 64 M:F = 9:25	Cancer of VA (7) Pancreatic cancer (21) CCC (6)	None	NA	Complete (except for one case)
2010	Suyama et al.	Case	78/M	Gallbladder cancer	Radical cholecystectomy with R-Y	NA	Complete
2011	Itoi et al.	Case	60/F	CCC	Expanded left lobectomy with R-Y	2	Complete
2014	Jang et al.	Case series	49/M	Pancreatic NET	PPPD with HJstomy	5	Complete
			27/M	Choledochal cyst	Excision of cyst with R-Y	5	Complete
			63/F	Pancreatic NET	Whipple operation with R-Y	77	Complete
2015	Rei et al.	Case	16/F	Type I biliary atresia	Cyst-jejunostomy	NA	Complete

B-II Billroth II, *CCC* cholangiocellular carcinoma, *HCC* hepatocellular carcinoma, *LC* liver cirrhosis, *LDLT* living-donor liver transplantation, *NA* not available, *NET* neuroendocrine tumor, *PPPD* pylorus-preserving pancreaticoduodenectomy, *R-Y* Roux-en-Y anastomosis, *VA* Vater's ampulla

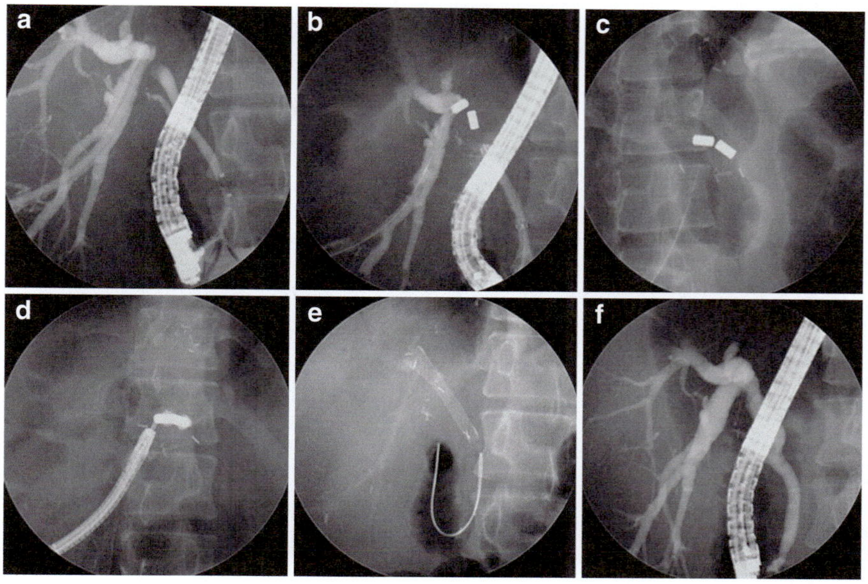

Fig. 3.8 Cholangiograms showing magnetic compression anastomosis (MCA) for a biliary stricture developing after left trisectionectomy performed due to hepatocellular carcinoma. (**a**) Right intrahepatic duct stricture after hepatic surgery. (**b**) One magnet was delivered through the percutaneous transhepatic biliary drainage (PTBD) tract, and a second was approximated using a duodenoscope to form an MCA, leading to successful recanalization. (**c**) The magnets were approximated, and the PTBD catheter was inserted. (**d**) After 8 weeks, the approximated magnets were removed by percutaneous transhepatic cholangioscopy through the PTBD tract. (**e**) A retrievable, fully covered self-expandable metal stent (FCSEMS) and a plastic stent were inserted for 6 months. (**f**) Finally, the FCSEMS was removed and a new fistula formed

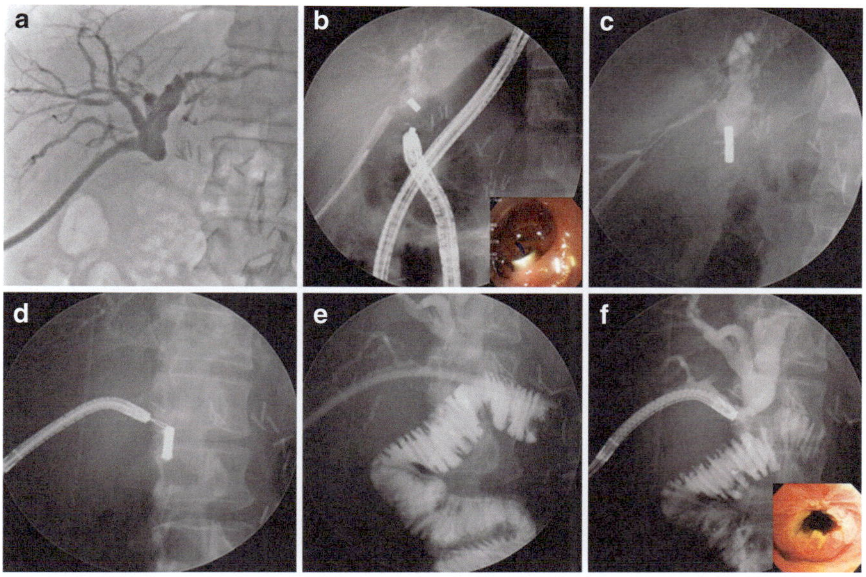

Fig. 3.9 Cholangiograms showing magnetic compression anastomosis for a bilioenteric stricture that developed after Whipple's operation with Roux-en-Y anastomosis for pancreatic cancer. (**a**) A percutaneous transhepatic biliary drainage (PTBD) catheter was inserted because the anastomosis site was completely obstructed, and the tract was dilated to 16 Fr. (**b**) A magnet attached to a polypectomy snare was delivered using a colonoscope with a transparent cap, and a second magnet was delivered through the PTBD tract. (**c**) The magnets were successfully approximated, and a PTBD catheter was inserted. (**d**) After 8 weeks, the approximated magnets were removed by percutaneous transhepatic cholangioscopy through the PTBD tract. (**e**) An internal drainage catheter (16 Fr) was inserted and maintained in situ for 6 months. (**f**) Finally, the catheter was removed, and the development of a new fistula was confirmed

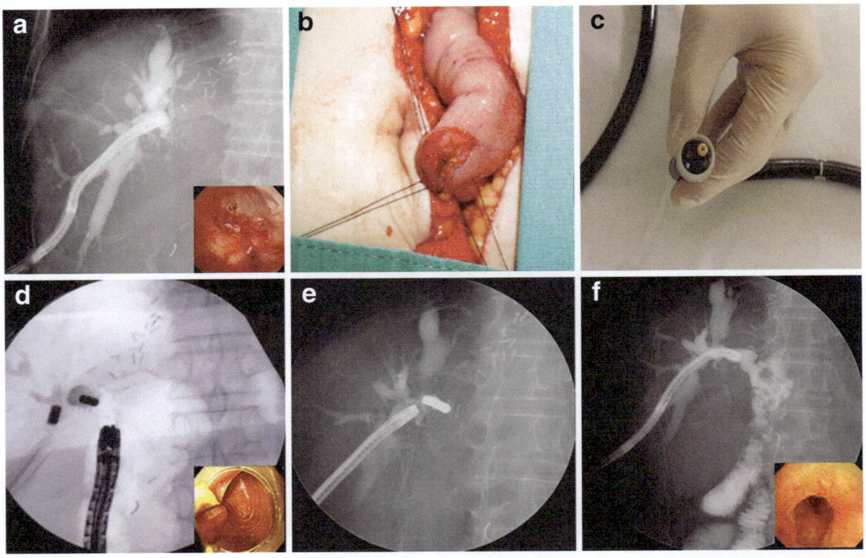

Fig. 3.10 Magnetic compression anastomosis for a bilioenteric stricture that developed after left lobectomy with Roux-en-Y anastomosis performed to treat intrahepatic stones. (**a**) A cholangiogram showing the completely obstructed anastomosis site (color photograph is of the anastomotic site). (**b**) A surgically formed percutaneous–jejunum tract was prepared in the operating room. (**c**) A magnet was attached to a polypectomy snare using a colonoscope with a transparent cap for delivery through the surgically formed percutaneous–jejunum tract. (**d**) The magnets were successfully approximated, and a percutaneous transhepatic biliary drainage (PTBD) catheter was inserted. (**e**) After 4 weeks, the approximated magnets were removed by percutaneous transhepatic cholangioscopy through the PTBD tract. An internal drainage catheter (16 Fr) was then inserted and maintained for 6 months. (**f**) Finally, the catheter was removed and development of a new fistula was confirmed

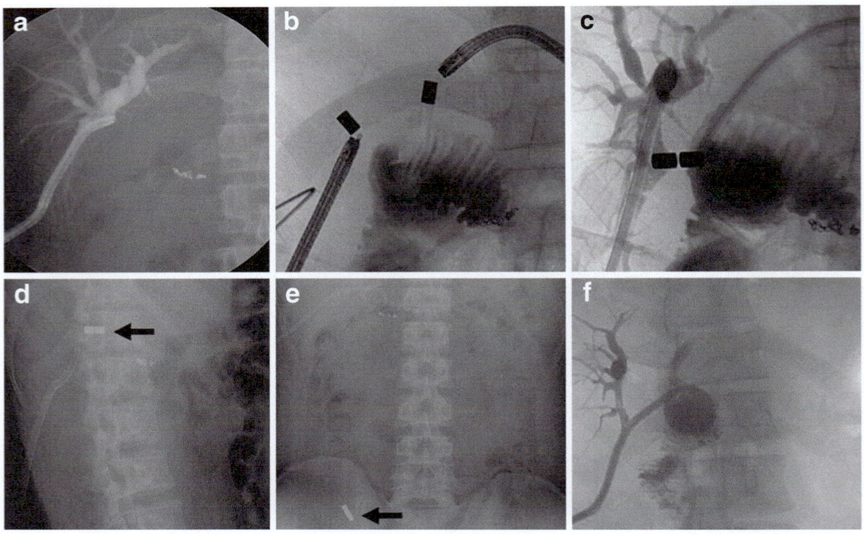

Fig. 3.11 Cholangiograms showing magnetic compression anastomosis for a bilioenteric stricture that developed after choledochal cyst excision with Roux-en-Y anastomosis. (**a**) Cholangiogram showing the completely obstructed anastomosis site. (**b**) One magnet was delivered via the right percutaneous transhepatic biliary drainage (PTBD) tract using a percutaneous transhepatic cholangioscopy (PTCS) scope, and a second magnet was delivered via the left PTBD tract using another PTCS scope, which moved to the stricture site due to magnetic attraction. (**c**) The magnets were successfully approximated, and a PTBD catheter was inserted. (**d**) Simple abdominal X-ray showing the approximated magnets at the stricture site. (**e**) After 2 weeks, the approximated magnets moved spontaneously into the intestine. (**f**) After removal of the approximated magnets, an internal drainage catheter (16 Fr) was inserted and maintained in situ for 6 months

between the two magnets was 4 mm (range, 2–7 mm), and the time to magnet removal was 7–40 days. Of the 42 subjects, 41 (97.6%) developed complete anastomoses and no MCA-related complication was noted. During the follow-up period (mean, 40 months; range, 2–53 months), restenosis occurred in a single case 6 days after drainage tube removal, but re-cannulation after balloon dilation was carried out without difficulty [32].

Pratical Tips for Difficult Cases

The difficulties associated with MCA in practice are caused by lengthy strictures, unsuitable magnet alignment, and difficult bile duct shapes. The following sections present some practical tips to improve MCA performance.

MCA Using Multiple Paired Magnets

A long stricture weakens the magnetic power, preventing magnet approximation. Although two magnets are typically used in MCA, multiple paired magnets can be applied to increase the magnetic power and thereby promote approximation (Fig. 3.12). The number and size of magnets are determined by the operator according to the shape and degree of dilatation of the bile duct.

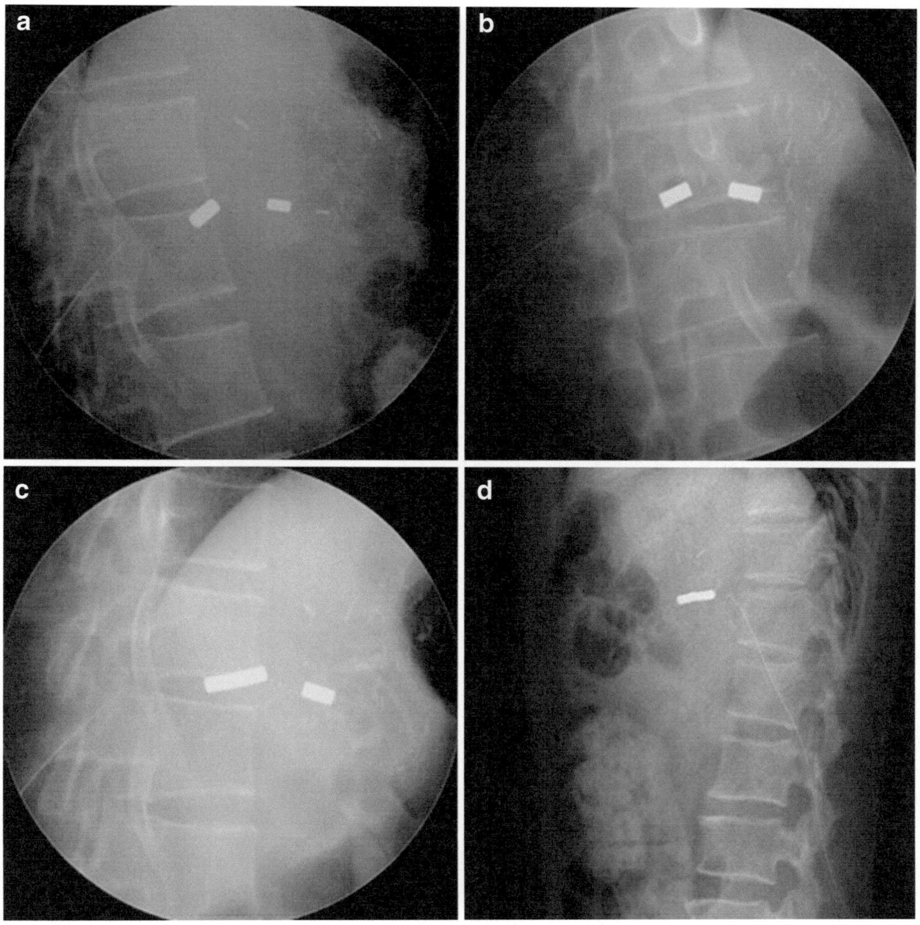

Fig. 3.12 Magnetic compression anastomosis using multiple paired magnets. (**a**) Magnet sizes (diameter × length), 4 × 8 and 2 × 6 mm. (**b**) Magnet size, 4 × 8 mm. The distance between the two magnets was not sufficient for approximation. (**c**) Magnet size, 4 × 8 mm. The two magnets were delivered via the percutaneous transhepatic biliary drainage tract and approximated more closely than in the previous procedure. (**d**) Magnet approximation was successful due to use of magnets of sufficient power

New Optimal Tract for MCA

Although the distance between the magnets is relatively short, their alignment axis should be suitable for approximation. Pre-evaluation of delivery routes using radiological modalities, such as computed tomography and/or magnetic resonance cholangiopancreatography, is essential; in some cases, the PTBD tract is unsuitable for magnet approximation. In such cases, a new PTBD tract is formed to correct the axis of alignment after consultation with radiologists (Fig. 3.13).

Optimal Size of Magnet

The magnets usually used are 4 mm in diameter and 8 mm in length. When the duct is insufficiently dilated or tortuous, magnets of this size cannot be delivered. Therefore, magnet size is determined by the operator according to the

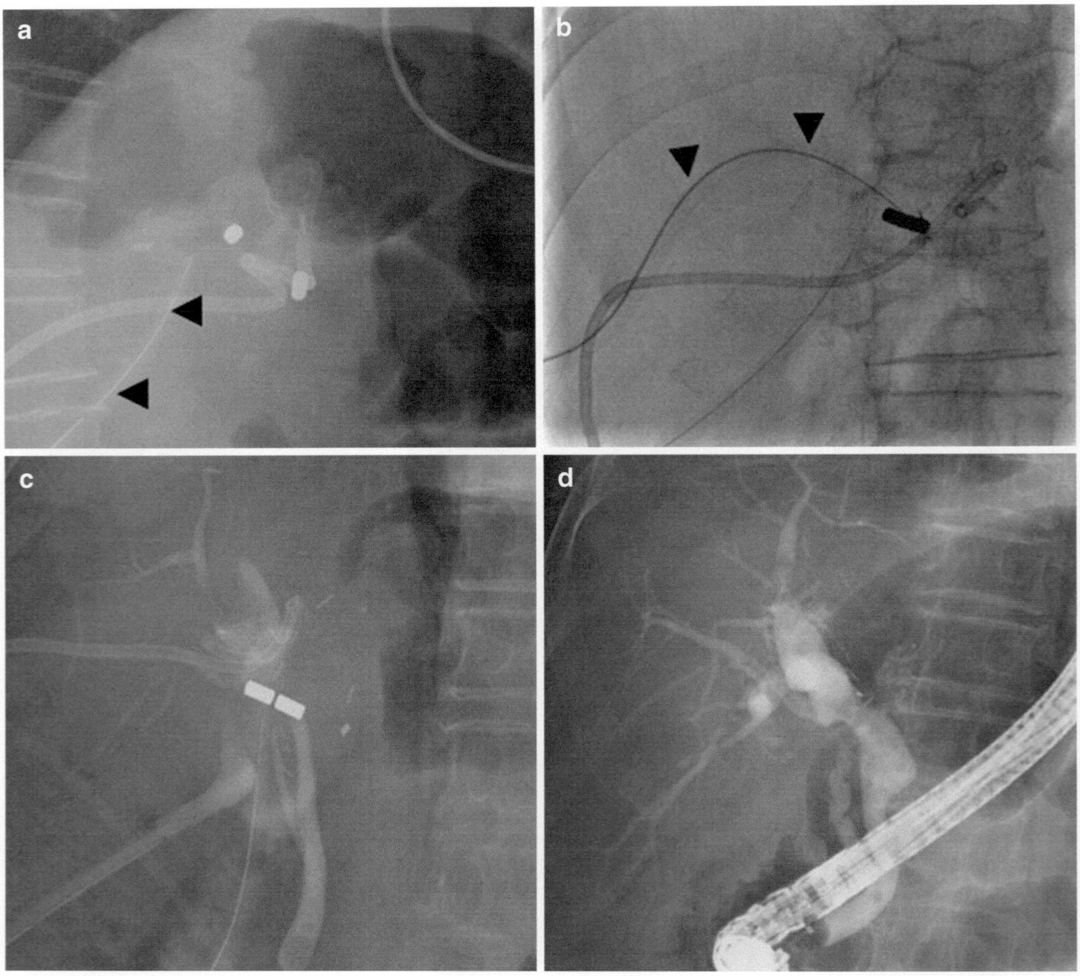

Fig. 3.13 New optimal tract for magnetic compression anastomosis. (**a**) The previous percutaneous transhepatic biliary drainage (PTBD) tract for insertion via the right inferior duct (arrowheads). The two magnets were aligned in parallel, so magnet approximation failed. (**b**) A new PTBD tract was formed via the right superior duct (arrowheads); the magnet was delivered using this tract. (**c**) The two magnets were aligned linearly, so magnet approximation was successful. (**d**) After magnet removal, a fully covered self-expandable metal stent (FCSEMS) was inserted for 6 months. Cholangiogram showing the new fistula that formed after FCSEMS removal

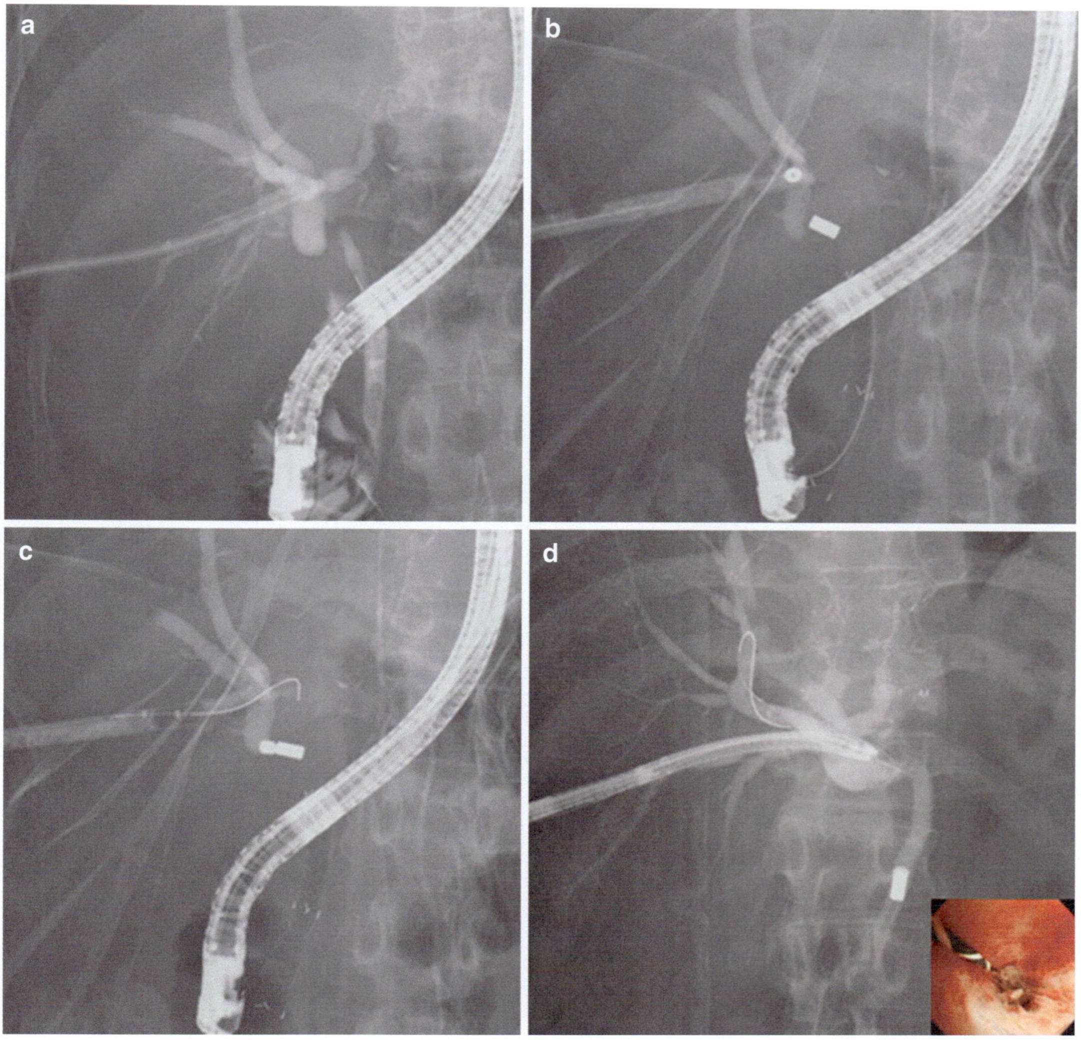

Fig. 3.14 Optimal magnet size. (**a**) The right intrahepatic duct was dilated and acutely angulated. (**b**) The magnet delivered via the percutaneous transhepatic biliary drainage (PTBD) tract could not move to the stricture site because its size (diameter × length, 4 × 8 mm) prohibited passage through the acutely angulated duct. (**c**) A smaller magnet (4 × 4 mm) could be delivered to the stricture site. (**d**) After magnet removal, a new fistula formed

shape and degree of dilatation of the bile duct (Fig. 3.14).

Bile Duct Dilation and Adjustment of Alignment Axis for MCA

Magnet delivery is typically successful in cases with sufficient ductal dilation. Moreover, duct dilation is required for magnet delivery to a position that allows adjustment of the alignment axis. An FCSEMS can be used to dilate a non-dilated bile duct (Fig. 3.15).

Summary

MCA is a non-surgical alternative for the treatment of completely obstructed or severe benign biliary strictures that cannot be resolved using conventional endoscopic or percutaneous methods. MCA is feasible and safe for BBSs and bil-

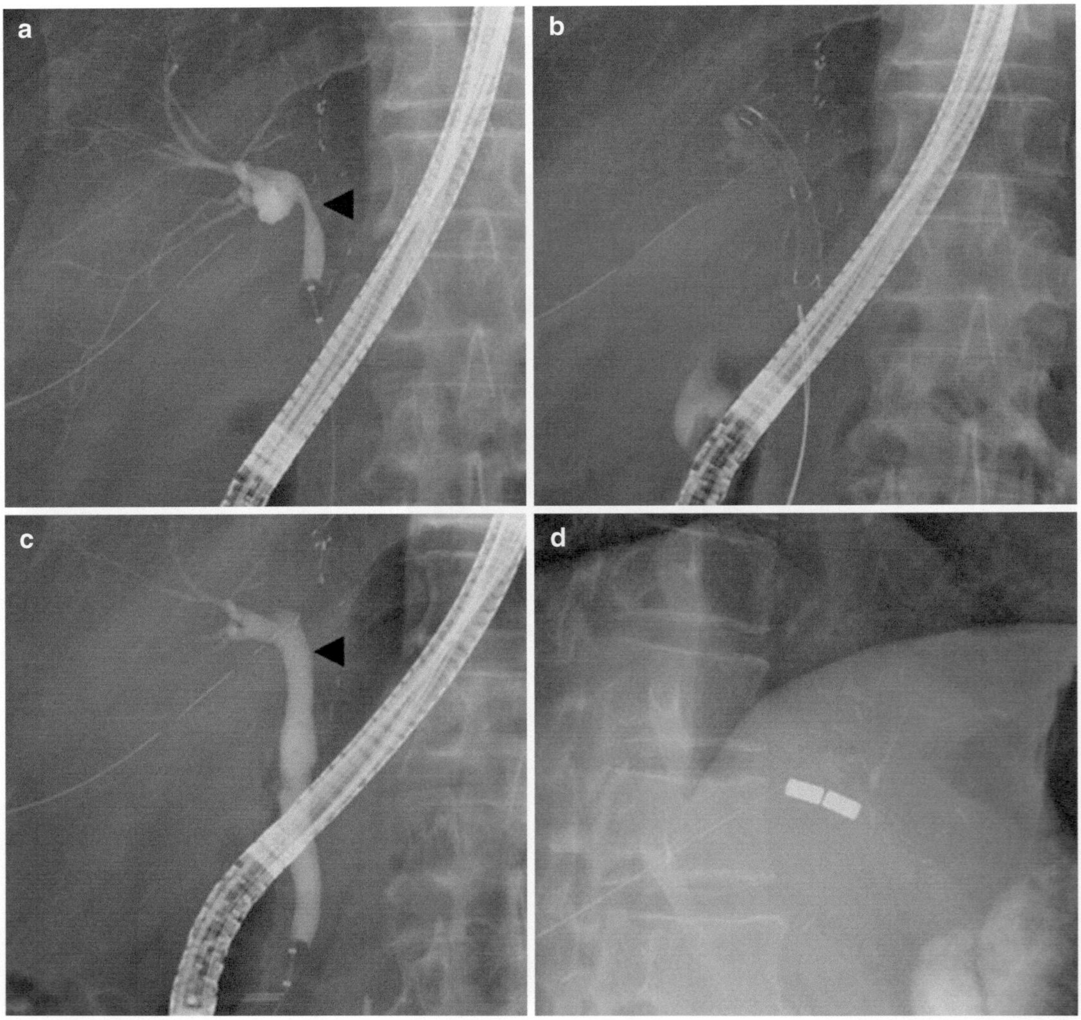

Fig. 3.15 Bile duct dilation and adjustment of the alignment axis for magnetic compression anastomosis. (**a**) Common hepatic duct (CHD) with a stricture (arrowhead), which prohibited magnet delivery and rotation to a suitable alignment axis. (**b**) A fully covered self-expandable metal stent (FCSEMS) was inserted for 2 months to dilate the CHD. (**c**) The CHD was sufficiently dilated after FCSEM removal (arrowhead). (**d**) Magnet approximation was successful after delivery of the magnets via the dilated CHD

ioenteric strictures caused by various surgeries. Although a pre-MCA assessment method that is predictive of the outcomes is needed for successful recanalization, smaller and more powerful magnets and an effective magnet delivery system have been developed. Endoscopists should understand the mechanisms and principles of MCA, and the clinical indications for MCA should be expanded to enable further application and development of the technique. MCA is effective and safe, has a low recurrence rate, and is less traumatic than other treatments for completely obstructed or severe benign biliary strictures.

References

1. Marcos A, et al. Liver regeneration and function in donor and recipient after right lobe adult to adult living donor liver transplantation. Transplantation. 2000;69(7):1375–9.
2. Sanchez-Urdazpal L, et al. Diagnostic features and clinical outcome of ischemic-type biliary com-

plications after liver transplantation. Hepatology. 1993;17(4):605–9.
3. Schwartz DA, et al. Endoscopic therapy of anastomotic bile duct strictures occurring after liver transplantation. Gastrointest Endosc. 2000;51(2):169–74.
4. Yoshimoto T, et al. Crane-neck deformity after right lobe living donor liver transplantation. Gastrointest Endosc. 2006;64(2):271.
5. Kim HJ, et al. Multidetector computed tomography cholangiography with multiplanar reformation for the assessment of patients with biliary obstruction. J Gastroenterol Hepatol. 2007;22(3):400–5.
6. Pasha SF, et al. Endoscopic treatment of anastomotic biliary strictures after deceased donor liver transplantation: outcomes after maximal stent therapy. Gastrointest Endosc. 2007;66(1):44–51.
7. Shah SA, et al. Biliary strictures in 130 consecutive right lobe living donor liver transplant recipients: results of a Western center. Am J Transplant. 2007;7(1):161–7.
8. Venu M, et al. Laboratory diagnosis and nonoperative management of biliary complications in living donor liver transplant patients. J Clin Gastroenterol. 2007;41(5):501–6.
9. Avaliani M, et al. Magnetic compression biliary-enteric anastomosis for palliation of obstructive jaundice: initial clinical results. J Vasc Interv Radiol. 2009;20(5):614–23.
10. Graziadei IW, et al. Long-term outcome of endoscopic treatment of biliary strictures after liver transplantation. Liver Transpl. 2006;12(5):718–25.
11. Wang SP, et al. Fast magnetic reconstruction of the portal vein with allogeneic blood vessels in canines. Hepatobiliary Pancreat Dis Int. 2015;14(3):293–9.
12. Matsuno N, et al. A nonsuture anastomosis using magnetic compression for biliary stricture after living donor liver transplantation. Hepato-Gastroenterology. 2009;56(89):47–9.
13. Yamanouchi E, et al. A new interventional method: magnetic compression anastomosis with rare-earth magnets. Cardiovasc Intervent Radiol. 1998;22(Suppl 1):S155.
14. Yamanouchi E, et al. Treatment for bowel or biliary obstruction by magnetic compression anastomosis development of Yamanouchi's method and its clinical evaluation. J Nippon Med Sch. 2002;69(5):471–5.
15. Mimuro A, et al. A novel technique of magnetic compression anastomosis for severe biliary stenosis. Gastrointest Endosc. 2003;58(2):283–7.
16. Itoi T, et al. Magnetic compression anastomosis: a novel technique for canalization of severe hilar bile duct strictures. Endoscopy. 2005;37(12):1248–51.
17. Muraoka N, et al. Yamanouchi magnetic compression anastomosis for bilioenteric anastomotic stricture after living-donor liver transplantation. J Vasc Interv Radiol. 2005;16(9):1263–7.
18. Yukawa N, et al. A case of magnetic compression anastomosis between the common bile duct and the duodenum after distal gastrectomy with Roux-Y reconstruction and cholecystectomy. Nihon Shokakibyo Gakkai Zasshi. 2008;105(10):1523–8.
19. Takao S, et al. Magnetic compression anastomosis for benign obstruction of the common bile duct. Endoscopy. 2001;33(11):988–90.
20. Jang SI, et al. Magnetic compression anastomosis is useful in biliary anastomotic strictures after living donor liver transplantation. Gastrointest Endosc. 2011;74(5):1040–8.
21. Jang SI, et al. Recanalization of refractory benign biliary stricture using magnetic compression anastomosis. Endoscopy. 2014;46(1):70–4.
22. Jang SI, et al. Treatment of completely obstructed benign biliary strictures with magnetic compression anastomosis: follow-up results after recanalization. Gastrointest Endosc. 2017;85(5):1057–66.
23. Sharma S, Gurakar A, Jabbour N. Biliary strictures following liver transplantation: past, present and preventive strategies. Liver Transpl. 2008;14(6):759–69.
24. Kim ES, et al. Percutaneous transhepatic biliary drainage may serve as a successful rescue procedure in failed cases of endoscopic therapy for a post-living donor liver transplantation biliary stricture. Gastrointest Endosc. 2009;69(1):38–46.
25. Weber A, et al. Long-term follow-up after endoscopic stent therapy for benign biliary strictures. J Clin Gastroenterol. 2014;48(1):88–93.
26. Dumonceau JM, et al. Biliary stenting: indications, choice of stents and results: European Society of Gastrointestinal Endoscopy (ESGE) clinical guideline. Endoscopy. 2012;44(3):277–98.
27. Schumacher B, et al. Long-term follow-up of percutaneous transhepatic therapy (PTT) in patients with definite benign anastomotic strictures after hepaticojejunostomy. Endoscopy. 2001;33(5):409–15.
28. Weber A, et al. Long-term follow-up of percutaneous transhepatic biliary drainage (PTBD) in patients with benign bilioenterostomy stricture. Endoscopy. 2009;41(4):323–8.
29. Bonnel DH, Fingerhut AL. Percutaneous transhepatic balloon dilatation of benign bilioenteric strictures: long-term results in 110 patients. Am J Surg. 2012;203(6):675–83.
30. Costamagna G, Boskoski I. Current treatment of benign biliary strictures. Ann Gastroenterol. 2013;26(1):37–40.
31. Curcio G, et al. Intraperitoneal rendezvous: a mini-invasive biliary reconstruction. Gastrointest Endosc. 2016;84(1):184–5.
32. Jang SI, Choi J, Lee DK. Magnetic compression anastomosis for treatment of benign biliary stricture. Dig Endosc. 2015;27(2):239–49.
33. Sugawara Y, Makuuchi M. Advances in adult living donor liver transplantation: a review based on reports from the 10th anniversary of the adult-to-adult living donor liver transplantation meeting in Tokyo. Liver Transpl. 2004;10(6):715–20.
34. Liu CL, et al. Operative outcomes of adult-to-adult right lobe live donor liver transplantation: a compara-

tive study with cadaveric whole-graft liver transplantation in a single center. Ann Surg. 2006;243(3):404–10.
35. Soejima Y, et al. Biliary strictures in living donor liver transplantation: incidence, management, and technical evolution. Liver Transpl. 2006;12(6):979–86.
36. Wadhawan M, Kumar A. Management issues in post living donor liver transplant biliary strictures. World J Hepatol. 2016;8(10):461–70.
37. Rao HB, et al. Endoscopic therapy for biliary strictures complicating living donor liver transplantation: factors predicting better outcome. World J Gastrointest Pathophysiol. 2017;8(2):77–86.
38. Gondolesi GE, et al. Biliary complications in 96 consecutive right lobe living donor transplant recipients. Transplantation. 2004;77(12):1842–8.
39. Kasahara M, et al. Biliary reconstruction in right lobe living-donor liver transplantation: comparison of different techniques in 321 recipients. Ann Surg. 2006;243(4):559–66.
40. Tsujino T, et al. Endoscopic management of biliary complications after adult living donor liver transplantation. Am J Gastroenterol. 2006;101(10):2230–6.
41. Yazumi S, et al. Endoscopic treatment of biliary complications after right-lobe living-donor liver transplantation with duct-to-duct biliary anastomosis. J Hepato-Biliary-Pancreat Surg. 2006;13(6):502–10.
42. Tashiro H, et al. Biliary complications after duct-to-duct biliary reconstruction in living-donor liver transplantation: causes and treatment. World J Surg. 2007;31(11):2222–9.
43. Londono MC, Balderramo D, Cardenas A. Management of biliary complications after orthotopic liver transplantation: the role of endoscopy. World J Gastroenterol. 2008;14(4):493–7.
44. Kato H, et al. Long-term outcomes of endoscopic management for biliary strictures after living donor liver transplantation with duct-to-duct reconstruction. Transpl Int. 2009;22(9):914–21.
45. Chang JH, et al. Biliary stricture after adult right-lobe living-donor liver transplantation with duct-to-duct anastomosis: long-term outcome and its related factors after endoscopic treatment. Gut Liver. 2010;4(2):226–33.
46. Duffy JP, et al. Long-term patient outcome and quality of life after liver transplantation: analysis of 20-year survivors. Ann Surg. 2010;252(4):652–61.
47. Melcher ML, et al. Comparison of biliary complications in adult living-donor liver transplants performed at two busy transplant centers. Clin Transpl. 2010;24(5):E137–44.
48. Kim PT, et al. Long-term follow-up of biliary complications after adult right-lobe living donor liver transplantation. Clin Transpl. 2015;29(5):465–74.
49. Ohkubo M, et al. Surgical anatomy of the bile ducts at the hepatic hilum as applied to living donor liver transplantation. Ann Surg. 2004;239(1):82–6.
50. Pesce A, et al. Bile duct injury during laparoscopic cholecystectomy without intraoperative cholangiography: a retrospective study on 1,100 selected patients. Dig Surg. 2012;29(4):310–4.
51. Archer SB, et al. Bile duct injury during laparoscopic cholecystectomy: results of a national survey. Ann Surg. 2001;234(4):549–58; discussion 558–9.
52. Bismuth H, Majno PE. Biliary strictures: classification based on the principles of surgical treatment. World J Surg. 2001;25(10):1241–4.
53. Strasberg SM, Hertl M, Soper NJ. An analysis of the problem of biliary injury during laparoscopic cholecystectomy. J Am Coll Surg. 1995;180(1):101–25.
54. Way LW, et al. Causes and prevention of laparoscopic bile duct injuries: analysis of 252 cases from a human factors and cognitive psychology perspective. Ann Surg. 2003;237(4):460–9.
55. Pesce A, et al. Iatrogenic bile duct injury: impact and management challenges. Clin Exp Gastroenterol. 2019;12:121–8.
56. Fiocca F, et al. Complete transection of the main bile duct: minimally invasive treatment with an endoscopic-radiologic rendezvous. Gastrointest Endosc. 2011;74(6):1393–8.
57. Deviere J. Benign biliary strictures and leaks. Gastrointest Endosc Clin N Am. 2015;25(4):713–23.

Percutaneous Intervention for Refractory Benign Biliary Strictures

4

Hans-Ulrich Laasch, Shofiq Al-Islam, and Raman Uberoi

Introduction

There are many different causes for benign bile duct strictures, and their management requires good cross-disciplinary collaboration between endoscopists, surgeons, and radiologists to provide an optimal solution for the myriad of different challenges they can present [1].

The change from open to laparoscopic cholecystectomy led to an increase in iatrogenic strictures by direct injury to the bile duct, inadvertent clipping of the duct, or ischemia. Although the initial learning curve of the new technique has been overcome, the volume of laparoscopic cholecystectomy has dramatically increased, with this now being the standard approach. More cholecystectomy procedures have led to more patients being discovered with aberrant anatomy and thus increasing the number of iatrogenic injuries [2, 3]. Iatrogenic bile duct injury is reported to occur in up to 0.5% of laparoscopic cholecystectomy procedures [4].

H.-U. Laasch (✉)
Department of Radiology,
The Christie NHS Foundation Trust, Manchester, UK
e-mail: HUL@christie.nhs.uk

S. Al-Islam
Department of Radiology, East Lancashire Hospitals
NHS Trust, Blackburn, UK

R. Uberoi
Department of Radiology, John Radcliffe Hospital,
Oxford, UK

It is a disastrous event for patients causing long-term morbidity, often requiring numerous procedures with high cost to the health system, and it needs rapid management in a specialist center [5].

The majority of benign biliary strictures with normal anatomy are accessible for treatment with endoscopic retrograde cholangiopancreatography (ERCP), and treatment strategies for dealing with these are well described. Options for the extra-hepatic bile duct include balloon dilatation, stenting with plastic stents or fully covered removable metal stents. In most of these cases, an endoscopic approach is preferable to a percutaneous approach, as the patients do not need a medium- or long-term trans-hepatic catheter.

However, for strictures of the intrahepatic bile ducts and particularly where endoscopic access is not possible, such as after a pancreatico-duodenectomy and Roux-en-Y gastric bypass, a percutaneous approach offers success rates of over 60% [4] and a number of technical advantages:

The access route is much shorter than through a duodenoscope, and therefore catheter manipulation is much easier. Access tracts of a diameter larger than those of the working channel of a therapeutic endoscope can be easily and safely created, and the range of available equipment is much greater. Furthermore, biliary drainage is secured, avoiding the risk of intercurrent sepsis,

D. K. Lee (ed.), *Advanced ERCP for Complicated and Refractory Biliary and Pancreatic Diseases*,
https://doi.org/10.1007/978-981-13-0608-2_4

and this process is easily maintained through an external drainage catheter. The access provided by the external drain also allows for quick and easy repeat interventions, whereas with repeat endoscopy, the procedure is essentially started afresh every time. Additional tools for dealing with the refractory stricture are available for percutaneous use, notably self-expanding biodegradable stents, which cannot be placed endoscopically at present.

In case of obstruction of the afferent biliary loop (bilio pancreatic limb) after biliary bypass surgery, balloon dilatation or stent insertion can be performed percutaneously, either by a transhepatic route or direct percutaneous puncture of the obstructed bowel.

Diagnostic Work-Up

Baseline blood and biochemical test are required to assess liver function, clotting and latent sepsis. In untreated strictures, a malignant cause tends to result in more extensive derangement of liver function tests, than a benign cause. Bilirubin levels approaching or exceeding 100 μmol/l (5.8 mg/dl) should prompt a review of the diagnosis of assumed benign disease [6, 7].

Adequate diagnostic imaging is essential to plan a successful procedure [8] and should involve different modalities due to their different strengths (Fig. 4.1). Ultrasound (US) is the cheapest and quickest method to confirm biliary dilatation and to assess for the existence of

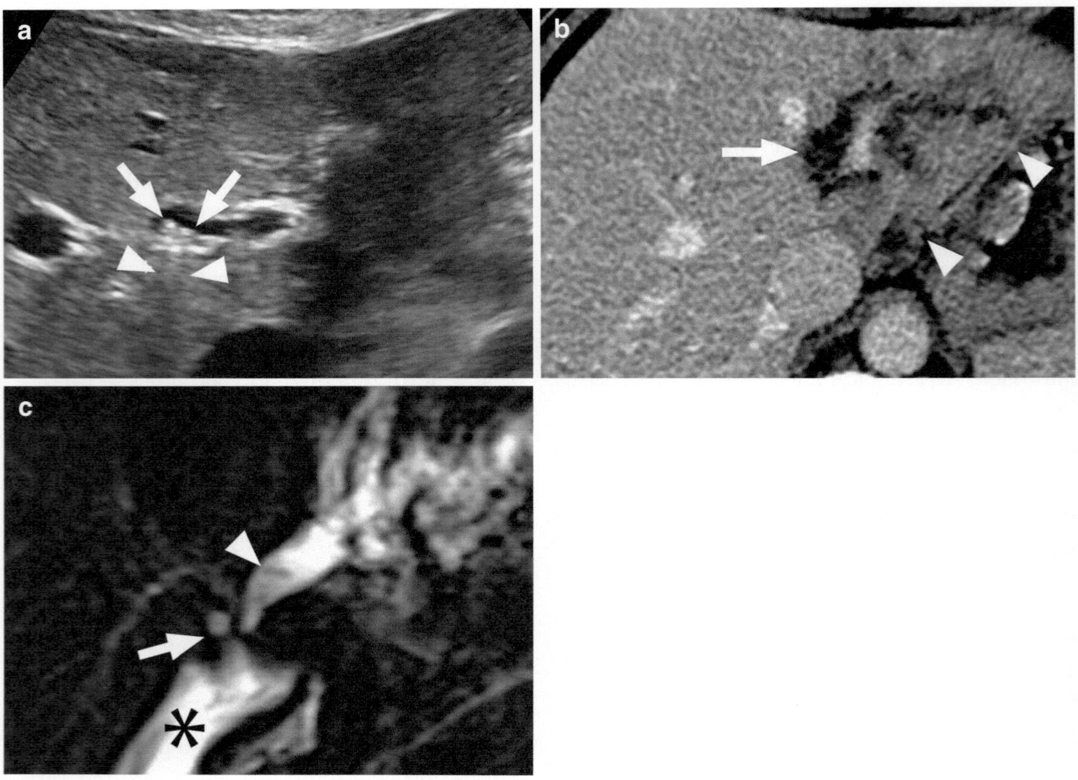

Fig. 4.1 (**a**) Patient with recurrent episodes of cholangitis after hepaticojejunostomy for choledochal cyst. Transaxial US scan shows dilated left-sided ducts containing small gallstones (arrows) with their characteristic "acoustic shadows" (arrowheads). (**b**) Transaxial CT shows not only left biliary dilatation (arrow) but also marked atrophy and irregular perfusion of the left lobe (arrowheads). The gallstones are not calcified and not apparent. (**c**) MRCP demonstrates the anatomy of the stricture at the anastomosis with the Roux loop below (asterisk), which is occluding the left hepatic duct and just starting to involve the right posterior sectoral duct (arrow). The bile duct stones are just appreciated (arrowhead)

stones above the stricture and to plan the optimal access path.

Computed tomography (CT) has its strength in excellent spatial resolution and the ability to look for unsuspected lymph node enlargement or other distant metastases, but may not identify associated gall stones.

Magnetic resonance imaging (MRI) with or without liver-specific contrast agents, which are excreted by the biliary system allows for better soft tissue discrimination [9] and the ability to accurately assess the biliary tree. The special sequences of magnetic resonance cholangiopancreatography (MRCP) depict the bile-filled ducts only, offering a 3D cholangiogram by non-invasive means (Fig. 4.2) [10].

Technetium Tc99m hepato-biliary iminodiacetic acid (HIDA) scan (Fig. 4.3) allows visualization of the liver's excretory function and is a sensitive way of demonstrating impediment to flow by a stricture [11, 12].

If the patient has a background of malignancy, for example, a previous Whipple's procedure, then it is important to exclude recurrent disease. MRI may be sufficient for this, but if percutaneous biliary drainage is required, intraductal biopsy can be readily undertaken. A dedicated transluminal biliary biopsy system is available (Cook Medical, Limerick, Ireland), which is a reduced version of endoscopic biopsy forceps, redesigned for percutaneous use. It allows formal histological examination yielding results

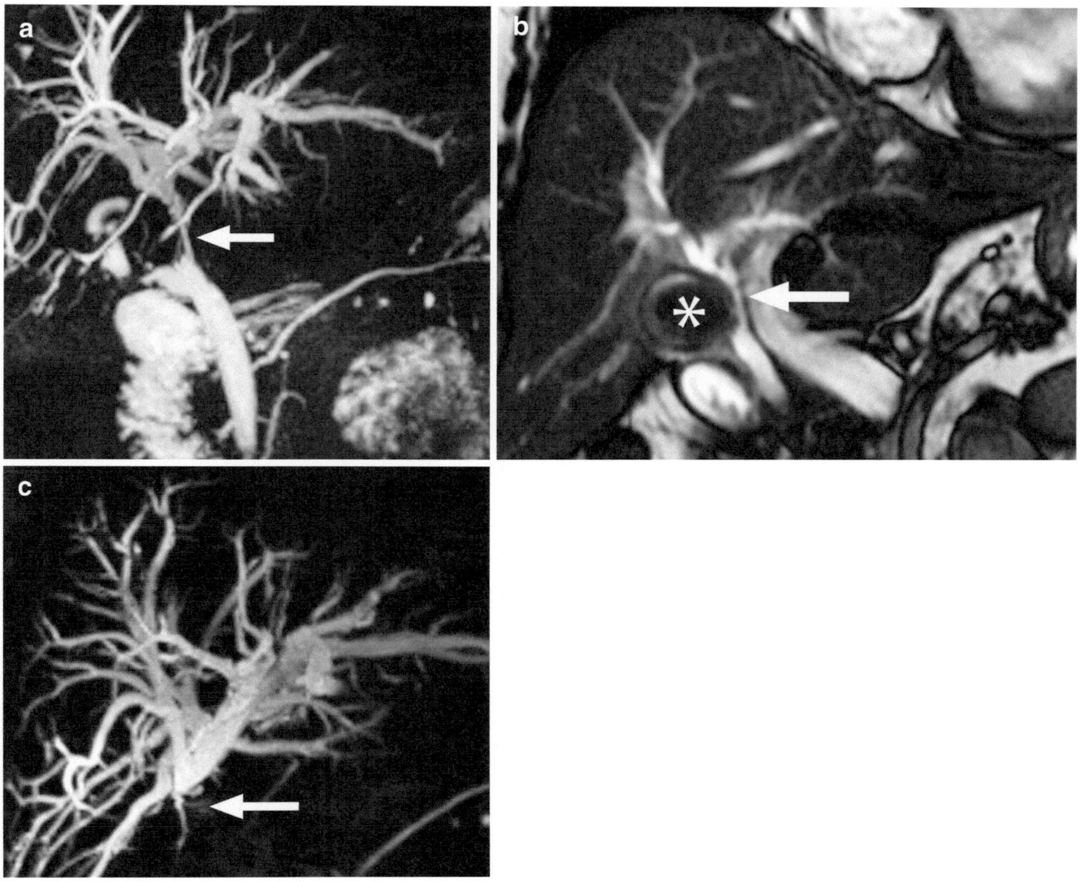

Fig. 4.2 (**a**) Patient with Mirizzi (type 1) syndrome. Maximum intensity projection (MIP) image from an MRCP shows dilated bile ducts above a high-grade stricture of the common hepatic duct (arrow). (**b**) T2-weighted, coronal image showing a large gallbladder stone (asterisk) compressing the common hepatic duct (arrow). Complications during cholecystectomy resulted in a surgical bypass. (**c**) Subsequent development of anastomotic stricture. MIP image from MRCP showing dilated intrahepatic ducts with no flow through the hepaticojejunostomy (arrow)

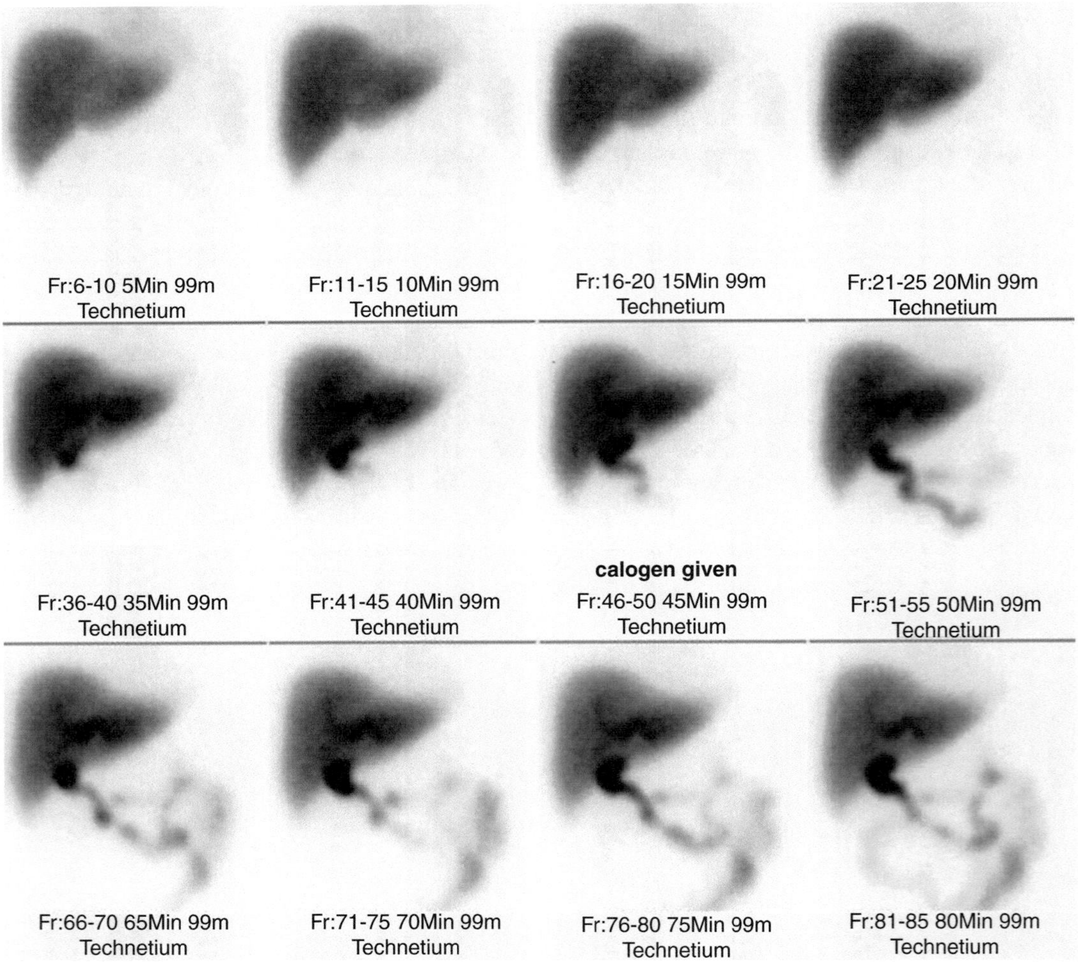

Fig. 4.3 HIDA scan showing prompt biliary uptake and good excretion of tracer through a hepaticojejunostomy into an afferent Roux loop (arrow)

superior to brush cytology and as good as EUS-FNA [13]. Sensitivity is reported to be 75–90% [14, 15], increased to over 90% with specific technique [16] and with a specificity approaching 100%.

Patients with benign strictures need to be counselled carefully to give them realistic expectations of the course of the treatment, which can take many months and will involve repeat procedures and the presence of an external biliary drain, which will impact on the patient's quality of life.

A multidisciplinary discussion between the various specialties is essential to evaluate all possible options, notably of combined radiologic and endoscopic procedures, which are often underutilized. For example, it might be difficult to selectively cannulate a strictured segmental duct retrogradely, but a percutaneously placed guidewire can be easily retrieved through duodenoscope and then act as a railroad to access the target duct from below (Fig. 4.4). The development of low-profile cholangioscopes offers further percutaneous treatment strategies by combining the expertise from both disciplines [17–20]. The benefit of combined procedures are well described across the literature of both specialties [21, 22] but often underused. Combining the skills of both teams significantly extends the options for strictures that cannot be managed by one of the disciplines alone [23–25].

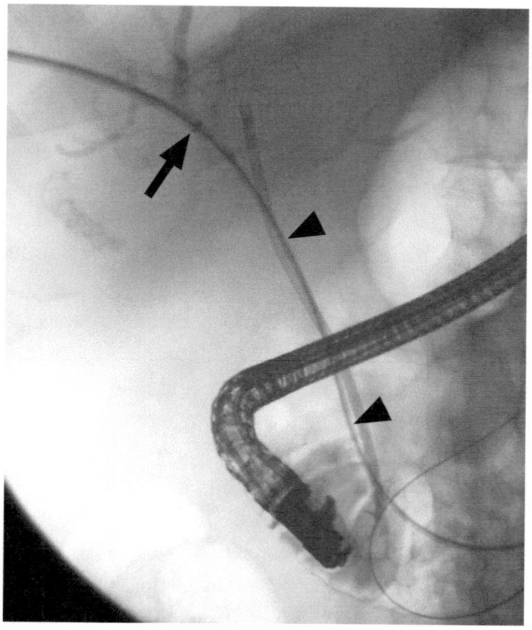

Fig. 4.4 Combined ("rendez-vous") procedure. A percutaneous sheath with radiopaque marker (arrow) has been placed, through which a catheter and guidewire were inserted alongside a plastic stent to facilitate endoscopic access

Percutaneous Intervention: Technical Aspects and Devices

One of the great advantages of percutaneous trans-hepatic cholangiography (PTC) is the ability to selectively access an obstructed segment. The "downstream" approach ensures that the desired duct is punctured for optimum access to the stricture. The correct duct is entered at the outset, avoiding contamination of obstructed segments, which may need to be left alone. There is also a greater choice of devices available than for ERCP, which are shorter and much easier to manipulate than through-the-scope devices, which are 5–6 times longer, and their manipulation is hampered by the passage through a potentially tortuous working channel. Catheter exchange and manipulation, balloon dilatation, and stent deployment using a 40–50 cm long device in a straight access route is naturally easier than undertaking the same with a 180–240 cm device, passed through an acute angle into the papilla. Furthermore, there are more options for dealing with technical difficulties, but this matter needs to be balanced with the additional risks of hepatic puncture, as both affect the outcome of two interventions with the identical goal [26, 27].

Routine use of antibiotics in de novo obstruction presenting for ERCP is not recommended [28]. By contrast, this process is usually suggested for percutaneous procedures, although the ideal regime cannot be specified, as it depends on local bacterial resistance [29].

Referral for percutaneous intervention is often only done after ERCP has failed, in which case the patients have to be assumed to have latent biliary sepsis due to contamination of the obstructed system by contrast injection or guidewire manipulation. In any situation where the natural barrier of the sphincter of Oddi has been breached, either by a trans-papillary stent or a bilio-enteric anastomosis, the biliary tree has been colonized with gut flora. Subsequent obstruction creates an ideal breeding ground for bacteria, and intervention in these can quickly lead to bacteremia, sepsis, and multi-organ failure.

Where cholangitis is present, the initial procedure should only aim to place a percutaneous drain and not undertake any other therapeutic maneuvers, which increase biliary pressure and the risk of bacteremia [30, 31]. In these cases, antibiotic therapy prior to the procedure is essential and should aim to create good levels in the obstructed biliary tree prior to the procedure as well as therapeutic plasma levels at the time of the drainage procedure in order to maximize antibiosis in both compartments. At the time of puncture, a bile sample should be sent for culture to confirm pathogens and their sensitivity.

The initial PTC and drain placement may be performed under sedation, but manipulation of the stricture and dilatation can be exceptionally painful and is best done under deep sedation performed by an anesthetist or even general anesthesia. For the initial treatment, the external access is ideally secured by insertion of a vascular access sheath (Fig. 4.5), which allows atraumatic exchange of therapeutic devices through this. These sheaths have a side arm with a tap, which allows decompression of the system or further contrast injection without the need to remove the catheter inserted through the sheath.

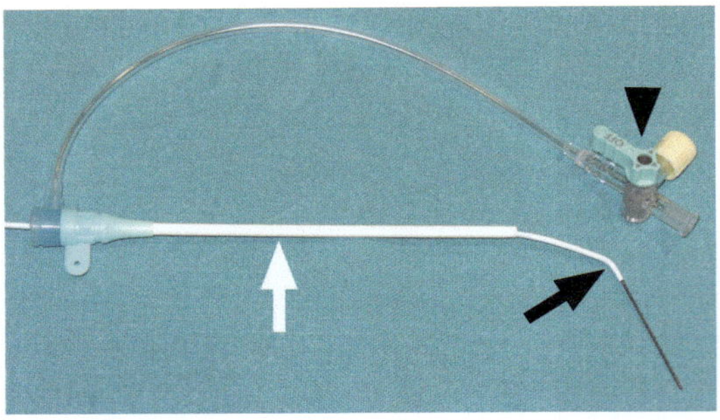

Fig. 4.5 8Fr Radiofocus vascular access sheath (white arrow; Terumo, Tokyo, Japan) with side arm for injection and decompression (arrowhead). A biliary manipulation catheter (Cook Medical, Limerick, Ireland) and a hydrophilic wire (Laureate, Merit Medical, Galway, Ireland) have been inserted through it

Drainage Catheters

Percutaneous catheters for temporary drainage either drain bile externally only or provide additional internal drainage by extending through the obstruction ("internal/external drain"). The latter have the benefit of not only conserving bile, with the obvious benefits of absorbing fat-soluble vitamins to produce clotting factors and preventing maldigestion and malnutrition, but also improving the general homeostasis of the patient.

Percutaneous drains offer several advantages and allow for different treatment strategies:

- In patients with biliary sepsis, they allow drainage of infected bile before attempting any therapeutic maneuvers, which may cause bacteremia and septic crisis.
- Drains provide an easy access route for repeat procedures and allow step-wise dilatation of the trans-hepatic track if larger access is required for managing stones, recalcitrant benign strictures, or performing cholangioscopy. While the latter is a standard technique during ERCP for diagnostic purposes, resulting in increased biopsy yield and potential for lithotripsy [32], a cholangioscope can also be inserted percutaneously for managing difficult situations [17, 33–35].
- External catheters usually have a retaining "pigtail" to provide anchoring in the bile duct. These may be secured by an additional "locking" string, which prevents the pigtail from unraveling inadvertently.
- Internal/external catheters conserve bile. They may also have a locking pigtail, but also exist in a variety of other configurations, which may provide a better profile at skin level if longer-term placement is required (Fig. 4.6).
- For short-term drainage (<2 weeks), sizes of 6–8 Fr (2–2.7 mm) are adequate. If longer-term drainage is required, then larger sizes should be considered to prevent tube blockage.
- Regular flushing of drains (e.g. 2–3 times/week) is desirable to prevent occlusion, although there are no agreed protocols. If the drain blocks, then the patient is at risk of biliary sepsis, and the situation should be treated as an emergency.

Dilatation Balloons

Initial treatment—endoscopic or radiologic—of a benign stricture will usually be performed by balloon dilatation, and a large number of balloons are available for this purpose. In general, an 8–10 mm balloon is sufficient for an extrahepatic stricture and 6–8 mm or less for strictures in the more proximal branches. It is worth noting that smaller diameter balloons tend to have a higher-rated burst pressure. Balloon dilatation should be performed using a pressure inflator with an attached manometer, which allows this process to be done slowly and with great control. The pressure required to dilate tough strictures, for example, calcified strictures in chronic pancreatitis, may exceed the rated burst pressure of standard dilating balloon, and occasionally high-pressure balloons with burst pressures of >20 atmospheres may be required. Following dilatation, insertion of an internal/external drain secures internal drainage, and maintains a minimum lumen through the stenosis (Fig. 4.7).

Primary success rates with balloon dilatation alone range between 85% and 95%, but several

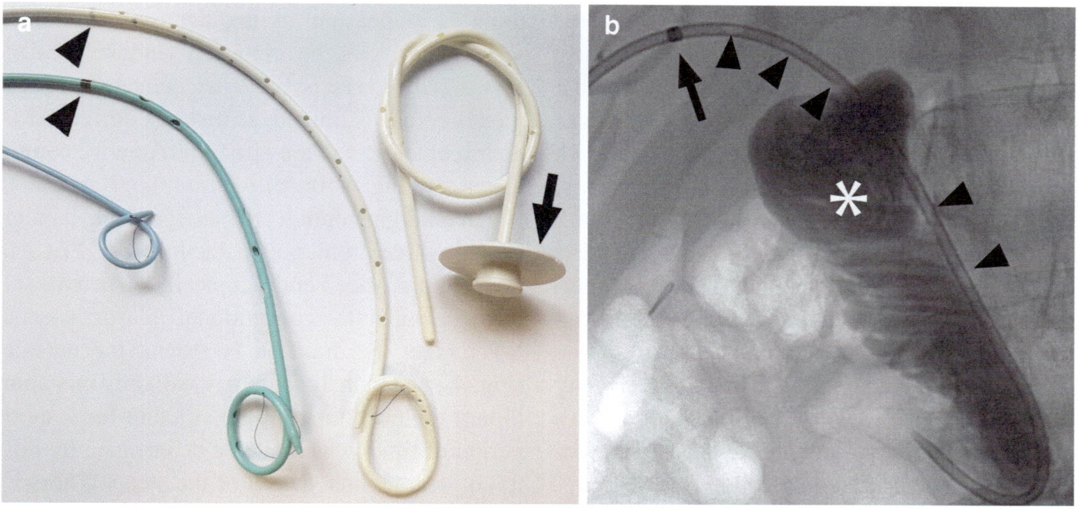

Fig. 4.6 (**a**) From left: 7Fr locked external drain, two 8 Fr internal/external drains (UK Medical, Sheffield, UK & Cook Medical, Limerick, Ireland) with metal markers (arrowheads) identifying the uppermost drainage hole which must not be placed outside the liver, 10 Fr straight internal/external "Munich" drain (Pflugbeil GmbH, Munich, Germany) with skin level fixation disc (arrow). (**b**) Internal/external drain sited through an anastomotic stricture into the afferent loop (asterisk). Note the radiopaque marker (arrow). The side holes are difficult to identify (arrowheads)

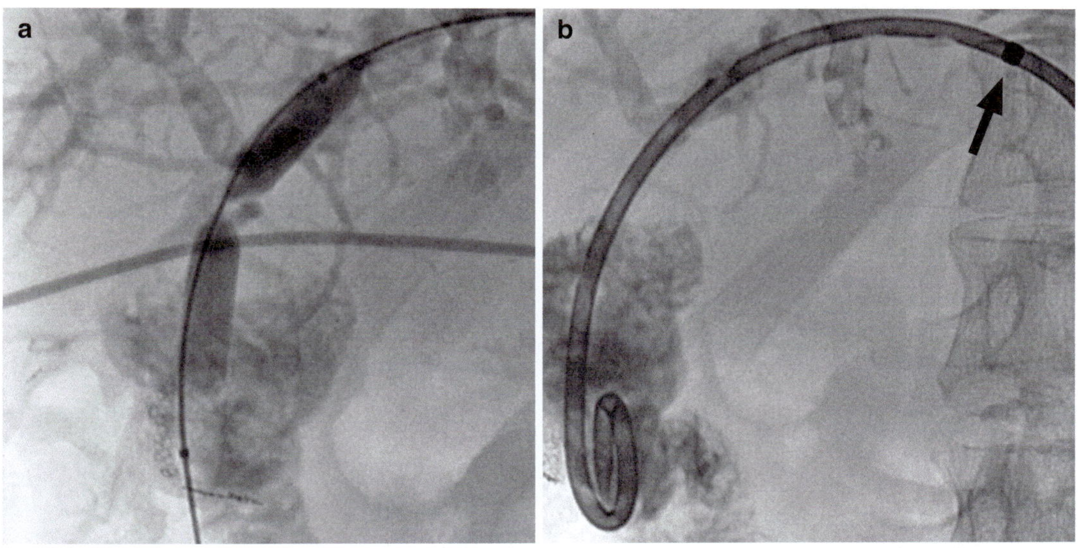

Fig. 4.7 (**a**) Balloon dilatation of an anastomotic stricture: At the beginning of the inflation, a tight waste is evident on the balloon. (**b**) Subsequent insertion of an internal/external drain to maintain stricture patency and antegrade drainage. Note the radiopaque marker indicating the position of the uppermost side hole (arrow)

weeks of external drainage is often required. Late recurrence (>3 years) is as high as 10–20% and depends on the underlying process [36–39]. A more aggressive approach with three long dilatation session within 1 week had similar initial results, avoided long-term trans-hepatic catheter, but had primary and secondary patency rates of 36% and 64%, respectively at 3 years [40].

Cutting Balloons

Cutting balloons are dilatation balloons that incorporate several small blades or plastic ridges (Fig. 4.8) and score the mucosa and submucosa of the dilated segment during inflation. In theory, this has two advantages: Firstly, there is better control over the trauma applied to the stenosis than with conventional dilatation. Several superficial incisions are made into the constricting tissue, whereas simple dilatation relies on random tearing of the fibrous tissues. Secondly, healing of the tissues treated with a cutting balloon is in a longitudinal fashion rather than recurrent circumferential scarring after simple radial dilatation.

Cutting balloons are not commonly used but may be helpful in tough and recurrent strictures. There are only few publications on their use in refractory strictures, most of which demonstrate good results in very small number of cases [41–43].

The largest series with 22 patients reported an over 90% success rate after 1–2 sessions using cutting balloon dilatation followed by conventional balloon dilatation [44].

Percutaneous Tubular Stents

Standard tubular plastic stents designed for placement during ERCP can be readily inserted percutaneously over a guidewire [45], but there are dedicated shorter systems available for percutaneous insertion (Fig. 4.9). Plastic stents have a place in the treatment of stone disease, and as a temporary measure in undiagnosed strictures, where they can be removed endoscopically. However, if there is only percutaneous access, then their use is limited, as they are designed for endoscopic use and are difficult to remove percutaneously (Fig. 4.10a–c).

An emerging option are biodegradable tubular stents. Made from poly-L-lactic acid (PLLA), they can be placed endoscopically or percutaneously similar to conventional plastic stents, except that the drainage is around the outside (Fig. 4.11). On their own, they will only maintain biliary drainage through the stricture for a short period of time, which can be determined by different degradation speeds of the stents. There is however the option to place several side by side as with plastic stents during ERCP.

Self-Expanding Metal Stents

Metal stents are easy to place and have a larger diameter than plastic stents, achieving an adequate lumen with a single procedure. They appear more successful than multiple plastic stents as a treatment strategy, reducing the number of procedures and complications [46], notably in strictures caused by chronic pancreatitis [12]. Successful outcomes are better for intrinsic biliary disease than for external processes [47], reflecting the hostile territory of calcified chronic

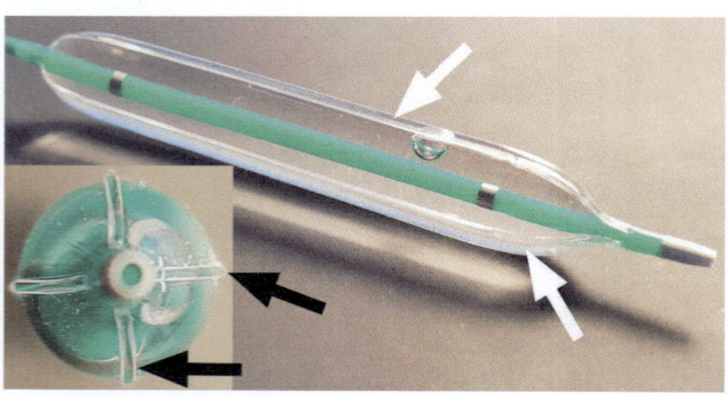

Fig. 4.8 Cutting balloon with four composite blades (arrows), (Enforcer, Boston Scientific, Hemel Hempstead, UK)

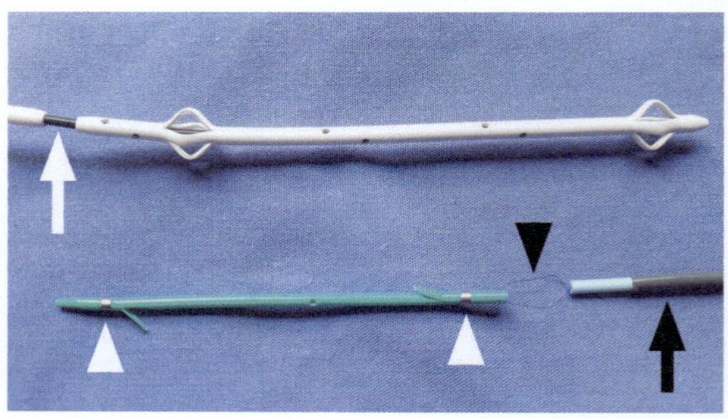

Fig. 4.9 Dedicated percutaneous plastic stents: Top: 10 Fr "double mushroom" stent (Cook Medical, Limerick, Ireland) with guiding catheter (white arrow) and pusher. Bottom: 8 Fr "EndoStay" stent (Pflugbeil GmbH, Munich, Germany) with radiopaque marker bands (white arrowheads), repositioning thread (black arrowhead) and insertion sheath (black arrow) and pusher

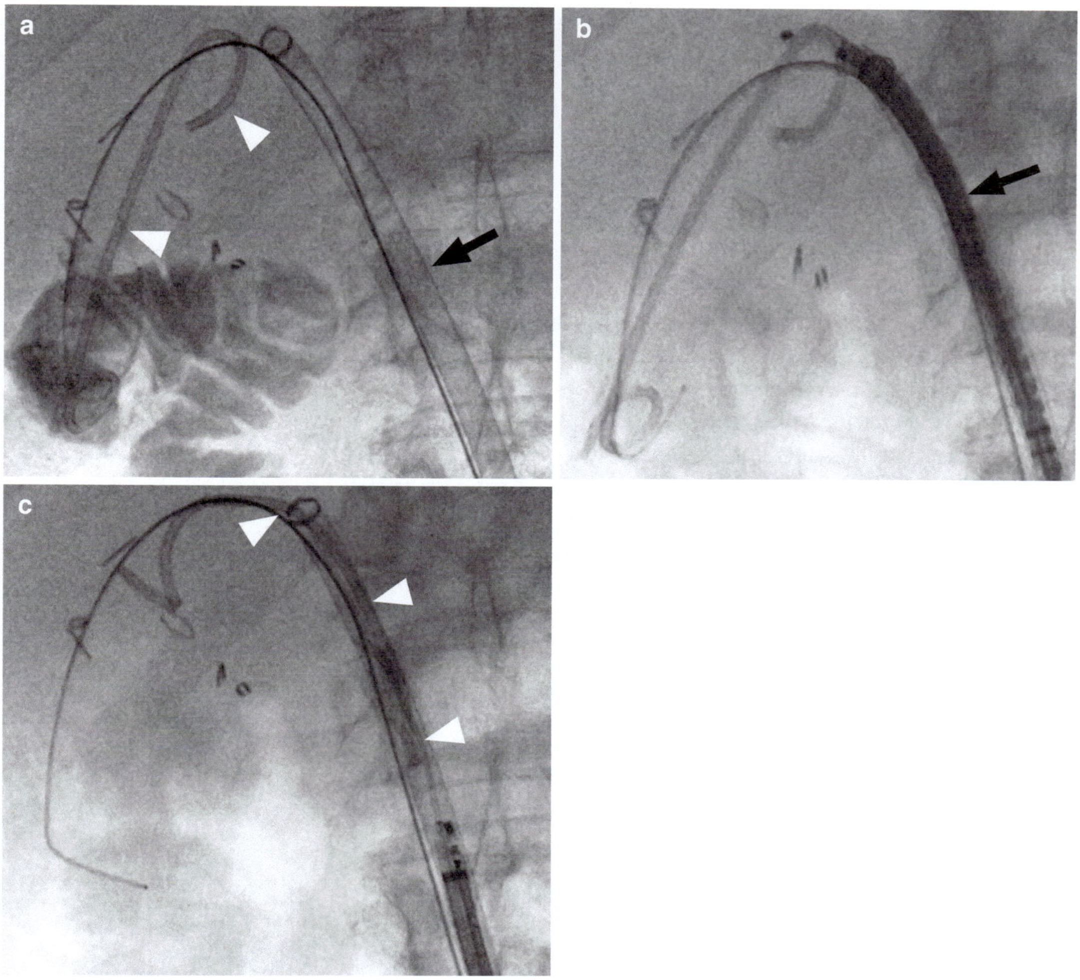

Fig. 4.10 (**a**) A transhepatic sheath (arrow) inserted from the left to retrieve a 7Fr double J plastic stent (arrow heads) placed in error across an anastomotic stricture of a hepaticojejunostomy. (**b**) A cholangioscope (arrow) is inserted and the stent captured with forceps. (**c**) The plastic stent (arrowheads) is withdrawn into the sheath

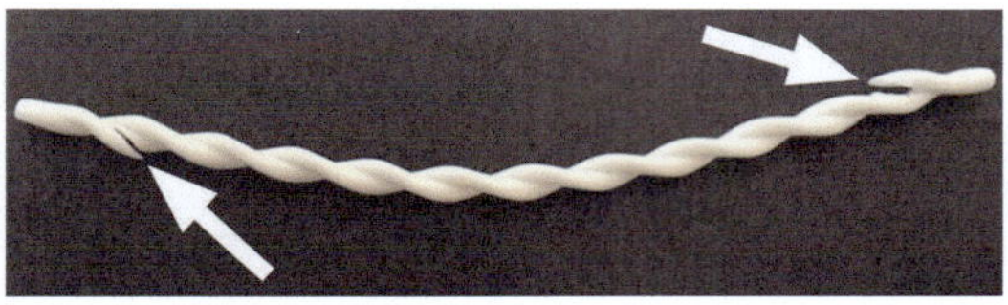

Fig. 4.11 10 Fr biodegradable "Archimedes" stent (AMG GI, Winsen, Germany) with fixation flaps (arrows). The helical structure facilitates drainage around the *outside* of the stent

pancreatitis. A multicenter trial assessing the success of fully covered stents in different etiologies reported the best outcomes for iatrogenic injury (92% resolution), followed by gallstone-related strictures (84%) and chronic pancreatitis (81%) with anastomotic strictures being the most difficult to treat (61.2%). Key features for success are the stent staying in correct position for more than 3 months [48].

It cannot be overemphasized that the stent must be fully covered to ensure it is removable, and stent placement must only be short-term as removal becomes more difficult with length of dwell time [49]. Bare or partially covered stents will induce endothelial hyperplasia, and the overgranulation tissue will fix the bare metal mesh of the stent, render it permanent, and cause subsequent occlusion.

Some fully covered metal stents are available for percutaneous removal with a dedicated hook, but these are not licensed or available in many countries. Fully covered metal stents can be easily removed by endoscopic extraction, if the patient's anatomy allows for access.

Removable, fully covered metal stents have become a main endoscopic strategy temporary stenting of benign strictures and a number are available for percutaneous placement [50]. Most require endoscopic removal, but some have a purse string at the proximal end which allows percutaneous extraction (Fig. 4.12a). The purse string is offset into the lumen of the stent, allowing this string to be captured like the arresting wires on an aircraft carrier. The hook is inserted through a sheath and the stent withdrawn through this. Reported results are good with 16% displacement, all other stents being retrieved and primary patency at 5 years of 68% [51]. Other stents have a retrieval suture, which is left to exit through the skin, thus facilitating removal at a later date (Fig. 4.12b).

Other centers have reported success with placing fully covered metal stents and awaiting their spontaneous displacement. This scenario forfeits the operator's control over the removal process and carries the inherent risk of long-term complications should the stents unexpectedly stay in place, such as secondary stricture formation and perforation.

Self-Expanding Biodegradable Stents

In 2019, only one biodegradable self-expanding biliary stent was commercially available. The SX-Ella BD stent (Ella-CS, Hradec Kralové,

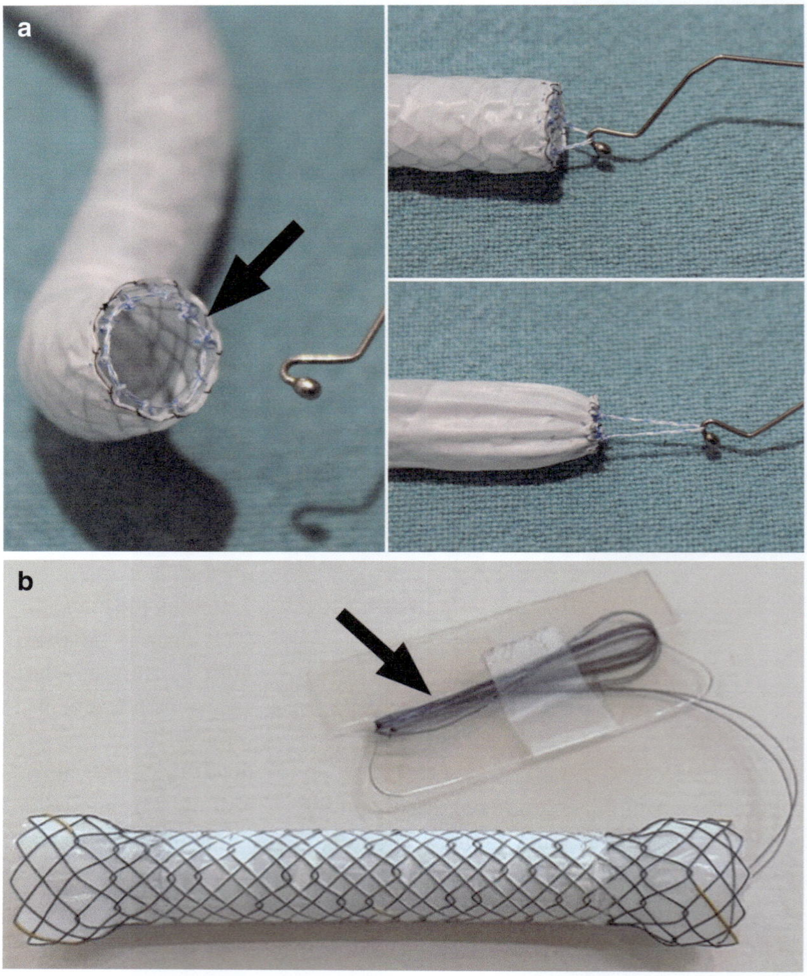

Fig. 4.12 (**a**) Fully covered, removable PD stent (TaeWoong Medical, Gyeonggi-do, Republic of Korea). The retrieval suture is set into the lumen (arrows) to allow percutaneous removal with a hook. (**b**) Fully covered Hilzo stent (BCM, Gyeonggi-do, Republic of Korea) with percutaneous removal string (arrow)

Czech Republic) is a self-expanding stent woven from a polydioxanone monofilament (Fig. 4.13). The long-term elasticity is not as well maintained as with shape-memory superalloys such as nitinol. For that reason, the stent is delivered unconstrained and is hand-loaded into an 11.5 Fr delivery system prior to deployment. Degradation is via hydrolysis leading to swelling of the filament in the first 6 weeks, loss of radial force after 2 months and beginning fragmentation after 3 months. Of note is that the stent does not dissolve, but breaks up into little pieces, which can cause biliary colic and or sepsis if the sphincter of Oddi is intact below. This issue is not relevant in anastomotic strictures of a biliary bypass, as the fragments of the degrading stent pass into the larger lumen of the afferent loop (Fig. 4.14).

A small number of studies have reported very high success rates in strictures refractory to conventional treatment [52–54]. In 2019, full licens-

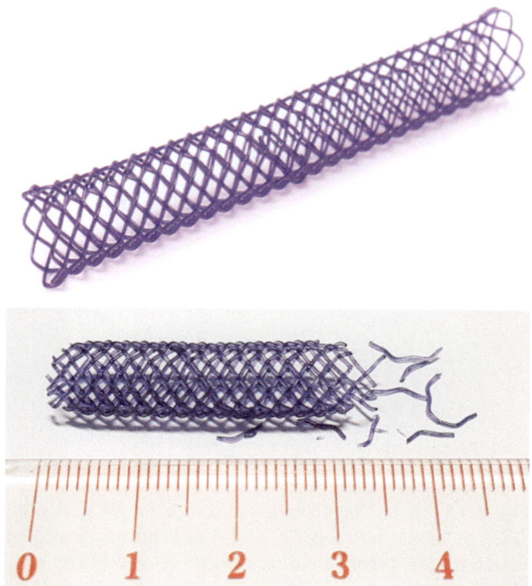

Fig. 4.13 SX-Ella BD stent intact (top) and fragmenting after 15 months exposure to room air (bottom)

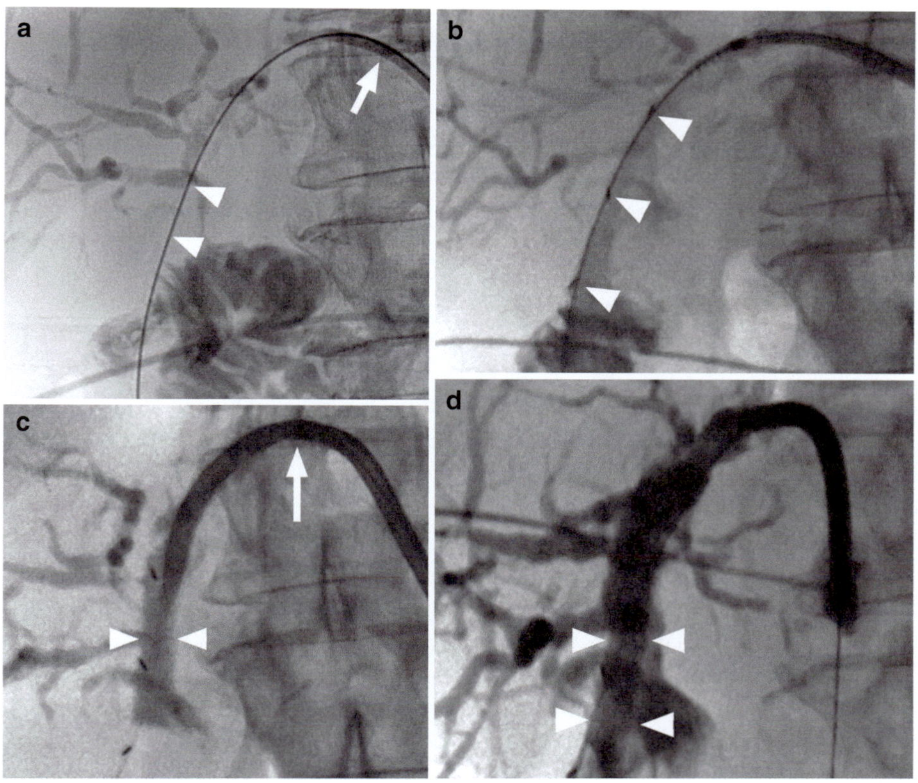

Fig. 4.14 (**a**) Cholangiogram taken through a vascular access sheath (arrow) placed into the biliary tree from the left. A guidewire has been placed across the stricture (arrowheads) at the hepaticojejunostomy. (**b**) Biodegradable stent placed across the stricture, prior to deployment. Note the radiopaque markers (arrows). (**c**) Biodegradable stent deployed (arrowheads) with an external drain left above (arrow). (**d**) Cholangiogram after stent degradation: The anastomosis is widely patent (arrowheads)

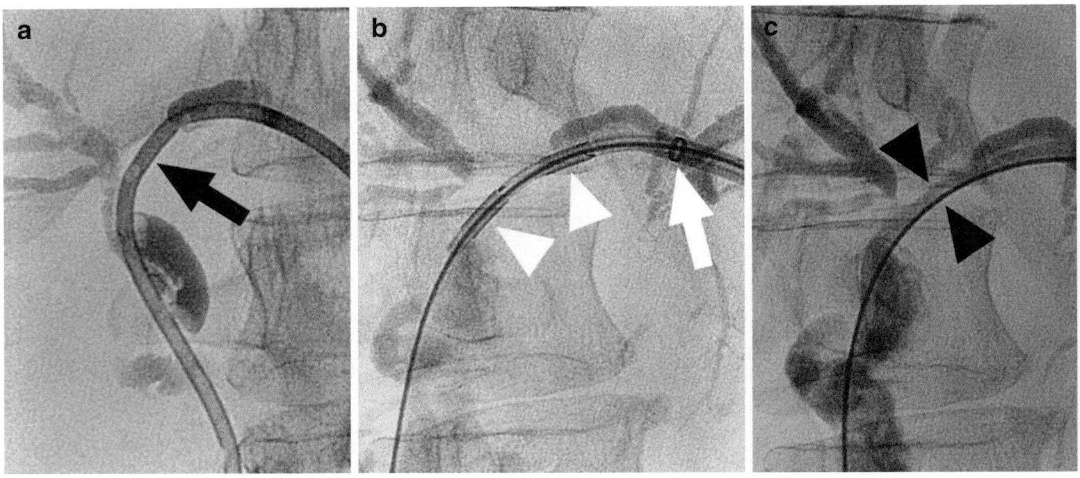

Fig. 4.15 (**a–c**) Percutaneous transluminal RFA. A tight stricture of the left hepatic duct (black arrow) is treated with a bipolar Habib ablation catheter (Boston Scientific, Hemel Hempstead, UK). The two electrodes (white arrowheads) are placed across the stricture through a sheath with a radiopaque marker (white arrow). Following treatment, there is immediate flow of contrast through the ablated segment (black arrowheads)

ing of this device is only available for the esophageal configuration, but the biliary version is readily available on a named patient basis.

Percutaneous Endobiliary Radiofrequency Ablation

As of 2019, there are two devices available for percutaneous endobiliary radiofrequency ablation (RFA) of the biliary tract. These devices are the Habib RFA Catheters (Boston Scientific, MA, United States) and the ELRA RFA catheter (Taewoong Medical, Gyeonggi-do, South Korea).

Their initial indication was for the treatment of malignant biliary strictures via the endoscopic route. Shorter versions of these catheters can easily be inserted via a vascular sheath into the biliary tree to treat the strictured segment (Fig. 4.15). It is important to oversize the sheath by 1 Fr in relation to the catheter to accommodate for the external electrodes. The area to be ablated is determined by fluoroscopy. The duration, burn rate, and depth are controlled by standard external RF generators as for endoscopic application.

Technical feasibility for endoscopic use in benign biliary strictures has been confirmed [55]. The first study treating refractory strictures percutaneously reported 100% technical success in 29 strictures in 18 patients, with a clinical success of 89% [8]. While very encouraging, thermal injury itself can cause stricture formation [11, 56]. More experience, notably around the perforation risk and the likelihood of stricture recurrence, is required before this method can be adopted as a standard option.

Treatment Strategies

Normal Biliary Anatomy

Initial treatment of benign de novo bile duct strictures, particularly of inflammatory origin, is by endoscopic means, and these treatments are well established [57, 58].

Where endoscopic access to these is precluded by adverse anatomy (e.g. a large peri-ampullary diverticulum), PTC may be used to allow retrograde placement of a stent through a combined procedure where an ultra-long (400–450 cm) guidewire is inserted percutaneously and retrieved endoscopically. The through-and-through guidewire allows greater purchase for advancing a biliary catheter or a stent retrogradely across the stenosis, particularly if traction is applied on the percutaneous end. Depending on the intended course of treatment, it may be sensible to maintain the external access after a combined procedure by percutaneous insertion of a locked pigtail catheter. This may be capped off if internal drainage is established. That way the access route to the stricture is maintained, but the patient does not suffer the inconvenience of an external drainage bag filling with bile [59].

Percutaneous Intervention After Biliary Bypass

If a pancreatico-duodenectomy has been performed resulting in a formal Roux-en-Y reconstruction, then endoscopic access to treat an anastomotic stricture is often impossible. The same applies to bilio-enteric anastomoses after liver transplantation.

PTC for these patients allows very direct access to the stricture as well as placement of an external drain to control any existing biliary sepsis and to allow for repeat procedures.

The conventional initial treatment is with pneumatic balloon dilatation to 8–12 mm depending on the level of anastomosis and postsurgical anatomy. Biliary dilatation can be extremely painful and should only be performed with good sedation or ideally under general anesthesia. This issue is not significant with a denervated liver after transplantation.

Short fibrotic strictures have the best response to dilatation, whereas longer ischemic segments or areas of dehiscence have a higher recurrence rate. Not much evidence exists on safety, and efficacy of cutting balloons and stent insertion would normally be considered the next step if stricturing recurs after balloon dilatation.

However, stricture recurrence may be subclinical and slowly lead to hepatic fibrosis or precipitate cholangitis, which may be life-threatening. Balloon dilatation may be repeated several times in the same session or performed with prolonged duration of the inflation, but temporary stenting secures the lumen for several weeks with a much higher chance of permanent stricture remodeling.

Placement of multiple plastic stents, as used as a treatment strategy during ERCP [60] is not a great option, as endoscopic access is not readily available and percutaneous removal is difficult.

Self-expanding biodegradable stents have been used successfully in this context, and the altered anatomy avoids the issues with fragmentation, which can cause a problem in a normal bile duct. This scenario presents an elegant option, as removal is not required and external access does not need to be maintained for this option. Biodegradable stents have a lower radial expansion force than shape-memory metal stents and benefit from balloon dilatation, ideally before stent placement, as this avoids damaging the stent by dilatation after deployment.

It is a difficult decision whether a percutaneous drain should be left in situ and if so for how long. Long-term drains are very inconvenient for the patient and carry a risk of bile leakage and displacement. Skin-level drains are an acceptable compromise for the medium term. When capped off they have a low profile, which is less obtrusive than drains with a conventional hub with a Luer lock, but they do represent an ongoing challenge to the patient in terms of body image, potential pain and skin care in the long term.

If a cholangiogram at 1 week demonstrates adequate stent expansion and drainage, then removal of the external access is acceptable. However, in complex strictures, which may represent a "floppy" segment from anastomotic dehiscence, rather than focal fibrosis, this may collapse again after stent degradation and ultimately require surgical revision [61].

Only few studies report on the use of percutaneously removable fully covered metal stents. Reported clinical success is 87% with 5-year patency of 68%, but stent migration remains a problem, occurring in around 20% of cases [51]. With further device development, they are likely to become a mainstream treatment, reflecting their success in endoscopic use.

Afferent Loop Obstruction

It is rare for the biliary limb of the reconstructive surgery to occlude from benign causes. This phenomenon is mostly due to recurrence of the original cancer. In either case, the bile is colonized with gut flora, and manipulation carries a very high risk of bacteremia and life-threatening sepsis.

If a Roux-en-Y reconstruction has been fashioned, access to the obstructed segment is not usually possible using conventional endoscopes. Stent insertion may be performed with the help of a double-balloon enteroscope [62, 63] or by EUS-guided puncture and a lumen-apposing stent [64]. However, the former is not widely available, and the latter leaves no room for error with regard to perforation, bile leakage, stent misplacement, or stent migration.

Percutaneous drainage has the great advantage of easily being performed as a staged procedure, with initial drainage relieving jaundice and sepsis. A percutaneous drain provides easy repeat access for subsequent stent insertion, once the patient is resuscitated.

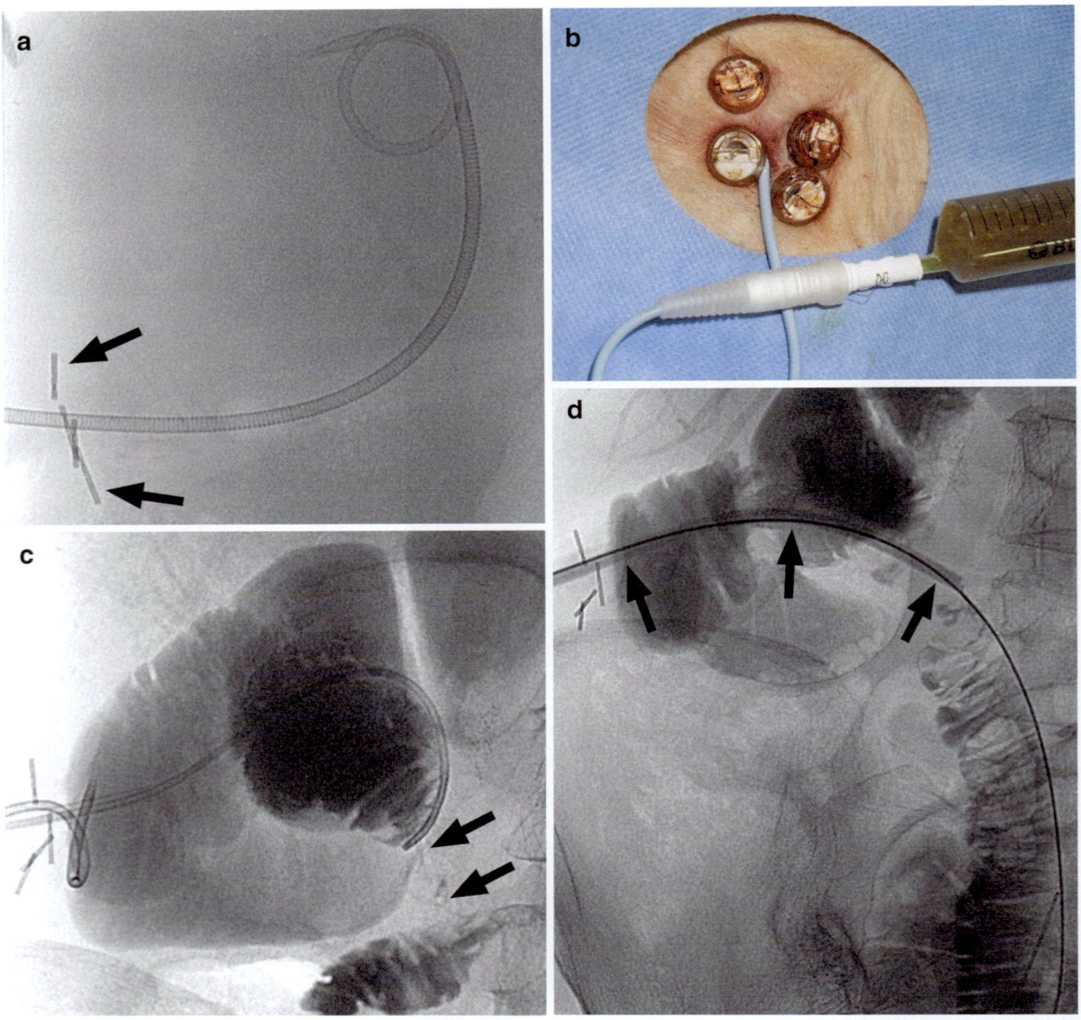

Fig. 4.16 (**a**) Percutaneous afferent loop stent. US-guided jejunopexy was performed with four T-fasteners (arrows), followed by insertion of an external locked pigtail drain. (**b**) External drain and the button fixators of the MIC Safe-T-pexy T-fasteners designed for gastropexy during radiological gastrostomy (O&M Halyard, Apeldoorn, The Netherlands). (**c**) After resolution of sepsis, a catheter was inserted alongside the drain, demonstrating the stricture (arrows) by injection of contrast. (**d**) A stiff guidewire was placed across the stricture, followed by a 10 Fr sheath (arrows). (**e**) A 24 × 100mm-covered double Egis enteral stent (S&G BioTech, Yongin-Si, Republic of Korea) was deployed

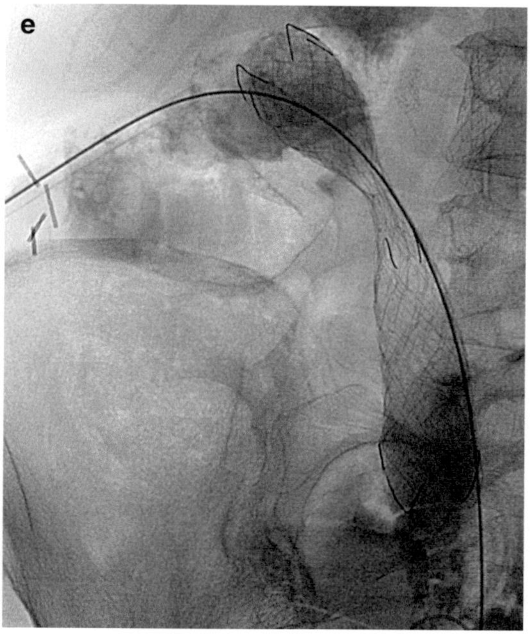

Fig. 4.16 (continued)

If the obstruction is close to the liver, a trans-hepatic route is feasible [65, 66], but if the stricture is too distal to be reached via a trans-hepatic route, then a direct puncture into the dilated afferent loop may be an option. Sometimes during the initial operation, the afferent limb is marked by the surgeon to give a fluoroscopic target for percutaneous access. However, the obstructed loop is usually easily identified on CT and USS.

Direct percutaneous puncture into an afferent loop should only be done after fashioning of a jejunopexy, similar to a gastropexy during radiologically inserted gastrostomy [67, 68]. A total of three or four T-fasteners are placed using ultrasound guidance, and a locked pigtail catheter is inserted as a first step. This action allows initial drainage of the biliary obstruction and resolution of sepsis. Percutaneous insertion of a stent is performed in a secondary step (Fig. 4.16). While 10 mm biliary stents are more than adequate to drain bile from the liver, an enteral stent of 18 mm or larger is more appropriate for insertion into a loop of small bowel. Not only does this process allow for better fixation but also the larger diameter will guarantee longer patency. As no food material are passed through this loop, even fully covered stents are very unlikely to be displaced, but the ideal stent would be a partially covered, knitted stent.

Follow-Up and Monitoring

Early detection of stricture recurrence is important to avoid complications of stone formation, cholangitis and cirrhosis. In combination with the patient's biochemistry, ultrasound is a cheap and available modality for monitoring the biliary tree. It needs to be borne in mind that liver parenchyma, which has undergone several insults such as ischemia and inflammation, may have become fibrotic and be less compliant, thus preventing biliary dilatation, even in complete obstruction. MR scanning and MRCP is a sensitive way to assess for patency and recurrent strictures, has a high correlation with direct cholangiography and avoids the high radiation burden associated with CT scanning [69].

Conclusion

The percutaneous approach to refractory benign biliary strictures offers several significant advantages:

- External or internal biliary drainage is readily established and can be monitored and controlled.
- A percutaneous drain provides an easy access route for repeat procedures.
- Monitoring of progress and response to treatment is simple and cheap.
- Self-expanding biodegradable stents are easily placed and obviate the need for maintaining an access track for later removal.
- It is essential that all patients are given the benefit of a multidisciplinary approach to offer each and every one the most appropriate treatment with the highest chance of success. While repeat surgery has traditionally been regarded as the gold standard, this method is not without risks, and the aim of the combined endoscopic/radiologic options should endeavor to remove the need for this.

References

1. Cotton PB. Endoscopic management of bile duct stones; (apples and oranges). Gut. 1984;25(6):587–97.
2. Lau WY, Lai EC, Lau SH. Management of bile duct injury after laparoscopic cholecystectomy: a review. ANZ J Surg. 2010;80(1-2):75–81. https://doi.org/10.1111/j.1445-2197.2009.05205.x. ANS5205 [pii].
3. Nagral S. Anatomy relevant to cholecystectomy. J Minim Access Surg. 2005;1(2):53–8. https://doi.org/10.4103/0972-9941.16527.
4. Weber A, Rosca B, Neu B, Rosch T, Frimberger E, Born P, Schmid RM, Prinz C. Long-term follow-up of percutaneous transhepatic biliary drainage (PTBD) in patients with benign bilioenterostomy stricture. Endoscopy. 2009;41(4):323–8. https://doi.org/10.1055/s-0029-1214507.
5. Hariharan D, Psaltis E, Scholefield JH, Lobo DN. Quality of life and medico-legal implications following iatrogenic bile duct injuries. World J Surg. 2017;41(1):90–9. https://doi.org/10.1007/s00268-016-3677-9. [pii].
6. Garcea G, Ngu W, Neal CP, Dennison AR, Berry DP. Bilirubin levels predict malignancy in patients with obstructive jaundice. HPB (Oxford). 2011;13(6):426–30. https://doi.org/10.1111/j.1477-2574.2011.00312.x. S1365-182X(15)30446-9 [pii].
7. Vasilieva L, Alexopoulou A, Papadhimitriou SI, Romanos A, Xynopoulos D, Dourakis SP. Total bilirubin is a good discriminator between benign and malignant biliary strictures. HPB (Oxford). 2012;14(1):71. https://doi.org/10.1111/j.1477-2574.2011.00400.x.
8. Thomas S, Jahangir K. Noninvasive imaging of the biliary system relevant to percutaneous interventions. Semin Interv Radiol. 2016;33(4):277–82. https://doi.org/10.1055/s-0036-1592328. 00976 [pii].
9. Katabathina VS, Dasyam AK, Dasyam N, Hosseinzadeh K. Adult bile duct strictures: role of MR imaging and MR cholangiopancreatography in characterization. Radiographics. 2014;34(3):565–86. https://doi.org/10.1148/rg.343125211.
10. Chung YH, Kim DJ, Kim IG, Kim HJ, Chon SE, Jeon JY, Jung JP, Jeong JC, Kim JS, Yun EJ. Relationship between the risk of bile duct injury during laparoscopic cholecystectomy and the types of preoperative magnetic resonance cholangiopancreatography (MRCP). Korean J Hepatobiliary Pancreat Surg. 2012;16(1):17–23. https://doi.org/10.14701/kjhbps.2012.16.1.17.
11. Ziessman HA. Nuclear medicine hepatobiliary imaging. Clin Gastroenterol Hepatol. 2010;8(2):111–6. https://doi.org/10.1016/j.cgh.2009.10.017. S1542-3565(09)01076-3 [pii].
12. Kim YJ, Lee KT, Jo YC, Lee KH, Lee JK, Joh JW, Kwon CH. Hepatobiliary scintigraphy for detecting biliary strictures after living donor liver transplantation. World J Gastroenterol. 2011;17(21):2626–31. https://doi.org/10.3748/wjg.v17.i21.2626.
13. Mohkam K, Malik Y, Derosas C, Isaac J, Marudanayagam R, Mehrzad H, Mirza DF, Muiesan P, Roberts KJ, Sutcliffe RP. Percutaneous transhepatic cholangiographic endobiliary forceps biopsy versus endoscopic ultrasound fine needle aspiration for proximal biliary strictures: a single-centre experience. HPB (Oxford). 2017;19(6):530–7. https://doi.org/10.1016/j.hpb.2017.02.001. S1365-182X(17)30066-7 [pii].
14. Inchingolo R, Spiliopoulos S, Nestola M, Nardella M. Outcomes of percutaneous transluminal biopsy of biliary lesions using a dedicated forceps system. Acta Radiol. 2018;60(5):602–7. https://doi.org/10.1177/0284185118795319. 284185118795319.
15. Park JG, Jung GS, Yun JH, Yun BC, Lee SU, Han BH, Ko JH. Percutaneous transluminal forceps biopsy in patients suspected of having malignant biliary obstruction: factors influencing the outcomes of 271 patients. Eur Radiol. 2017;27(10):4291–7. https://doi.org/10.1007/s00330-017-4796-x.
16. Patel P, Rangarajan B, Mangat K. Improved accuracy of percutaneous biopsy using "cross and push" technique for patients suspected with malignant biliary strictures. Cardiovasc Intervent Radiol. 2015;38(4):1005–10. https://doi.org/10.1007/s00270-014-0976-0.
17. Bukhari MA, Haito-Chavez Y, Ngamruengphong S, Brewer Gutierrez O, Chen YI, Khashab MA. Rendezvous biliary recanalization of complete biliary obstruction with direct peroral and percutaneous transhepatic cholangioscopy. Gastroenterology. 2018;154(1):23–5. https://doi.org/10.1053/j.gastro.2017.09.050. S0016-5085(17)36301-1 [pii].
18. Itoi T, Shinohara Y, Takeda K, Nakamura K, Sofuni A, Itokawa F, Moriyasu F, Tsuchida A. A novel technique for endoscopic sphincterotomy when using a percutaneous transhepatic cholangioscope in patients with an endoscopically inaccessible papilla. Gastrointest Endosc. 2004;59(6):708–11. https://doi.org/10.1016/s0016-5107(04)00170-1. S0016-5107(04)00170-1 [pii].
19. Kawakami H, Ban T, Kubota Y, Ashizuka S, Sannomiya I, Imamura N, Hamada T. Rendezvous biliary recanalization with combined percutaneous transhepatic cholangioscopy and double-balloon endoscopy. Endoscopy. 2018;50(7):E146–8. https://doi.org/10.1055/a-0591-2109.
20. Yoshida M, Morimoto M, Kato A, Hayashi K, Naitoh I, Miyabe K, Matsuo Y. Recanalization of postoperative biliary disconnection with intraductal cholangioscopy-assisted forceps retrieval of rendezvous guidewire. Endoscopy. 2018;50(12):E338–9. https://doi.org/10.1055/a-0667-7751.
21. Gordon RL, Ring EJ. Combined radiologic and retrograde endoscopic and biliary interventions. Radiol Clin N Am. 1990;28(6):1289–95.
22. Kerr RM, Gilliam JH 3rd. The team approach to biliary tract intervention: current status of combined percutaneous-endoscopic techniques. Gastrointest Endosc. 1988;34(5):432–4. https://doi.org/10.1016/

s0016-5107(88)71413-3.S0016-5107(88)71413-3 [pii].

23. Curcio G, Traina M, Miraglia R, Tarantino I, Barresi L, Granata A, Luca A, Gridelli B. Endoscopy after radiology: two-step combined therapy for biliary stricture after Roux-en-Y hepaticojejunostomy. Dig Endosc. 2012;24(4):271–4. https://doi.org/10.1111/j.1443-1661.2011.01203.x.
24. Khashab M, Perez-Miranda M. Finding the middle ground in bile duct injury: the evolving role of biliary rendezvous. Endoscopy. 2018;50(6):559–60. https://doi.org/10.1055/a-0580-7144.
25. Verstandig AG, Goldin E, Sasson T, Weinberger G, Wengrower D, Fich A, Lax E. Combined transhepatic and endoscopic procedures in the biliary system. Postgrad Med J. 1993;69(811):384–8.
26. Gwon DI, Ko GY, Kim JH, Shin JH, Kim KA, Yoon HK, Sung KB. Percutaneous bilateral metallic stent placement using a stentin-stent deployment technique in patients with malignant hilar biliary obstruction. AJR Am J Roentgenol. 2013a;200(4):909–14. https://doi.org/10.2214/AJR.12.8780.
27. Yang MJ, Kim JH, Hwang JC, Yoo BM, Lee SH, Ryu JK, Kim YT, Woo SM, Lee WJ, Jeong S, Lee DH. Prospective multicenter study of the challenges inherent in using large cell-type stents for bilateral stent-in-stent placement in patients with inoperable malignant hilar biliary obstruction. Gut Liver. 2018;12(6):722–7. https://doi.org/10.5009/gnl17468.gnl17468 [pii].
28. Domagk D, Oppong KW, Aabakken L, Czako L, Gyokeres T, Manes G, Meier P, Poley JW, Ponchon T, Tringali A, Bellisario C, Minozzi S, Senore C, Bennett C, Bretthauer M, Hassan C, Kaminski MF, Dinis-Ribeiro M, Rees CJ, Spada C, Valori R, Bisschops R, Rutter MD. Performance measures for endoscopic retrograde cholangiopancreatography and endoscopic ultrasound: a European Society of Gastrointestinal Endoscopy (ESGE) Quality Improvement Initiative. United European Gastroenterol J. 2018;6(10):1448–60. https://doi.org/10.1177/2050640618808157.
29. Chehab MA, Thakor AS, Tulin-Silver S, Connolly BL, Cahill AM, Ward TJ, Padia SA, Kohi MP, Midia M, Chaudry G, Gemmete JJ, Mitchell JW, Brody L, Crowley JJ, Heran MKS, Weinstein JL, Nikolic B, Dariushnia SR, Tam AL, Venkatesan AM. Adult and pediatric antibiotic prophylaxis during vascular and IR procedures: a Society of Interventional Radiology Practice Parameter Update Endorsed by the Cardiovascular and Interventional Radiological Society of Europe and the Canadian Association for Interventional Radiology. J Vasc Interv Radiol. 2018;29(11):1483–1501 e1482. https://doi.org/10.1016/j.jvir.2018.06.007. S1051-0443(18)31259-4 [pii].
30. Huang SY, Philip A, Richter MD, Gupta S, Lessne ML, Kim CY. Prevention and management of infectious complications of percutaneous interventions. Semin Interv Radiol. 2015;32(2):78–88. https://doi.org/10.1055/s-0035-1549372.
31. Pitt HA. Does cholangiovenous reflux cause cholangitis? HPB Surg. 1990;2(3):220–3.
32. Thaker AT, Muthusamy VR. The role and utility of cholangioscopy for diagnosing indeterminate biliary strictures. Gastrointest Interv. 2017;6(1):2–8. https://doi.org/10.18528/gii160035.
33. Mendonca EQ, de Oliveira JF, Baba ER, Dias AR, Maluf-Filho F. Percutaneous transhepatic cholangioscopy for the diagnosis of biliary obstruction in a patient with Roux-en-Y partial gastrectomy. Gastrointest Endosc. 2017;85(1):255–6. https://doi.org/10.1016/j.gie.2016.07.057. S0016-5107(16)30442-4 [pii].
34. Peck JR, Spain J, Al Taani J, McCarthy ST. Percutaneous antegrade digital cholangioscopy in the management of biliary disorders. VideoGIE. 2017;2(6):145–6. https://doi.org/10.1016/j.vgie.2017.03.001. S2468-4481(17)30060-7 [pii].
35. Weigand K, Kandulski A, Zuber-Jerger I, Mueller M, Goessmann H. Cholangioscopy-guided electrohydraulic lithotripsy of large bile duct stones through a percutaneous access device. Endoscopy. 2018;50(5):E111–2. https://doi.org/10.1055/s-0044-101015.
36. Bonnel DH, Fingerhut AL. Percutaneous transhepatic balloon dilatation of benign bilioenteric strictures: long-term results in 110 patients. Am J Surg. 2012;203(6):675–83. https://doi.org/10.1016/j.amjsurg.2012.02.001. S0002-9610(12)00169-9 [pii].
37. Janssen JJ, van Delden OM, van Lienden KP, Rauws EA, Busch OR, van Gulik TM, Gouma DJ, Lameris JS. Percutaneous balloon dilatation and long-term drainage as treatment of anastomotic and nonanastomotic benign biliary strictures. Cardiovasc Intervent Radiol. 2014;37(6):1559–67. https://doi.org/10.1007/s00270-014-0836-y.
38. Kocher M, Cerna M, Havlik R, Kral V, Gryga A, Duda M. Percutaneous treatment of benign bile duct strictures. Eur J Radiol. 2007;62(2):170–4.
39. Zajko AB, Sheng R, Zetti GM, Madariaga JR, Bron KM. Transhepatic balloon dilation of biliary strictures in liver transplant patients: a 10-year experience. J Vasc Interv Radiol. 1995;6(1):79–83.
40. Dhondt E, Vanlangenhove P, Van Vlierberghe H, Troisi R, De Bruyne R, Huyck L, Defreyne L. Benign anastomotic biliary strictures untreatable by ERCP: a novel percutaneous balloon dilatation technique avoiding indwelling catheters. Eur Radiol. 2019;29(2):636–44. https://doi.org/10.1007/s00330-018-5526-8.
41. Atar E, Bachar GN, Bartal G, Mor E, Neyman H, Graif F, Belenky A. Use of peripheral cutting balloon in the management of resistant benign ureteral and biliary strictures. J Vasc Interv Radiol. 2005;16(2 Pt 1):241–5. https://doi.org/10.1097/01.RVI.0000143767.87399.9C. 16/2/241 [pii].
42. Mukund A, Rajesh S, Agrawal N, Arora A. Percutaneous management of resistant biliary-enteric anastomotic strictures with the use of a combined cutting and conventional balloon cholangioplasty protocol: a single-center experience. J Vasc Interv Radiol. 2015;26(4):560–5. https://

doi.org/10.1016/j.jvir.2014.12.011. S1051-0443(14)01182-8 [pii].
43. Sheridan JS, Maclennan AC. Percutaneous transhepatic use of a cutting balloon in the treatment of a benign common bile duct stricture. Cardiovasc Intervent Radiol. 2007;30(2):346. https://doi.org/10.1007/s00270-006-0248-8.
44. Saad WE, Davies MG, Saad NE, Waldman DL, Sahler LG, Lee DE, Kitanosono T, Sasson T, Patel NC. Transhepatic dilation of anastomotic biliary strictures in liver transplant recipients with use of a combined cutting and conventional balloon protocol: technical safety and efficacy. J Vasc Interv Radiol. 2006;17(5):837–43. https://doi.org/10.1097/01.RVI.0000209343.80105. B4. 17/5/837 [pii].
45. Lee ES, Han JK, Baek JH, Suh SW, Joo I, Yi NJ, Lee KW, Suh KS. Long-term efficacy of percutaneous internal plastic stent placement for non-anastomotic biliary stenosis after liver transplantation. Cardiovasc Intervent Radiol. 2016;39(6):909–15. https://doi.org/10.1007/s00270-016-1297-2.
46. Kaffes A, Griffin S, Vaughan R, James M, Chua T, Tee H, Dinesen L, Corte C, Gill R. A randomized trial of a fully covered self-expandable metallic stent versus plastic stents in anastomotic biliary strictures after liver transplantation. Ther Adv Gastroenterol. 2014;7(2):64–71. https://doi.org/10.1177/1756283X13503614.
47. Sung RS, Campbell DA Jr, Rudich SM, Punch JD, Shieck VL, Armstrong JM, Ford E, Sullivan P, Dasika NL, Magee JC. Long-term follow-up of percutaneous transhepatic balloon cholangioplasty in the management of biliary strictures after liver transplantation. Transplantation. 2004;77(1):110–5. https://doi.org/10.1097/01.TP.0000101518.19849.C8.
48. Kahaleh M, Brijbassie A, Sethi A, Degaetani M, Poneros JM, Loren DE, Kowalski TE, Sejpal DV, Patel S, Rosenkranz L, McNamara KN, Raijman I, Talreja JP, Gaidhane M, Sauer BG, Stevens PD. Multicenter trial evaluating the use of covered self-expanding metal stents in benign biliary strictures: time to revisit our therapeutic options? J Clin Gastroenterol. 2013;47(8):695–9. https://doi.org/10.1097/MCG.0b013e31827fd311.
49. Chaput U, Vienne A, Audureau E, Bauret P, Bichard P, Coumaros D, Napoleon B, Ponchon T, Duchmann JC, Laugier R, Lamouliatte H, Vedrenne B, Gaudric M, Chaussade S, Robin F, Leblanc S, Prat F. Temporary placement of fully covered self-expandable metal stents for the treatment of benign biliary strictures. United European Gastroenterol J. 2016;4(3):403–12. https://doi.org/10.1177/2050640615606550.
50. Gwon DI, Laasch HU. Radiological approach to benign biliary strictures. Gastrointest Interv. 2015;4:9–14.
51. Gwon DI, Ko GY, Ko HK, Yoon HK, Sung KB. Percutaneous transhepatic treatment using retrievable covered stents in patients with benign biliary strictures: mid-term outcomes in 68 patients. Dig Dis Sci. 2013b;58(11):3270–9. https://doi.org/10.1007/s10620-013-2784-9.
52. Gimenez ME, Palermo M, Houghton E, Acquafresca P, Finger C, Verde JM, Cuneo JC. Biodegradable biliary stents: a new approach for the management of hepaticojejunostomy strictures following bile duct injury. Prospective study. Arq Bras Cir Dig. 2016;29(2):112–6. https://doi.org/10.1590/0102-6720201600020012. S0102-67202016000200112 [pii].
53. Mauri G, Michelozzi C, Melchiorre F, Poretti D, Tramarin M, Pedicini V, Solbiati L, Cornalba G, Sconfienza LM. Biodegradable biliary stent implantation in the treatment of benign bilioplastic-refractory biliary strictures: preliminary experience. Eur Radiol. 2013;23(12):3304–10. https://doi.org/10.1007/s00330-013-2947-2.
54. Petrtyl J, Bruha R, Horak L, Zadorova Z, Dosedel J, Laasch HU. Management of benign intrahepatic bile duct strictures: initial experience with polydioxanone biodegradable stents. Endoscopy. 2010;42(Suppl 2):E89–90. https://doi.org/10.1055/s-0029-1243880.
55. Hu B, Gao DJ, Wu J, Wang TT, Yang XM, Ye X. Intraductal radiofrequency ablation for refractory benign biliary stricture: pilot feasibility study. Dig Endosc. 2014;26(4):581–5. https://doi.org/10.1111/den.12225.
56. Shin JU, Lee KH, Kim SA, Choi JH, Kim KM, Lee JK, Lee KT, Choi YL. Intraductal thermal injury using a heat probe and radiofrequency ablation electrode in a swine model of biliary stenosis. Clin Res Hepatol Gastroenterol. 2013;37(2):159–65. https://doi.org/10.1016/j.clinre.2012.04.013.
57. Baron TH Sr, Davee T. Endoscopic management of benign bile duct strictures. Gastrointest Endosc Clin N Am. 2013;23(2):295–311. https://doi.org/10.1016/j.giec.2013.01.001. S1052-5157(13)00002-0 [pii].
58. Costamagna G, Boskoski I. Current treatment of benign biliary strictures. Ann Gastroenterol. 2013;26(1):37–40.
59. Gwon DI, Shim HJ, Kwak BK. Retrievable biliary stent-graft in the treatment of benign biliary strictures. J Vasc Interv Radiol. 2008;19(9):1328–35. https://doi.org/10.1016/j.jvir.2008.05.017. S1051-0443(08)00511-3 [pii].
60. Costamagna G, Shah SK, Tringali A. Current management of postoperative complications and benign biliary strictures. Gastrointest Endosc Clin N Am. 2003;13(4):635–48.
61. Mullan D, Shepherd D, Laasch HU. Percutaneous biodegradable stent insertion for a benign biliary stricture complicating choledochojejunostomy. Gastrointest Interv. 2015;4(1):58–60. https://doi.org/10.1016/j.gii.2015.03.001.
62. Fujii M, Ishiyama S, Saito H, Ito M, Fujiwara A, Niguma T, Yoshioka M, Shiode J. Metallic stent insertion with double-balloon endoscopy for malignant afferent loop obstruction. World J Gastrointest Endosc. 2015;7(6):665–9. https://doi.org/10.4253/wjge.v7.i6.665.

63. Sasaki T, Isayama H, Kogure H, Yamada A, Aoki T, Kokudo N, Koike K. Double-balloon enteroscope-assisted enteral stent placement for malignant afferent-loop obstruction after Roux-en-Y reconstruction. Endoscopy. 2014;46(Suppl 1 UCTN):E541–2. https://doi.org/10.1055/s-0034-1377633.
64. Taunk P, Cosgrove N, Loren DE, Kowalski T, Siddiqui AA. Endoscopic ultrasound-guided gastroenterostomy using a lumen-apposing self-expanding metal stent for decompression of afferent loop obstruction. Endoscopy. 2015;47(Suppl 1 UCTN):E395–6. https://doi.org/10.1055/s-0034-1392564.
65. Caldicott DG, Ziprin P, Morgan R. Transhepatic insertion of a metallic stent for the relief of malignant afferent loop obstruction. Cardiovasc Intervent Radiol. 2000;23(2):138–40.
66. Hosokawa I, Kato A, Shimizu H, Furukawa K, Miyazaki M. Percutaneous transhepatic metallic stent insertion for malignant afferent loop obstruction following pancreaticoduodenectomy: a case report. J Med Case Rep. 2012;6:198. https://doi.org/10.1186/1752-1947-6-198. 1752-1947-6-198 [pii].
67. Brown AS, Mueller PR, Ferrucci JT Jr. Controlled percutaneous gastrostomy: nylon T-fastener for fixation of the anterior gastric wall. Radiology. 1986;158(2):543–5. https://doi.org/10.1148/radiology.158.2.2934763.
68. Laasch HU. Obstructive jaundice after bilioenteric anastomosis: transhepatic and direct percutaneous enteral stent insertion for afferent loop occlusion. Gut Liver. 2010;4(Suppl 1):S89–95. https://doi.org/10.5009/gnl.2010.4.S1.S89.
69. Katz LH, Benjaminov O, Belinki A, Geler A, Braun M, Knizhnik M, Aizner S, Shaharabani E, Sulkes J, Shabtai E, Pappo O, Atar E, Tur-Kaspa R, Mor E, Ben-Ari Z. Magnetic resonance cholangiopancreatography for the accurate diagnosis of biliary complications after liver transplantation: comparison with endoscopic retrograde cholangiography and percutaneous transhepatic cholangiography – long-term follow-up. Clin Transpl. 2010;24(5):E163–9. https://doi.org/10.1111/j.1399-0012.2010.01300.x.

SEMS Insertion for Hilar Stricture: Who, When, and Why?

5

Osman Ahmed and Jeffrey H. Lee

Introduction

Hilar, or perihilar, strictures are narrowings that occur at or around the bifurcation of the left and right hepatic ducts. There are a variety of causes of hilar strictures with the most common being malignant strictures due to cholangiocarcinoma. Other less common etiologies include primary sclerosing cholangitis, infectious etiologies, and postoperative strictures [1].

Cholangiocarcinoma is an epithelial cancer that arises from the cells lining the bile ducts. They represent roughly 3% of all gastrointestinal cancers, although there has been a recent increase in their incidence [2]. The majority of the increase can be attributed in the rise of intrahepatic cholangiocarcinomas (ICC) where there has been an almost 165% increase in ICCs in the previous decades. Interestingly, the incidence of extrahepatic cholangiocarcinoma (ECC) is actually decreasing worldwide [3]. Unfortunately, the prognosis of patients with cholangiocarcinoma that are not surgical candidates remains dismal, with a less than 5% rate of overall survival after 5 years [4].

There are different methods of classifying cholangiocarcinomas, with the most recent AJCC eighth edition now subdividing cholangiocarcinoma into intrahepatic and extrahepatic cholangiocarcinoma. The tumors can also be further divided anatomically into three groups: the intrahepatic, the perihilar (or hilar), and the distal (extrahepatic) groups of cholangiocarcinoma. The proportion of cholangiocarcinomas in each group is roughly 50% in the perihilar group, roughly 40% in the distal (extrahepatic) group, and less than 10% in the intrahepatic group [5].

The hilar group of cholangiocarcinomas (previously known as Klatskin tumors) represent tumors that arise at or near the confluence of the right and left hepatic duct. These tumors are further subclassified based on a system designed by Bismuth et al. in 1992 and known as the Bismuth–Corlette classification. This classification was made to aid in decision-making about surgical resection options in patients. There are four types of hilar tumors in the Bismuth–Corlette classification: type 1 are tumors that arise just distal to the bifurcation, type 2 arise at the bifurcation but do not extend into either right or left hepatic duct, type 3 arise either into the right hepatic duct (type 3a) or the left hepatic duct (type 3b), and finally type 4 involve the right, left, and hilar regions of the biliary tree (Fig. 5.1) [6].

Although the presentation of hilar strictures are varied, the most common reason for presentation is development of obstructive jaundice, with more than 80% of patients presenting with the symptom [7]. Other methods of presentation

O. Ahmed · J. H. Lee (✉)
Department of Gastroenterology, Hepatology and Nutrition, University of Texas MD Anderson Cancer Center, Houston, TX, USA
e-mail: jefflee@mdanderson.org

D. K. Lee (ed.), *Advanced ERCP for Complicated and Refractory Biliary and Pancreatic Diseases*,
https://doi.org/10.1007/978-981-13-0608-2_5

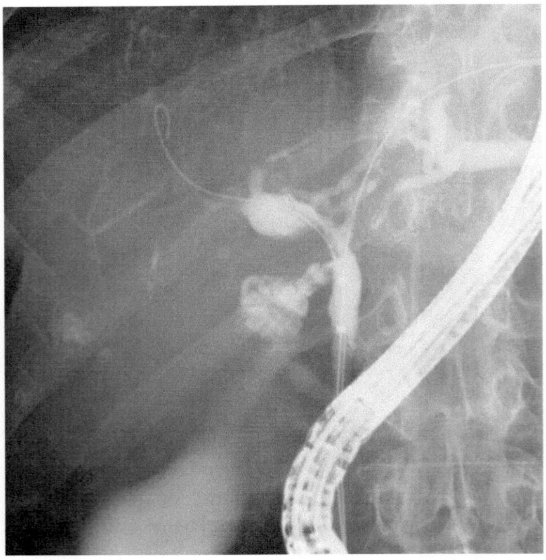

Fig. 5.1 Bismuth–Corlette type 4 hilar stricture

include abdominal pain, weight loss, and fever. When patients with known risk factors for cholangiocarcinoma present with obstructive jaundice and a hilar stricture is discovered, they should be investigated appropriately to rule out malignancy. In patients with a strong suspicion for malignancy who are potentially surgical or liver transplant candidates, the decision to pursue endoscopic investigation or management should be done in conjunction with the surgical and transplant team as there remains a risk of tumor seeding that might make someone ineligible for transplant [8].

Although surgery and liver transplant remain the only curative treatment option for patients with malignant hilar strictures, the majority of patients will not be candidates either due to progression of disease, metastases, or comorbidities precluding intervention. In one study, only half the patients diagnosed with hilar cholangiocarcinoma were deemed to be candidates for either surgical resection or liver transplant [9]. In patients with unresectable hilar obstructions, the role for endoscopic management of symptoms becomes essential. In this chapter, we will provide an overview on why patients with hilar strictures should undergo endoscopic management, the role of self-expandable metal stents (SEMS) in biliary drainage, methods of placing SEMS in patient with hilar obstruction, and finally review the evidence behind recent controversies and advancements in metal stent placements.

Biliary Decompression

In patients who are potential surgical candidates, the role of preoperative biliary drainage remains controversial. Three previous randomized controlled trials failed to demonstrate any difference in perioperative outcomes with preoperative biliary drainage. However, all three of these trials are dated and included patients where the purpose of surgery was palliative and not curative [10–12]. Similarly, a systematic review and meta-analysis on preoperative biliary drainage which included 11 studies and 711 cases found no clinical benefit to preoperative biliary drainage but an increased risk of infectious complications. The main limitation of the review was that it included both randomized controlled trials and retrospective studies [13]. Some proponents suggest that preoperative biliary drainage be reserved for patients with cholangitis, markedly high bilirubin, and low liver remnant function anticipation [14, 15].

In patients with unresectable hilar cholangiocarcinoma, or in those with benign hilar strictures, the indication to decompress is more straightforward. Decompression of the biliary tree is important to prevent cholangitis, to prevent the worsening of liver function, and to relieve symptoms associated with hyperbilirubinemia. Similarly, a recent study demonstrated that patients who achieved biliary decompression had improved outcomes compared with patients where it was unsuccessful [16]. A similar study demonstrated not only that drainage in inoperable patients increased survival, but that baseline bilirubinemia was the only factor affecting successful biliary decompression [17]. Therefore, in patients who are deemed nonsurgical, it is recommended to proceed with biliary decompression.

Method of Drainage

Once the decision to pursue biliary drainage has been made, the next issue is to determine which method of biliary drainage to perform.

Traditionally, there have been two methods of biliary drainage, endoscopic and percutaneous. Although previously surgical biliary drainage was performed as well, this method has fallen out of favor due to worse outcomes. The main surgical biliary drainage method was the creation of a biliary-enteric anastomosis though this led to an increase in postoperative mortality, increased procedure-related complications, and increased length of stay compared with endoscopic stenting. The only advantage of surgical bypass drainage was a lower rate of recurrence [18].

Although endoscopic decompression with the use of endoscopic retrograde cholangiopancreatography is the generally accepted first-line method, its role at the top of the algorithm is not without controversy. Two older randomized controlled trials comparing endoscopic vs. percutaneous biliary decompression found mixed results. Both studies included all types of biliary obstruction and not necessarily only hilar malignancies. In the first study, percutaneous placement had similar technical success rates, but higher therapeutic success rates (defined as decrease in bilirubin of at least 20%). Endoscopic placement had fewer periprocedural complications but increased overall mortality [19]. In the second study, endoscopic intervention had higher clinical success and decreased mortality rates, though this was limited by being an older study [20].

There has been more recent data on the use of percutaneous compared with endoscopic drainage specifically in the setting of perihilar strictures. A meta-analysis published in 2017, consisting of four retrospective studies involving 433 patients, showed that percutaneous drainage was associated with lower overall-mortality, lower rate of conversion to the other method, and lower rates of cholangitis and pancreatitis. There was no difference in the rate of technical failure between the two groups [21–24]. The main limitation of percutaneous drainage is related to the quality of life for the patient as it initially involves a drainage that is external and attached to a bag (Fig. 5.2). Nonetheless, serious consideration should be given to percutaneous drainage depending on anatomy, and a low threshold should be available for crossing over to percutaneous drainage if endoscopic management is chosen as first-line therapy. In addition, a large-scale randomized controlled trial investigating percutaneous transhepatic drainage vs. ERCP is currently underway (INTERCPT trial) and hopefully will address which method should be performed first [25].

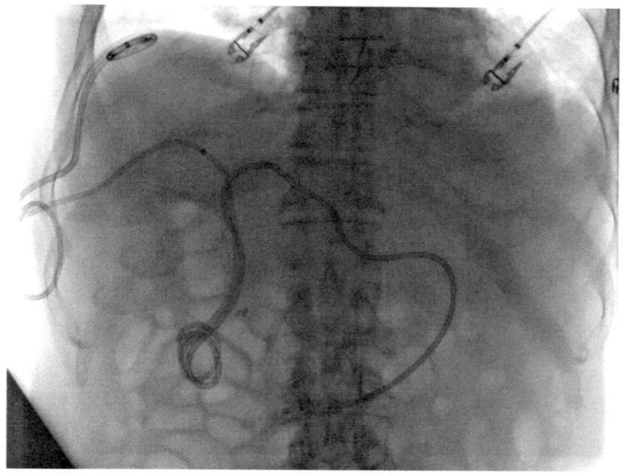

Fig. 5.2 Percutaneous bilateral external plastic stents

Finally, although stenting is the general consensus for biliary drainage (either endoscopically or percutaneous), other forms of decompression have been studied, including nasobiliary drainage. In this procedure, a drain is left in situ and continuously drained. This procedure is generally performed in the preoperative setting. The main limitation is patient discomfort. A recent study for hilar tumors showed that nasobiliary drainage had similar technical success rates to stenting with no difference in total complications [26].

Metal or Plastic Stent Insertion

After deciding to pursue biliary stenting for the purposes of biliary decompression, the next decision is usually whether to pursue a plastic stent or a metal stent. Plastic stents are generally considered to be cheaper; however, they require prophylactic routine replacements due to an increased risk of stent occlusion and biofilm formation. They are also easier to insert for proximal strictures and have smaller diameters with the most common size being 10 Fr. They can be straight with flaps or have a pigtail to prevent migration (Fig. 5.3). Metal stents, also known as self-expanding metal stents (SEMS), are generally thought to last longer, though they are more expensive (Fig. 5.4). There are different types of metal stents: covered, partially covered, and uncovered. Uncovered stents have the risk of tumor in-growth and are generally not removable post-insertion. Covered metal stents do not have the risk of tumor in-growth but do carry an increased risk of migration. SEMS come in larger diameters compared to plastic stents, with the most common size being 10 mm, though 8 mm and 6 mm SEMS are available as well [27].

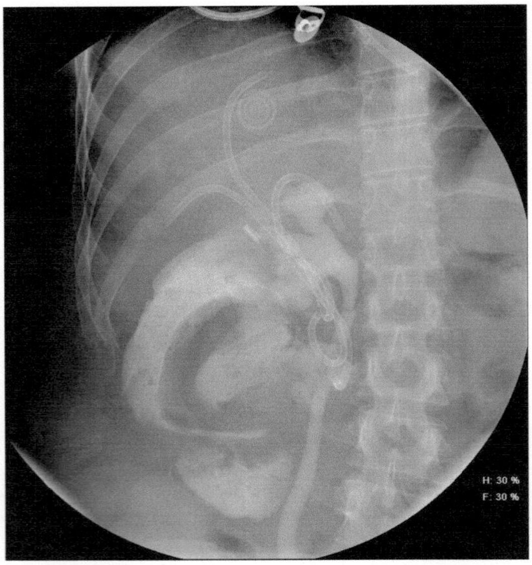

Fig. 5.3 Three double-pigtail internal plastic biliary stents

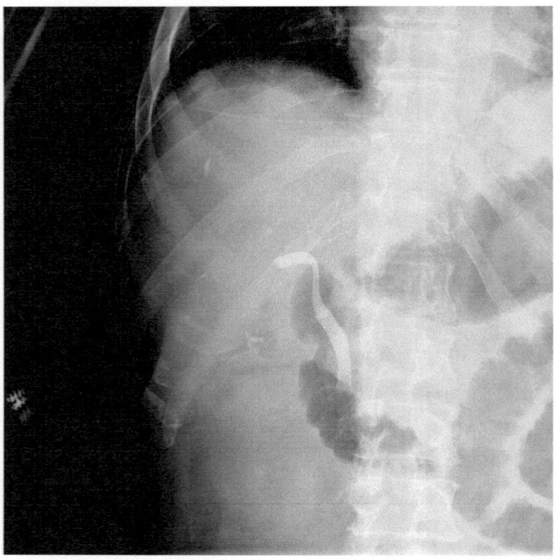

Fig. 5.4 Right hepatic duct self-expanding metal stent

Although SEMS placement has a large body of evidence in distal biliary obstructions, their role in hilar obstructions is not as well studied. Two previous randomized controlled studies have compared the efficacy of SEMS to plastic stents. The first, done in Japan, found that SEMS had longer patency and lower re-intervention rates [28]. In the second study, performed in Thailand, SEMS not only had better biliary drainage characteristic compared to plastic stents but also had higher overall survival rates [29]. The benefit of the latter study is that it included only endoscopic placement of SEMS rather than both endoscopic and percutaneous placement. In a prospective observational study, SEMS were associated with similar technical success, but lower rates of complications such as cholangitis, occlusion, and migration [30]. Similarly, systematic review and meta-analysis looked specifically at plastic compared to SMES insertion in hilar obstructions. They included ten studies and found that SEMS were associated with higher successful drainage rates, lower complication rates, longer patency, and longer overall survival.

There have been different recommendations in regards to appropriate stent type in biliary drainage. Some experts recommend that if a patient has longer than 3 months expected survival time, then they should receive SEMS drainage; otherwise, a plastic stent is reasonable. Others have suggested that initial placement should be done with a plastic stent (to ensure appropriate drainage can be achieved endoscopically), and then in subsequent ERCPs, the plastic stent can be changed to a SEMS [31]. However, if there are strictures involving the second-order branches of the biliary tree without significant proximal duct dilation, SEMS may not be ideal, as secondary branches may occlude with the increased radial force and pressure from SEMS on them. In these cases, we recommend double pigtail plastic stents which have multiple side holes facilitating drainage from the second-order branches.

Unilateral or Bilateral Drainage

Malignant hilar obstructions are challenging due to their location right at the bifurcation of the right and left hepatic ducts. It is thought that because of their anatomy, it is possible that hilar strictures cause biliary obstruction in both the left lobe and the right lobe of the liver. This has led many to question whether bilateral drainage is required so that one lobe of the liver does not atrophy (Fig. 5.5). A study based out of France examined the role of liver volume and successful clinical drainage. Successful biliary drainage was defined as a decrease in bilirubin to less than 50% of the pretreatment value. It was a retrospective study looking at 107 patients undergoing biliary drainage for malignant hilar strictures. Liver volume was assessed by computed tomography scans and divided into three groups: less than 30%, 30–50%, and greater than 50%. The study found that greater than 50% drainage of the liver was associated with an increase in rates of successful biliary drainage, decreased rates of cholangitis, and improvement in overall survival (determined by median survival in days) [32]. Nevertheless, this study was criticized due to its retrospective nature, large number of excluded patients, and large interval in time (1996–2005) which did not account for advancements in technology and technique [33]. A more recent study has suggested that patients without impaired liver function only require greater than 33% percent of liver volume drainage, whereas those with impaired liver function require greater than 50% [34].

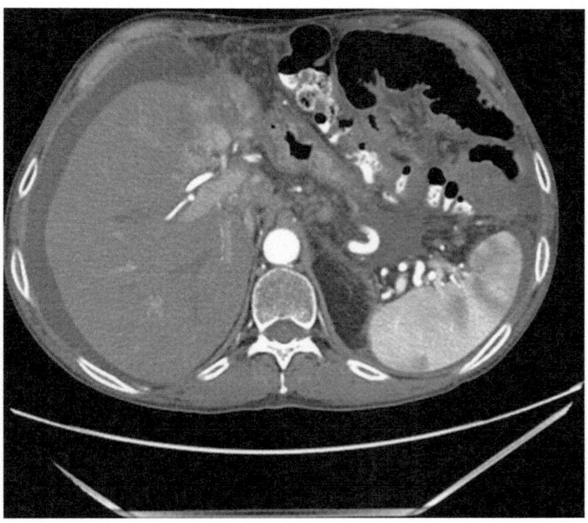

Fig. 5.5 Left lobe of liver atrophied. Plastic stent in right hepatic duct

The initial seminal study looking at unilateral compared to bilateral drainage was done in Canada and retrospectively showed that patients with hilar strictures that received bilateral drainage had improved survival rates compared to those that had unilateral drainage. Patients that had unilateral drainage but had both ducts opacified had the worse outcomes [35]. A subsequent prospective, randomized study showed no difference in mortality, complications, or technical success between unilateral and bilateral drainage using a per-protocol analysis, but higher rates of successful drainage and lower complication rate with unilateral drainage in an intention-to-treat analysis [36].

The most recent study examining unilateral compared to bilateral stents was published in 2017 and was a prospective randomized controlled trial involving 133 patients. This study exclusively looked at self-expanding metal stents only. The study found no difference in technical success but a higher clinical success rate in the bilateral group. The bilateral group also has had more durable stent patency and fewer reinterventions. This study has led to an increase interest in the role of SEMS for bilateral drainage. Similar results have been published elsewhere as well [37, 38]. Finally, a systematic review and meta-analysis in 2015 included three randomized trials and seven observational studies and found no significant difference in drainage rate or patient survival. However, the bilateral group did have longer stent patency compared to the unilateral group [39].

Overall, the decision to pursue unilateral or bilateral drainage should be individualized. The location of the stricture (based on Bismuth–Corlette classification) and the amount of liver volume that can be drained should direct therapy. Ideally, greater than 50% of liver volume should be drained if possible with the use of either unilateral or bilateral stents. If doing unilateral stenting, care should be taken so that contrast is only injected into the side that will be stented [31].

Stent-in-Stent or Side-by-Side Insertion

The challenging aspect with placing bilateral SEMS is the method in which the stents are placed. There are two widely accepted methods for bilateral SEMS placement: the stent-in-stent and the side-by-side. In the stent-in-stent method (also known as Y-stent), one stent is deployed (generally into the left hepatic duct first due to the greater angulation), and a second stent is then deployed through the mesh of the first stent into the other duct (Figs. 5.6 and 5.7). The advantage of this method is that it allows physiological drainage as well as having a smaller diameter and not over-dilating the biliary tree. The main disadvantage is the technical difficulty in performing the insertion, and the difficulty in adjusting the stents post-deployment. In side-by-side stenting, the two SEMS are separately placed into the two ducts side-by-side, similar to a double barrel. The advantage of this method is that it is easier to place, with the disadvantage being that it requires fairly dilated ducts; otherwise, the risk of over-dilation is increased (Figs. 5.8 and 5.9).

There is minimal evidence suggesting that one type of stent insertion is superior to the other. Three previous retrospective studies have compared the two methods. The first study by Naitoh et al. demonstrated that there was no significant difference in technical success, functional success, or complications between the two groups, but that side-by-side stenting had higher stent patency [40]. A similar study, around the same time, likewise showed no major differences between the two groups and no difference in stent patency [41]. The third study, done in the United States, also showed no difference between stent-in-stent or side-by-side deployment [42].

The main factor predicting failure of stent-in-stent placement was the angle between the stricture and the first SEMS placed [43]. Interestingly, the size of the cell in the stent did not change the rates of success in stent-in-stent placement [44]. Another study looked at using 10 mm diameter SEMS compared to 8 mm dimeter SEMS in patients with stent-in-stent placement and found no significant differences other than a higher success rate for revisionary stent in the 10 mm diameter stent group [45].

Additionally, there is also the question of whether malignant hilar strictures treated with

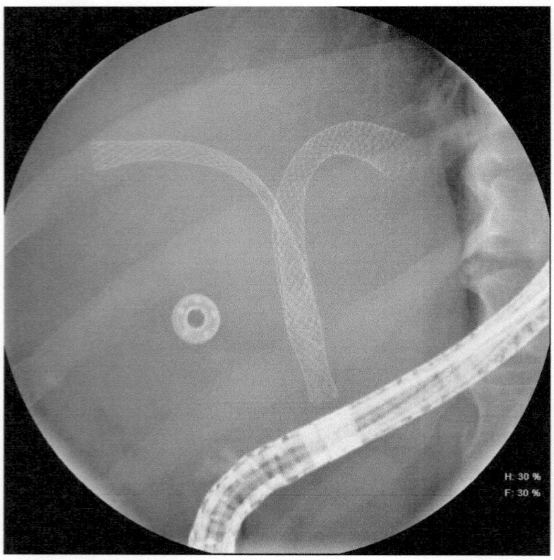

Fig. 5.6 Stent-in-stent SEMS insertion

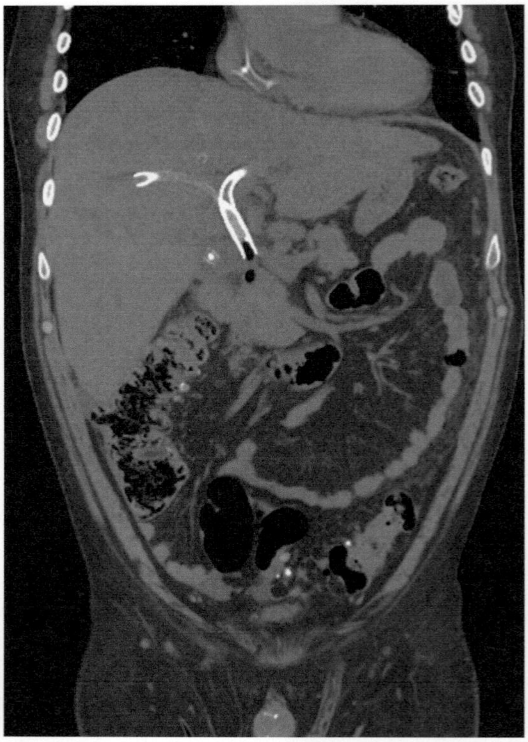

Fig. 5.7 CT image of stent-in-stent SEMS insertion

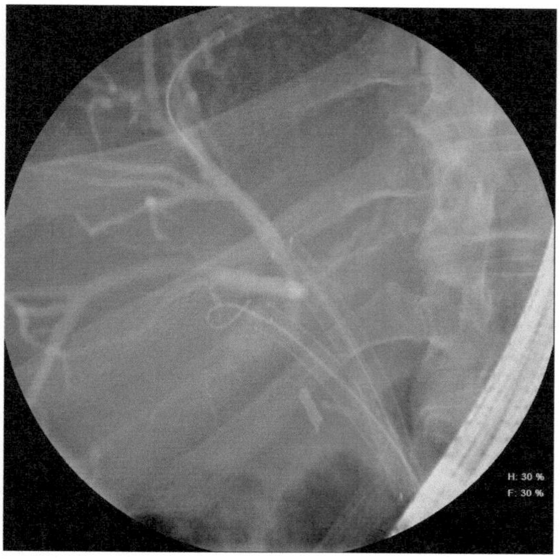

Fig. 5.8 Side-by-side SEMS insertion

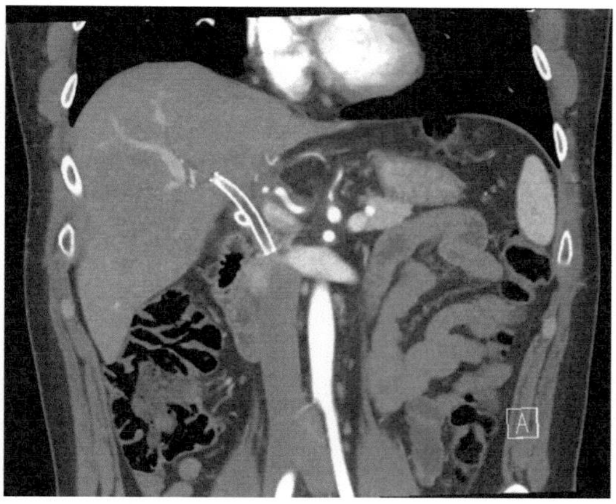

Fig. 5.9 CT image of side-by-side SEMS insertion

SEMS require the distal end of the metal stent to be above the ampulla or below. The advantage of being above the ampulla is that potentially a sphincterotomy is not required, and an intact sphincter of Oddi might reduce the rate of cholangitis. A study comparing above and across sphincter of Oddi SEMS deployment showed that placing the SEMS above led to fewer complications, including episodes of post-ERCP pancreatitis. There was no difference in stent patency or insertion rates [46].

In summary, the decision to pursue side-by-side vs. stent-in-stent insertion should be left to the clinician, and factors to be considered before deciding on any method should include anatomy, location of stricture, clinician preference, and tools available.

Advancements

Similar to the preceding decades, the rate of endoscopic technological advancement is exponentially increasing. Although improvements in endoscopic techniques, side-viewer endoscopes, and deployment devices have made insertion of SEMS easier, the constant improvement is expected to continue. One such potential is the use of a two-channel endoscope to place side-by-side SEMS. A recent study showed high technical and functional success rates with minimal complications [47].

Although the use of endoscopic ultrasound-guided biliary drainage (EUS-BD) is well established in distal extrahepatic strictures, its use in hilar strictures is controversial due to challenging anatomy and the fact that percutaneous drainage has strong evidence for its use (including as first-line drainage). Nonetheless, there have been reports about using EUS-BD to assist in hilar drainage using SEMS [48]. Another potential source of progress is the advent of smaller deployment devices, specifically 6 Fr SEMS delivery devices. These new smaller devices not only aid in placement of stent-in-stent insertion but also can allow simultaneous side-by-side deployment (rather than sequential) [49].

Conclusion

In conclusion, due to an increase in the incidence of cholangiocarcinoma and routine hepatobiliary surgeries, endoscopists will frequently encounter patients presenting with hilar obstructions. For those patients not presenting with cholangitis, the first decision should be to determine whether they are surgical resection candidates or liver transplant candidates, especially in patients with malignant hilar strictures. Depending on the timing of surgery, the decision to pursue preoperative biliary drainage should be individualized.

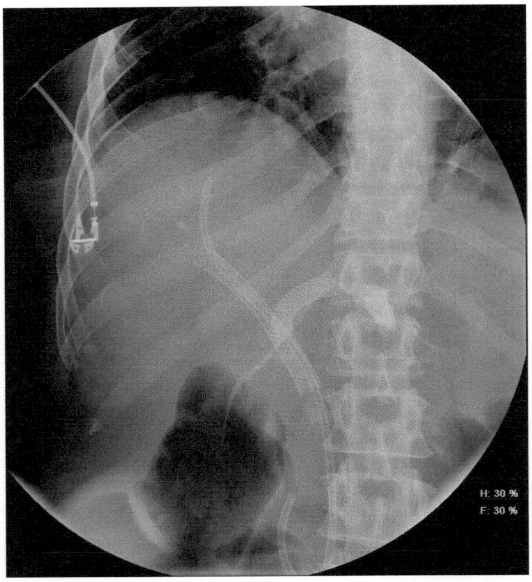

Fig. 5.10 Side-by-side SEMS bilaterally with double-pigtail plastic stent in right hepatic duct

For unresectable hilar obstructions, biliary decompression can be done endoscopically or percutaneously, though controversy exists in terms of which to perform first line. Although metal stents (or SEMS) are preferred over plastic stents, a trial of decompression with plastic stent can be considered prior to SEMS insertion. A goal of at least 50% of liver volume drainage should be sought with either unilateral or bilateral stent insertion, and contrast should be avoided in undrained bile ducts. Finally, the method of SEMS placement (stent-in-stent or side-by-side) is left to the clinician to decide based on a variety of factors and could potentially include a combination of SEMS and plastic stents (Fig. 5.10). With recent advancements and ongoing improvements in the tools available to endoscopists, the methods of drainage of hilar strictures will continue to evolve moving forward into the future.

References

1. Larghi A, Tringali A, Lecca PG, Giordano M, Costamagna G. Management of hilar biliary strictures. Am J Gastroenterol. 2008;103(2):458–73.
2. Vauthey JN, Blumgart LH. Recent advances in the management of cholangiocarcinomas. Semin Liver Dis. 1994;14(2):109–14.
3. Shaib Y, El-Serag HB. The epidemiology of cholangiocarcinoma. Semin Liver Dis. 2004;24(2):115–25.
4. Farley DR, Weaver AL, Nagorney DM. "Natural history" of unresected cholangiocarcinoma: patient outcome after noncurative intervention. Mayo Clin Proc. 1995;70(5):425–9.
5. Sharma P, Yadav S. Demographics, tumor characteristics, treatment, and survival of patients with Klatskin tumors. Ann Gastroenterol. 2018;31(2):231–6.
6. Bismuth H, Nakache R, Diamond T. Management strategies in resection for hilar cholangiocarcinoma. Ann Surg. 1992;215(1):31–8.
7. Nakeeb A, Pitt HA, Sohn TA, Coleman J, Abrams RA, Piantadosi S, et al. Cholangiocarcinoma. A spectrum of intrahepatic, perihilar, and distal tumors. Ann Surg. 1996;224(4):463–73; discussion 73–5.
8. Khashab MA, Fockens P, Al-Haddad MA. Utility of EUS in patients with indeterminate biliary strictures and suspected extrahepatic cholangiocarcinoma (with videos). Gastrointest Endosc. 2012;76(5):1024–33.
9. Klempnauer J, Ridder GJ, Werner M, Weimann A, Pichlmayr R. What constitutes long-term survival after surgery for hilar cholangiocarcinoma? Cancer. 1997;79(1):26–34.
10. Hatfield AR, Tobias R, Terblanche J, Girdwood AH, Fataar S, Harries-Jones R, et al. Preoperative external biliary drainage in obstructive jaundice. A prospective controlled clinical trial. Lancet. 1982;2(8304):896–9.
11. McPherson GA, Benjamin IS, Hodgson HJ, Bowley NB, Allison DJ, Blumgart LH. Pre-operative percutaneous transhepatic biliary drainage: the results of a controlled trial. Br J Surg. 1984;71(5):371–5.
12. Pitt HA, Gomes AS, Lois JF, Mann LL, Deutsch LS, Longmire WP Jr. Does preoperative percutaneous biliary drainage reduce operative risk or increase hospital cost? Ann Surg. 1985;201(5):545–53.
13. Liu F, Li Y, Wei Y, Li B. Preoperative biliary drainage before resection for hilar cholangiocarcinoma: whether or not? A systematic review. Dig Dis Sci. 2011;56(3):663–72.
14. Laurent A, Tayar C, Cherqui D. Cholangiocarcinoma: preoperative biliary drainage (Con). HPB. 2008;10(2):126–9.
15. Kennedy TJ, Yopp A, Qin Y, Zhao B, Guo P, Liu F, et al. Role of preoperative biliary drainage of liver remnant prior to extended liver resection for hilar cholangiocarcinoma. HPB. 2009;11(5):445–51.
16. Cassani LS, Chouhan J, Chan C, Lanke G, Chen HC, Wang X, et al. Biliary decompression in perihilar cholangiocarcinoma improves survival: a single-center retrospective analysis. Dig Dis Sci. 2019;64(2):561–9. https://doi.org/10.1007/s10620-018-5277-z.
17. Arvanitakis M, Van Laethem JL, Pouzere S, Le Moine O, Deviere J. Predictive factors for survival in patients with inoperable Klatskin tumors. Hepato-Gastroenterology. 2006;53(67):21–7.

18. Smith AC, Dowsett JF, Russell RC, Hatfield AR, Cotton PB. Randomised trial of endoscopic stenting versus surgical bypass in malignant low bileduct obstruction. Lancet. 1994;344(8938):1655–60.
19. Pinol V, Castells A, Bordas JM, Real MI, Llach J, Montana X, et al. Percutaneous self-expanding metal stents versus endoscopic polyethylene endoprostheses for treating malignant biliary obstruction: randomized clinical trial. Radiology. 2002;225(1):27–34.
20. Speer AG, Cotton PB, Russell RC, Mason RR, Hatfield AR, Leung JW, et al. Randomised trial of endoscopic versus percutaneous stent insertion in malignant obstructive jaundice. Lancet. 1987;2(8550):57–62.
21. Al Mahjoub A, Menahem B, Fohlen A, Dupont B, Alves A, Launoy G, et al. Preoperative biliary drainage in patients with resectable perihilar cholangiocarcinoma: is percutaneous transhepatic biliary drainage safer and more effective than endoscopic biliary drainage? A meta-analysis. J Vasc Interv Radiol. 2017;28(4):576–82.
22. Kloek JJ, van der Gaag NA, Aziz Y, Rauws EA, van Delden OM, Lameris JS, et al. Endoscopic and percutaneous preoperative biliary drainage in patients with suspected hilar cholangiocarcinoma. J Gastrointest Surg. 2010;14(1):119–25.
23. Kim KM, Park JW, Lee JK, Lee KH, Lee KT, Shim SG. A comparison of preoperative biliary drainage methods for perihilar cholangiocarcinoma: endoscopic versus percutaneous transhepatic biliary drainage. Gut Liver. 2015;9(6):791–9.
24. Paik WH, Park YS, Hwang JH, Lee SH, Yoon CJ, Kang SG, et al. Palliative treatment with self-expandable metallic stents in patients with advanced type III or IV hilar cholangiocarcinoma: a percutaneous versus endoscopic approach. Gastrointest Endosc. 2009;69(1):55–62.
25. Al-Kawas F, Aslanian H, Baillie J, Banovac F, Buscaglia JM, Buxbaum J, et al. Percutaneous transhepatic vs. endoscopic retrograde biliary drainage for suspected malignant hilar obstruction: study protocol for a randomized controlled trial. Trials. 2018;19(1):108.
26. Jo JH, Chung MJ, Han DH, Park JY, Bang S, Park SW, et al. Best options for preoperative biliary drainage in patients with Klatskin tumors. Surg Endosc. 2017;31(1):422–9.
27. Pfau PR, Pleskow DK, Banerjee S, Barth BA, Bhat YM, Desilets DJ, et al. Pancreatic and biliary stents. Gastrointest Endosc. 2013;77(3):319–27.
28. Mukai T, Yasuda I, Nakashima M, Doi S, Iwashita T, Iwata K, et al. Metallic stents are more efficacious than plastic stents in unresectable malignant hilar biliary strictures: a randomized controlled trial. J Hepatobiliary Pancreat Sci. 2013;20(2):214–22.
29. Sangchan A, Kongkasame W, Pugkhem A, Jenwitheesuk K, Mairiang P. Efficacy of metal and plastic stents in unresectable complex hilar cholangiocarcinoma: a randomized controlled trial. Gastrointest Endosc. 2012;76(1):93–9.
30. Perdue DG, Freeman ML, DiSario JA, Nelson DB, Fennerty MB, Lee JG, et al. Plastic versus self-expanding metallic stents for malignant hilar biliary obstruction: a prospective multicenter observational cohort study. J Clin Gastroenterol. 2008;42(9):1040–6.
31. Rerknimitr R, Angsuwatcharakon P, Ratanachu-ek T, Khor CJ, Ponnudurai R, Moon JH, et al. Asia-Pacific consensus recommendations for endoscopic and interventional management of hilar cholangiocarcinoma. J Gastroenterol Hepatol. 2013;28(4):593–607.
32. Vienne A, Hobeika E, Gouya H, Lapidus N, Fritsch J, Choury AD, et al. Prediction of drainage effectiveness during endoscopic stenting of malignant hilar strictures: the role of liver volume assessment. Gastrointest Endosc. 2010;72(4):728–35.
33. Kozarek RA. Malignant hilar strictures: one stent or two? Plastic versus self-expanding metal stents? The role of liver atrophy and volume assessment as a predictor of survival in patients undergoing endoscopic stent placement. Gastrointest Endosc. 2010;72(4):736–8.
34. Takahashi E, Fukasawa M, Sato T, Takano S, Kadokura M, Shindo H, et al. Biliary drainage strategy of unresectable malignant hilar strictures by computed tomography volumetry. World J Gastroenterol. 2015;21(16):4946–53.
35. Chang WH, Kortan P, Haber GB. Outcome in patients with bifurcation tumors who undergo unilateral versus bilateral hepatic duct drainage. Gastrointest Endosc. 1998;47(5):354–62.
36. De Palma GD, Galloro G, Siciliano S, Iovino P, Catanzano C. Unilateral versus bilateral endoscopic hepatic duct drainage in patients with malignant hilar biliary obstruction: results of a prospective, randomized, and controlled study. Gastrointest Endosc. 2001;53(6):547–53.
37. Liberato MJ, Canena JM. Endoscopic stenting for hilar cholangiocarcinoma: efficacy of unilateral and bilateral placement of plastic and metal stents in a retrospective review of 480 patients. BMC Gastroenterol. 2012;12:103.
38. Naitoh I, Ohara H, Nakazawa T, Ando T, Hayashi K, Okumura F, et al. Unilateral versus bilateral endoscopic metal stenting for malignant hilar biliary obstruction. J Gastroenterol Hepatol. 2009;24(4):552–7.
39. Li M, Wu W, Yin Z, Han G. Unilateral versus bilateral biliary drainage for malignant hilar obstruction: a systematic review and meta-analysis. Chin J Hepatol. 2015;23(2):118–23.
40. Naitoh I, Hayashi K, Nakazawa T, Okumura F, Miyabe K, Shimizu S, et al. Side-by-side versus stent-in-stent deployment in bilateral endoscopic metal stenting for malignant hilar biliary obstruction. Dig Dis Sci. 2012;57(12):3279–85.
41. Kim KM, Lee KH, Chung YH, Shin JU, Lee JK, Lee KT, et al. A comparison of bilateral stenting methods for malignant hilar biliary obstruction. Hepato-Gastroenterology. 2012;59(114):341–6.
42. Law R, Baron TH. Bilateral metal stents for hilar biliary obstruction using a 6Fr delivery system: outcomes

following bilateral and side-by-side stent deployment. Dig Dis Sci. 2013;58(9):2667–72.
43. Sugimoto M, Takagi T, Suzuki R, Konno N, Asama H, Watanabe K, et al. Predictive factors for the failure of endoscopic stent-in-stent self-expandable metallic stent placement to treat malignant hilar biliary obstruction. World J Gastroenterol. 2017;23(34):6273–80.
44. Lee JM, Lee SH, Chung KH, Park JM, Paik WH, Woo SM, et al. Small cell- versus large cell-sized metal stent in endoscopic bilateral stent-in-stent placement for malignant hilar biliary obstruction. Digest Endosc. 2015;27(6):692–9.
45. Naitoh I, Nakazawa T, Ban T, Okumura F, Hirano A, Takada H, et al. 8-mm versus 10-mm diameter self-expandable metallic stent in bilateral endoscopic stent-in-stent deployment for malignant hilar biliary obstruction. J Hepatobiliary Pancreat Sci. 2015;22(5):396–401.
46. Cosgrove N, Siddiqui AA, Adler DG, Shahid H, Sarkar A, Sharma A, et al. A comparison of bilateral side-by-side metal stents deployed above and across the sphincter of oddi in the management of malignant hilar biliary obstruction. J Clin Gastroenterol. 2017;51(6):528–33.
47. Okuwaki K, Yamauchi H, Kida M, Imaizumi H, Iwai T, Matsumoto T, et al. Efficacy and long-term outcomes of side-by-side self-expandable metal stent placement using a 2-channel endoscope for unresectable malignant hilar biliary obstruction occurring after Billroth II reconstruction (with video). Dig Dis Sci. 2018;63(6):1641–6.
48. Yamauchi H, Kida M, Miyazawa S, Okuwaki K, Iwai T, Imaizumi H, et al. Endoscopic ultrasound-guided antegrade metal stent placement using the stent-in-stent technique in a patient with malignant hilar biliary obstruction. Endosc Ultrasound. 2018;7(3):204–6.
49. Inoue T, Ishii N, Kobayashi Y, Kitano R, Sakamoto K, Ohashi T, et al. Simultaneous versus sequential side-by-side bilateral metal stent placement for malignant hilar biliary obstructions. Dig Dis Sci. 2017;62(9):2542–9.

SEMS Insertion for Hilar Stricture: Which Stent, How and Why?

6

Hiroyuki Isayama, Toshio Fujisawa, Shigeto Ishii, Hiroaki Saito, Akinori Suzuki, Yusuke Takasaki, Sho Takahashi, Hirofumi Kogure, and Yousuke Nakai

Background

Endoscopic stenting of hilar strictures remains challenging; many techniques are available but none is yet standard [1]. Such stenting is technically difficult; many strategies are very complicated (Table 6.1). Technically, it is important to consider both insertion and re-intervention, and patient status. In the palliative setting (patients with unresectable hilar malignancies), self-expandable metallic stents (SEMSs) have been reported to be superior as endoprostheses versus plastic stents (PSs) [2]. However, in cases with resectable hilar malignancies, PSs are preferred. In the palliative setting, it is important to consider both the technique and the long-term outcomes of SEMS placement. Prior to stent choice, it is essential to establish a drainage strategy.

H. Isayama (✉) · T. Fujisawa · S. Ishii · H. Saito
A. Suzuki · Y. Takasaki · S. Takahashi · H. Kogure
Y. Nakai
Department of Gastroenterology, Graduate School of Medicine, Juntendo University, Tokyo, Japan

Department of Gastroenterology, Graduate School of Medicine, The University of Tokyo, Tokyo, Japan
e-mail: h-isayama@juntendo.ac.jp

Drainage Volume and Stent Number

The optimal number of stents has been widely discussed; over 50% of the liver volume should be drained [3]. Takahashi and Fukasawa et al. reported that 33% drainage adequately improved jaundice if the liver was normal [4]; drainage of over 50% was required if liver function was impaired. Recently, Lee et al. conducted a randomized controlled trial comparing unilateral and bilateral stent placement [5]. Bilateral stenting was associated with longer stent patency than unilateral stenting; stents of larger diameter prolonged the time to occlusion caused by both tumor ingrowth and sludge accumulation. The recent literature suggests that at least two stents are required to ensure an adequate liver volume. However, there is no good evidence that the drained volume should be increased to over 50%. Some consider that complete drainage is better than incomplete drainage because it reduces the rate of cholangitis, which is more common in undrained areas. Uchida and Kato et al. reported that patients in whom more than three stents were placed to treat hilar strictures survived for longer than others [6]. However, discussion continues, and definitive evidence is lacking.

D. K. Lee (ed.), *Advanced ERCP for Complicated and Refractory Biliary and Pancreatic Diseases*,
https://doi.org/10.1007/978-981-13-0608-2_6

Table 6.1 Patient's condition of malignant hilar stricture

Patients' status
Bridge to surgery
Palliation
Tumorous status
Cancer type
Extra hepatic tumor
Extrahepatic cholangiocarcinoma (EHC)
Gallbladder cancer
Metastatic lymph node
Liver tumor
Intrahepatic cholangiocarcinoma (IHC)
Hepatocellular carcinoma
Metastatic liver tumor
Clinical stage
Resectable
Locally advanced
Metastatic
Stricture status
Bismuth type: 1–4
Portal perfusion
Normal
Impaired hemi lobe
Impaired both lobes
Basic liver function
Normal
Chronic liver disease
Liver cirrhosis
Atrophic liver lobe

Table 6.2 Relationship between stent type and stenting manner

	Side by side		Stent in stent	
	Above	Across	Above	Across
Stent type				
Braided	△	○	×	×
Knitted	△	△	×	×
Laser-cut	○	×	○	×
Special SEMS	×	×	○	△
Covered SEMS	○	○	×	×

Method of Stenting

Stent selection depends on the chosen technique: stent-in-stent (SIS) or side-by-side (SBS) [1]. A few reports have compared the two techniques, with differing results. Here, we outline the advantages and disadvantages of the two techniques, and suggest the available stent type (Table 6.2).

The Stent-in-Stent Technique

With this technique, two or more uncovered SEMSs are inserted through the mesh of an initially placed SEMS. An advantage is that the common bile duct (CBD) hosts only one SEMS and is thus not excessively dilated. The through-the-mesh (TTM) technique can be used to approach many bile duct branches. However, this technique is relatively difficult when used either for initial stent placement or re-intervention when stents become occluded. Many dedicated SEMSs are available; most have flexible mid-points to facilitate the TTM approach. For these SEMSs, only the central portion can be employed in the TTM approach; the SEMS length must be carefully chosen and the stent placed accurately. However, the Niti-S, a large-cell D-type stent (LCD; TaeWoong Medical Inc., Seoul, South Korea), is of uniform cell size throughout, and all SEMS regions can undergo TTM insertion [7, 8]. Figure 6.1 shows some of the available SEMSs. Laser-cut SEMSs with low axial forces and wide cells can also be used when employing the SIS technique (Fig. 6.2) [9–11]. SIS is the standard approach in Japan and Korea; however, endoscopists in other countries do not favor the procedure because it is technically difficult.

Stent-in-Stent Techniques

Magnetic resonance cholangiopancreatography (MRCP) and enhanced computed tomography are required prior to endoscopy. Drainage of over 50% of the liver volume is essential to retain liver function and avoid cholangitis of a small drained volume. Planning of drainage by reference to the cholangiogram and the use of guidewire (GW) manipulation to select the target biliary branch in the absence of contrast injection may minimize the incidence of cholangitis in the undrained area [12, 13]. After biliary cannulation, the GW is manipulated to select all target biliary branches: (1) SEMS are inserted into the first branch (that

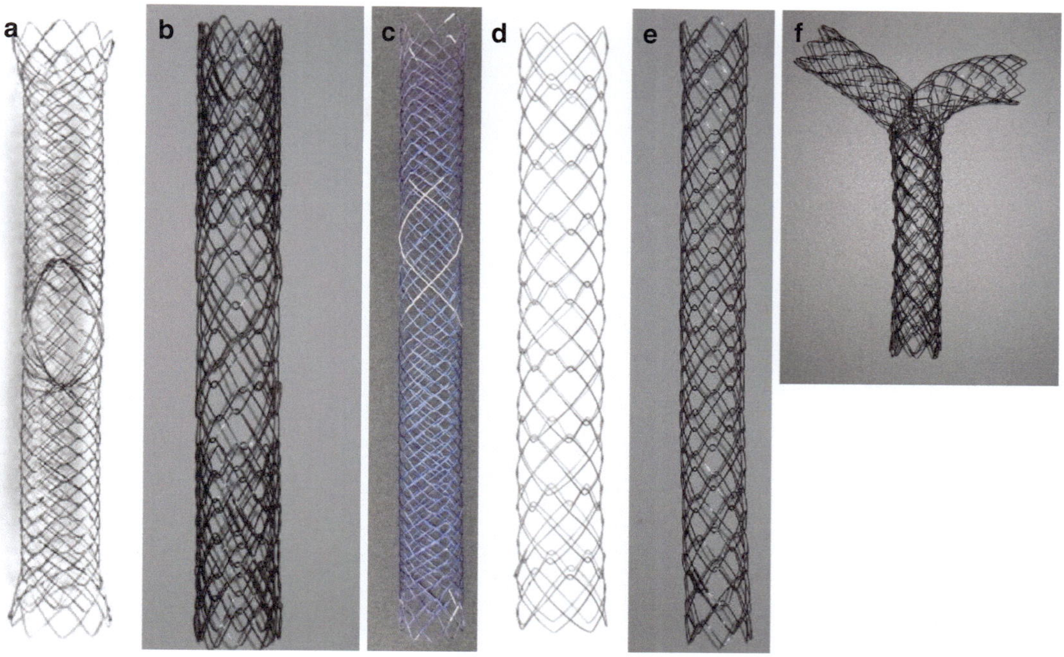

Fig. 6.1 Dedicated metal stents for repair of hilar biliary strictures. (**a**) The BONA stent, K-Hilar (Standard Sci Tech Inc., Seoul, South Korea). (**b**) The Niti-S stent, Y-Stent (TaeWoong Medical Inc., Seoul, South Korea). (**c**) The BONA stent, M-Hilar (Standard Sci Tech Inc.). (**d**) The Hilzo stent; moving cell type (BCM Medical Inc., Seoul, South Korea). (**e**) The Niti-S stent, large-cell D-type (LCD; TaeWoong Medical Inc.). (**f**) A partial stent-in-stent (SIS) pattern using LCD stents

nearest to the papilla), (2) another SEMS is inserted into the branch that is more angled at the branchpoint (usually the left hepatic bile duct), and (3) SEMSs are inserted into any branch into which it is difficult to insert a GW (Fig. 6.3). In terms of SEMS insertion and deployment in the initial branch, it is useful to try to insert a second GW into the next branch using the TTM technique. At this juncture, the previously placed GW serves as a good landmark of the branch point. Subsequently, a delivery system is inserted using the TTM approach. Figure 6.4 shows the use of the SIS technique to place LCD stents.

Troubleshooting the Second Stent Insertion

Sometimes, difficulties present during insertion of the second stent. The following tips can counter these problems: (1) balloon dilation of all branches prior to stenting, (2) balloon dilation of the stent cell; (3) balloon dilation of the initially placed SEMS, and (4) one-time GW withdrawal and reinsertion. Often, insufficient dilation of the first stent may cause cell narrowing; balloon dilation of both the stent cell and cavity dilates the targeted cell. Sometimes, the tip of the stent delivery system is obstructed by the GW; wire reinsertion may change the cell orientation and facilitate delivery system insertion. Use of a second SEMS with a sharp delivery system tip is helpful. Of course, balloon dilation aids all steps of the TTM technique.

Side-by-Side Stenting

SBS stenting is commonly employed because the spreading procedure is easier than that of SIS [14]. Several SEMSs are placed in parallel to drain biliary branches occluded by the malignant tumor. Some stents are placed in the CBD using this technique, at a risk of complications

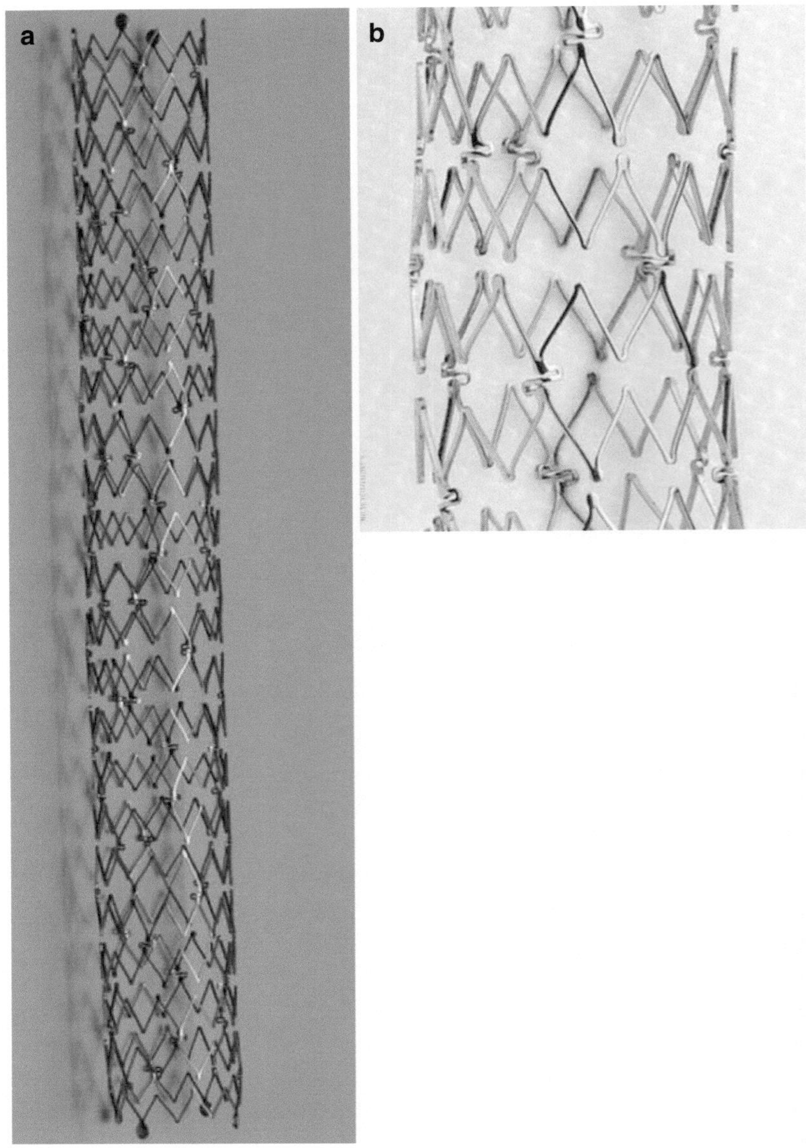

Fig. 6.2 A laser-cut self-expandable metallic stent suitable for use with the SIS technique. (**a**) The ZEO stent (Zeon Medical Inc., Tokyo, Japan). (**b**) There are only three binding points across the width of the cell; these points may reduce the axial force

caused by excessive dilation of the CBD. Thus, many Japanese endoscopists did not use this technique before recent SEMSs became available. Portal vein (PV) compression may injure the vein or cause a thrombosis; radiation therapy for patients who have undergone SBS placement may trigger bleeding caused by a PV-biliary fistula. Orifice compression may cause cholecystitis or pancreatitis. The variations of the technique include the above- and across-the-papilla approaches and use of uncovered or slim fully covered SEMSs.

Preservation of papillary function may reduce the incidence of cholangitis [15]. However, re-intervention when a SEMS becomes occluded is now difficult. The end of the SEMS may impact or become embedded in the bile duct wall. Re-intervention is easy if the SEMS is placed across the papilla, but controversy remains. It was earlier believed that covered SEMSs could not be used for hilar stenting; however, recently, slim (6-mm diameter)-covered SEMSs have been used to treat hilar obstructions [16] and were reportedly effective and safe. Some reports found

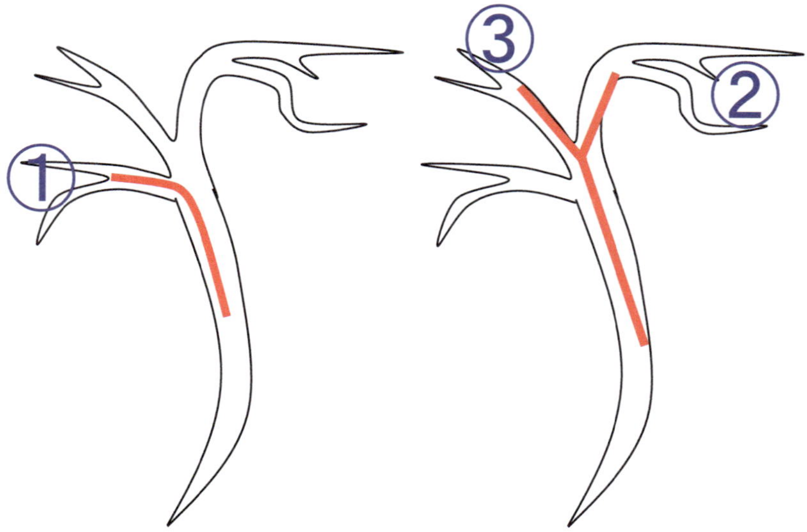

Fig. 6.3 Stent insertion using the SIS technique. (**a**) Insertion of the first stent into the distal branch. (**b**) At the same branch level, insertion of the stent into the acutely angled branch (i.e., the branch for which guidewire (GW) insertion is more difficult)

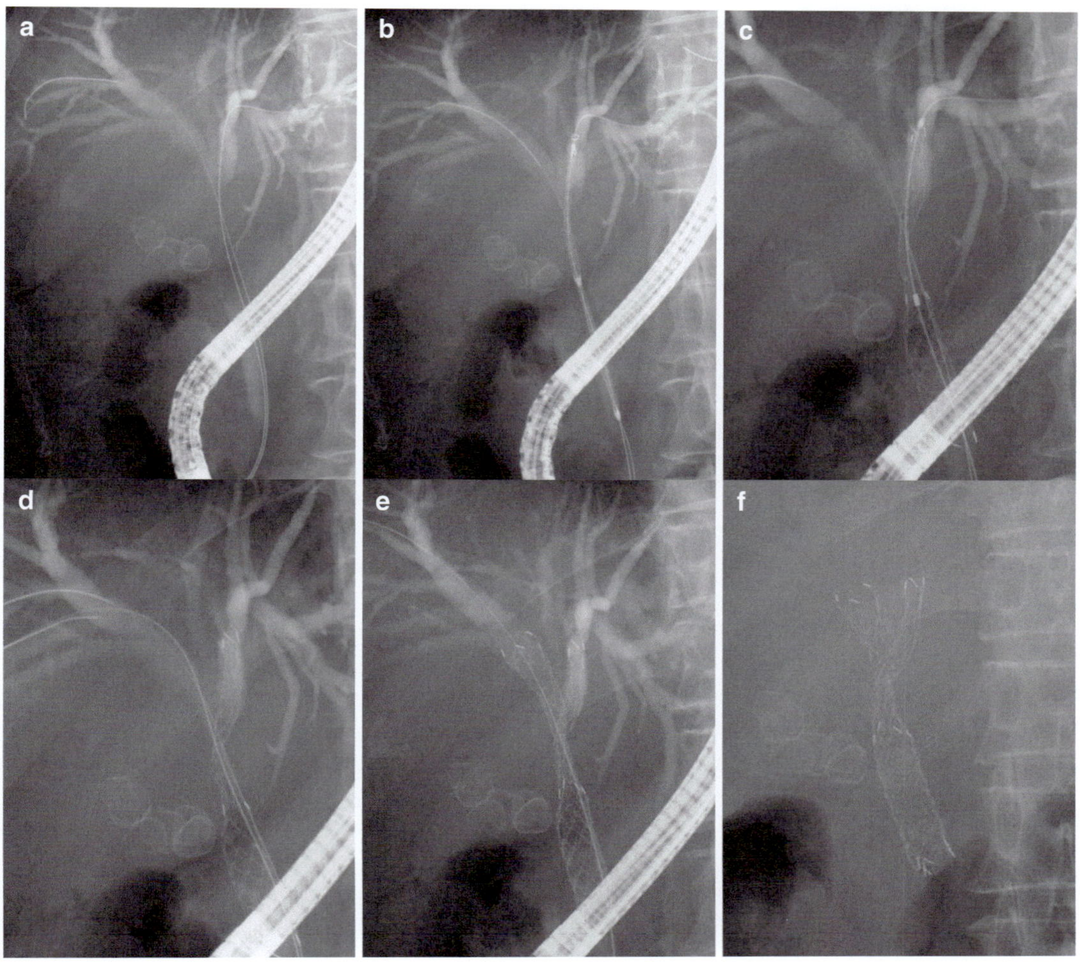

Fig. 6.4 SIS placement using Niti-S, an LCD stent (TaeWoong Medical Inc.). (**a**) After successful biliary cannulation, two GWs are inserted into the target hepatic ducts. (**b**) Insertion of an initial LCD stent into the left hepatic duct, the angle of which is more acute than that of the right hepatic duct, over one of the two GWs. (**c**) Deployment of the initial LCD. (**d**) Insertion of the GW used for initial stent insertion through the mesh of the first LCD. (**e**) Delivery system insertion and deployment of the LCD after withdrawal of the landmark GW. (**f**) After scope withdrawal

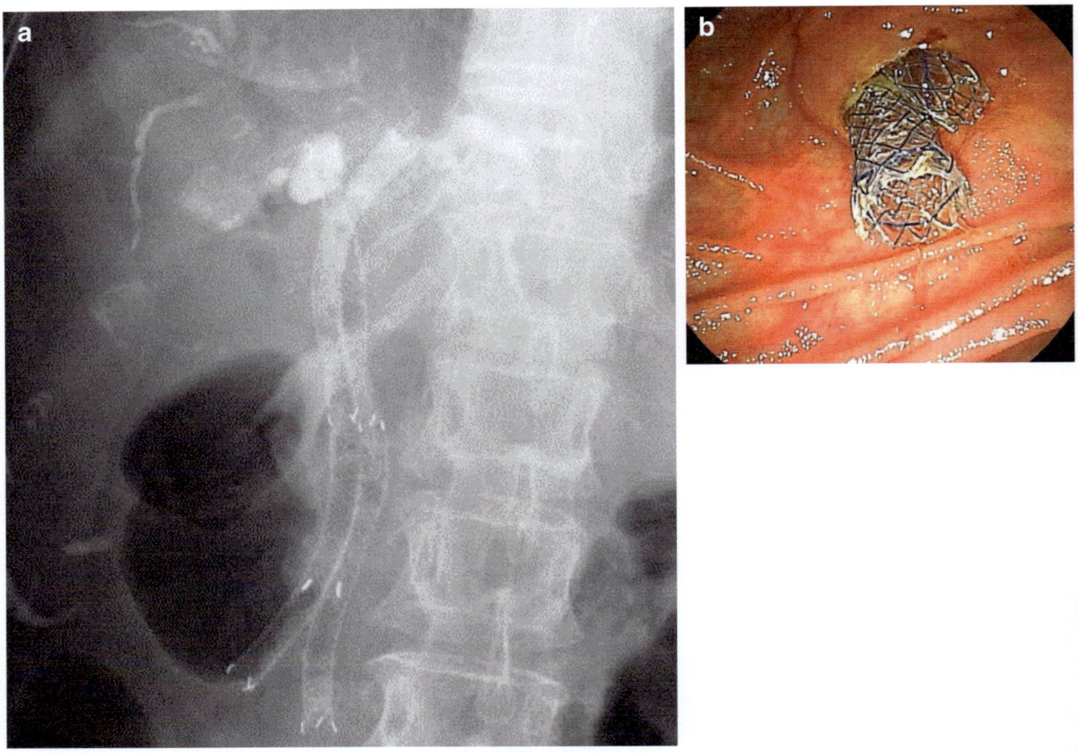

Fig. 6.5 Side-by-side across-the-papilla placement of slim (6-mm diameter), fully covered self-expandable metallic stents (FCSEMSs). (**a**) Two slim FCSEMSs (Hanaro stents; M.I. Tech Inc., Seoul, South Korea) placed in parallel. (**b**) Endoscopic view of FCSEMS placement across the papilla

that the Bismuth type 4 stent was unsuitable when used to place slim-covered SEMSs. A prospective multicenter comparative study is required.

Stent Selection for SBS

Stent selection depends on whether the above- or across-the-papilla approach is chosen and whether slim fully covered SEMSs are preferred. When using the above-the-papilla approach, uncovered SEMSs are appropriate. Especially, laser-cut structures with slim delivery systems can easily be placed in a single treatment (Fig. 6.5). The across-the-papilla approach requires very long braided stents; the final length is longer than expected when the stent is fully expanded. The relatively new slim covered SEMSs are under evaluation by many Japanese endoscopists. A braided fully covered SEMS of diameter 6 mm is available.

Side-by-Side Insertion Techniques

GW placement and other actions prior to stent insertion are the same as those of the SIS technique. SEMSs featuring slim delivery systems can be deployed simultaneously. Two delivery systems can be inserted into the bile duct at the same time, using the scope channel. Other SEMSs require sequential placement; a second delivery system must be inserted after initial SEMS deployment. Sometimes, insertion of a second or later delivery system is difficult; initial balloon dilation of every stricture for which SEMS placement is planned greatly aids insertion of the second delivery system. It is important to ensure that the stent ends are at the same level. If the stents are placed above the papilla, then the stent ends must be lined; otherwise, re-intervention is difficult because the approach to the cavity of the proximal stent is challenging.

Re-intervention is easier when stenting is performed across the papilla.

Tokyo Criteria 2014

No accepted system for evaluating biliary stenting is available. The relevant articles employed different definitions, rendering meta-analysis challenging; the results of published meta-analyses do not agree. Therefore, we created the Tokyo criteria 2014, a unified reporting system for biliary stenting [17]. Events related to stent quality are described and complications defined. We employ the term "recurrent biliary obstruction (RBO)" in preference to occlusion; we define stent dysfunction and other terms. RBO refers to both stent occlusion and migration; the interval between stent insertion and RBO is termed the "time to RBO (TRBO)." We hope that others will employ these criteria to facilitate meta-analysis.

Conclusion

No standard approach to manage hilar biliary obstructions is yet available. Here, we discuss the techniques and stent selection for hilar endoscopic stenting, where the aim is to achieve high clinical success rates and a good clinical course over the lifespan of our patients.

References

1. Moon JH, Rerknimitr R, Kogure H, Nakai Y, Isayama H. Topic controversies in the endoscopic management of malignant hilar strictures using metal stent: side-by-side versus stent-in-stent techniques. J Hepatobiliary Pancreat Sci. 2015;22(9):650–6.
2. Mukai T, Yasuda I, Isayama H, Nakashima M, Doi S, Iwashita T, et al. Comparison of axial force and cell width of self-expandable metallic stents: which type of stent is better suited for hilar biliary strictures? J Hepatobiliary Pancreat Sci. 2011;18:646–52.
3. Vienne A, Hobeika E, Gouya H, Lapidus N, Fritsch J, Choury AD, Chryssostalis A, Gaudric M, Pelletier G, Buffet C, Chaussade S, Prat F. Prediction of drainage effectiveness during endoscopic stenting of malignant hilar strictures: the role of liver volume assessment. Gastrointest Endosc. 2010;72(4):728–35.
4. Takahashi E, Fukasawa M, Sato T, Takano S, Kadokura M, Shindo H, Yokota Y, Enomoto N. Biliary drainage strategy of unresectable malignant hilar strictures by computed tomography volumetry. World J Gastroenterol. 2015;21(16):4946–53.
5. Lee TH, Kim TH, Moon JH, Lee SH, Choi HJ, Hwangbo Y, Hyun JJ, Choi JH, Jeong S, Kim JH, Park DH, Han JH, Park SH. Bilateral versus unilateral placement of metal stents for inoperable high-grade malignant hilar biliary strictures: a multicenter, prospective, randomized study (with video). Gastrointest Endosc. 2017;86(5):817–27.
6. Uchida D, Kato H, Muro S, Noma Y, Yamamoto N, Horiguchi S, Harada R, Tsutsumi K, Kawamoto H, Okada H, Yamamoto K. Efficacy of endoscopic over 3-branched partial stent-in-stent drainage using self-expandable metallic stents in patients with unresectable hilar biliary carcinoma. J Clin Gastroenterol. 2015;49(6):529–36.
7. Kogure H, Isayama H, Kawakubo K, Sasaki T, Yamamoto N, Hirano K, Sasahira N, Tsujino T, Tada M, Koike K. Endoscopic bilateral metallic stenting for malignant hilar obstruction using newly designed stents. J Hepatobiliary Pancreat Sci. 2011;18(5):653–7.
8. Kogure H, Isayama H, Nakai Y, Tsujino T, Matsubara S, Yashima Y, Ito Y, Hamada T, Takahara N, Miyabayashi K, Mizuno S, Mohri D, Kawakubo K, Sasaki T, Yamamoto N, Hirano K, Sasahira N, Tada M, Koike K. High single-session success rate of endoscopic bilateral stent-in-stent placement with modified large cell Niti-S stents for malignant hilar biliary obstruction. Dig Endosc. 2014;26(1):93–9.
9. Kawamoto H, Tsutsumi K, Harada R, Fujii M, Kato H, Hirao K, Kurihara N, Nakanishi T, Mizuno O, Ishida E, Ogawa T, Fukatsu H, Sakaguchi K. Endoscopic deployment of multiple JOSTENT SelfX is effective and safe in treatment of malignant hilar biliary strictures. Clin Gastroenterol Hepatol. 2008;6(4):401–8.
10. Kawamoto H, Tsutsumi K, Fujii M, Harada R, Kato H, Hirao K, Kurihara N, Nakanishi T, Mizuno O, Ishida E, Ogawa T, Fukatsu H, Sakaguchi K. Endoscopic 3-branched partial stent-in-stent deployment of metallic stents in high-grade malignant hilar biliary stricture (with videos). Gastrointest Endosc. 2007;66(5):1030–7.
11. Mukai T, Yasuda I, Isayama H, Nakashima M, Doi S, Iwashita T, Iwata K, Kato T, Tomita E, Moriwaki H. Comparison of axial force and cell width of self-expandable metallic stents: which type of stent is better suited for hilar biliary strictures? J Hepatobiliary Pancreat Sci. 2011;18(5):646–52.
12. Freeman ML, Overby C. Selective MRCP and CT-targeted drainage of malignant hilar biliary obstruction with self-expanding metallic stents. Gastrointest Endosc. 2003;58(1):41–9.
13. Chang WH, Kortan P, Haber GB. Outcome in patients with bifurcation tumors who undergo unilateral versus

bilateral hepatic duct drainage. Gastrointest Endosc. 1998;47(5):354–62.
14. Lee TH, Park DH, Lee SS, Choi HJ, Lee JK, Kim TH, Kim JH, Jeong S, Park SH, Moon JH. Technical feasibility and revision efficacy of the sequential deployment of endoscopic bilateral side-by-side metal stents for malignant hilar biliary strictures: a multicenter prospective study. Dig Dis Sci. 2013;58(2):547–55.
15. Okamoto T, Fujioka S, Yanagisawa S, Yanaga K, Kakutani H, Tajiri H, Urashima M. Placement of a metallic stent across the main duodenal papilla may predispose to cholangitis. Gastrointest Endosc. 2006;63(6):792–6.
16. Kitamura K, Yamamiya A, Ishii Y, Mitsui Y, Nomoto T, Yoshida H. Side-by-side partially covered self-expandable metal stent placement for malignant hilar biliary obstruction. Endosc Int Open. 2017;5(12):E1211–7.
17. Isayama H, Hamada T, Yasuda I, Itoi T, Ryozawa S, Nakai Y, Kogure H, Koike K. TOKYO criteria 2014 for transpapillary biliary stenting. Dig Endosc. 2015;27(2):259–64.

SEMS Insertion for Malignant Hilar Stricture: ERCP Versus the Percutaneous Approach

7

Yonsoo Kim, Sung Ill Jang, and Dong Ki Lee

Introduction

Hilar cholangiocarcinoma (HC) has a poor prognosis, with a 5-year survival rate <10%, and is a common cause of malignant biliary obstruction in Asian populations [1, 2]. Treatment of hilar obstruction of the liver caused by malignancy is difficult. Regardless of the tumor histology, curative resection is possible in <30% of patients with a malignant hilar stricture [3]. Because curative treatment is difficult and life expectancy is short, symptom relief is often the best option for these patients [4]. In addition, treating jaundice and cholangitis in patients with unresectable biliary carcinoma is important for chemotherapy [5]. Surgical bypass or nonsurgical methods can be used to perform biliary decompression. However, because of the high risk of surgical treatment, therapeutic endoscopy and interventional radiology are increasingly replacing surgical treatment. These noninvasive therapies are becoming the standard of care for obstructive jaundice [6, 7].

It is difficult to achieve effective drainage for a biliary obstruction of the hepatic hilum because of the anatomical complexity of the bile duct; thus, no consensus has been reached on the optimal drainage strategy. Various procedures have been performed for biliary drainage of a hilar biliary obstruction, including percutaneous and endoscopic approaches, use of plastic and metallic stents, and unilateral and bilateral hepatic duct drainage. Self-expandable metallic stents (SEMSs) are now used more frequently for endoscopic [1, 8–10] and percutaneous [11] insertion compared to plastic stents (PSs) [12–15].

Y. Kim · S. I. Jang · D. K. Lee (✉)
Department of Internal Medicine, Gangnam Severance Hospital, Yonsei University College of Medicine, Seoul, South Korea
e-mail: dklee@yuhs.ac

Biliary Stenting Strategy

Since SOHENDRA and Reyners-Frederix introduced transpapillary biliary drainage in 1980 [16], endoscopic biliary drainage through stenting has become increasingly popular [17]. Many changes have been made to the original PSs, including the introduction of large-bore PSs, non-expandable metallic stents, and SEMS, over the course of about 40 years. More than 20 years ago, only uncovered SEMSs were available, but in recent years additional types of SEMSs have been developed. Examples include SEMS almost completely covered by materials, internal stents, and anti-migration stents such as flare, professionally surfaced, anchoring-type, and anti-reflux valve stents [17]. Bioabsorbable and biodegradable stents have also been developed recently [18].

It is the most effective maximize drainage of the intact, but not the atrophied, liver. Right, left, and caudate lobes account for 55–60%, 30%,

D. K. Lee (ed.), *Advanced ERCP for Complicated and Refractory Biliary and Pancreatic Diseases*,
https://doi.org/10.1007/978-981-13-0608-2_7

and 10% of overall liver volume, respectively [19]. The liver volume that can be drained by deploying a stent can vary depending on the extent of the malignant biliary stricture [20]. In the case of a Bismuth type I stricture, both lobes can be drained with only a single stent. However, in the case of Bismuth types II–IV, multiple stents are required to drain both lobes. Although unilateral stenting may be a simpler and safer method than bilateral stenting, there is a limit to the drainage possible for an advanced stricture [20]. In a previous study, drainage of ≥25% of the liver volume was deemed sufficient [21]. However, recent studies suggest that survival can be prolonged with drainage of >50% of the liver volume. This scenario implies that the two hepatic sectors should be intubated separately in most cases, particularly in Bismuth type III patients [22].

The liver volume drainage required depends on liver function status. According to one study, >33% of the liver volume should be drained if the liver function is good, and >50% of the volume should be drained when the liver function is reduced (decompensated liver cirrhosis) [23].

Cholangitis is an important complication that may occur after stenting for a hilar biliary stricture. Injecting contrast into undrained sectors is a risk factor for cholangitis. In addition, atrophied areas, and inserting a stent into a small area, increase the frequency of cholangitis because bile excretory function decreases [15, 22, 24–26]. Cholangitis after endoscopic retrograde cholangiopancreatography (ERCP) is a known risk factor for early mortality [27]. Therefore, unilateral and bilateral stenting should be applied with consideration of the drainage volume and liver function status. Excessive multi-stenting, particularly of an atrophied area, should be avoided to reduce the risk of cholangitis.

In addition, several factors should be considered when choosing between a PS and SEMS, including the patient's prognosis, cause of stricture, location and length of the obstruction, diameter of the bile duct, site of the cystic duct, and whether the patient is receiving multidisciplinary therapy, including chemotherapy.

Endoscopic Biliary Drainage

Preprocedural Evaluation

Because of the diverse nature of the hilar bile duct, endoscopic management of hilar bile duct lesions is more difficult than for lesions of the distal bile duct. Freeman and Overby reported that computed tomography (CT) and magnetic resonance cholangiopancreatography (MRCP) are useful to confirm hilar obstruction lesions and locate a SEMS [28]. Vienna et al. reported that cross-sectional CT images help to identify the hepatic volume distribution, where this information could be used to optimize the endoscopic procedure. This scenario is because drainage of the bile ducts corresponding to >50% of the liver volume is important for effective drainage of malignant hilar biliary strictures, particularly Bismuth type III [22].

Plastic Stents Versus SEMS

The use of metal stents rather than PSs for treating hilar malignancy has resulted in longer stent patencies, fewer complications, fewer re-interventions, and improved cost-effectiveness in prospective multicenter studies [13, 15, 29]. Although a SEMS is more expensive than a PS, the former has better cost-effectiveness if the patient's expected survival is 4–6 months, because SEMS use is associated with fewer occlusions and re-interventions, shorter hospital stays, and less antibiotic use [20]. The Asia-Pacific Consensus also recommended biliary palliation via SEMS in cases of predicted survival >3 months and Bismuth type II–IV HC [30]. PSs are recommended for temporary drainage in patients with cholangitis for whom no treatment plan has yet been established [20] (Fig. 7.1).

However, the life span of a SEMS is often shorter than the life expectancy of a patient with an unresectable cholangiocarcinoma, and reintervention is often difficult if the SEMS becomes blocked [31]. The prognosis of patients with cholangiocarcinoma and gallbladder carcinoma has improved due to the development of chemotherapy

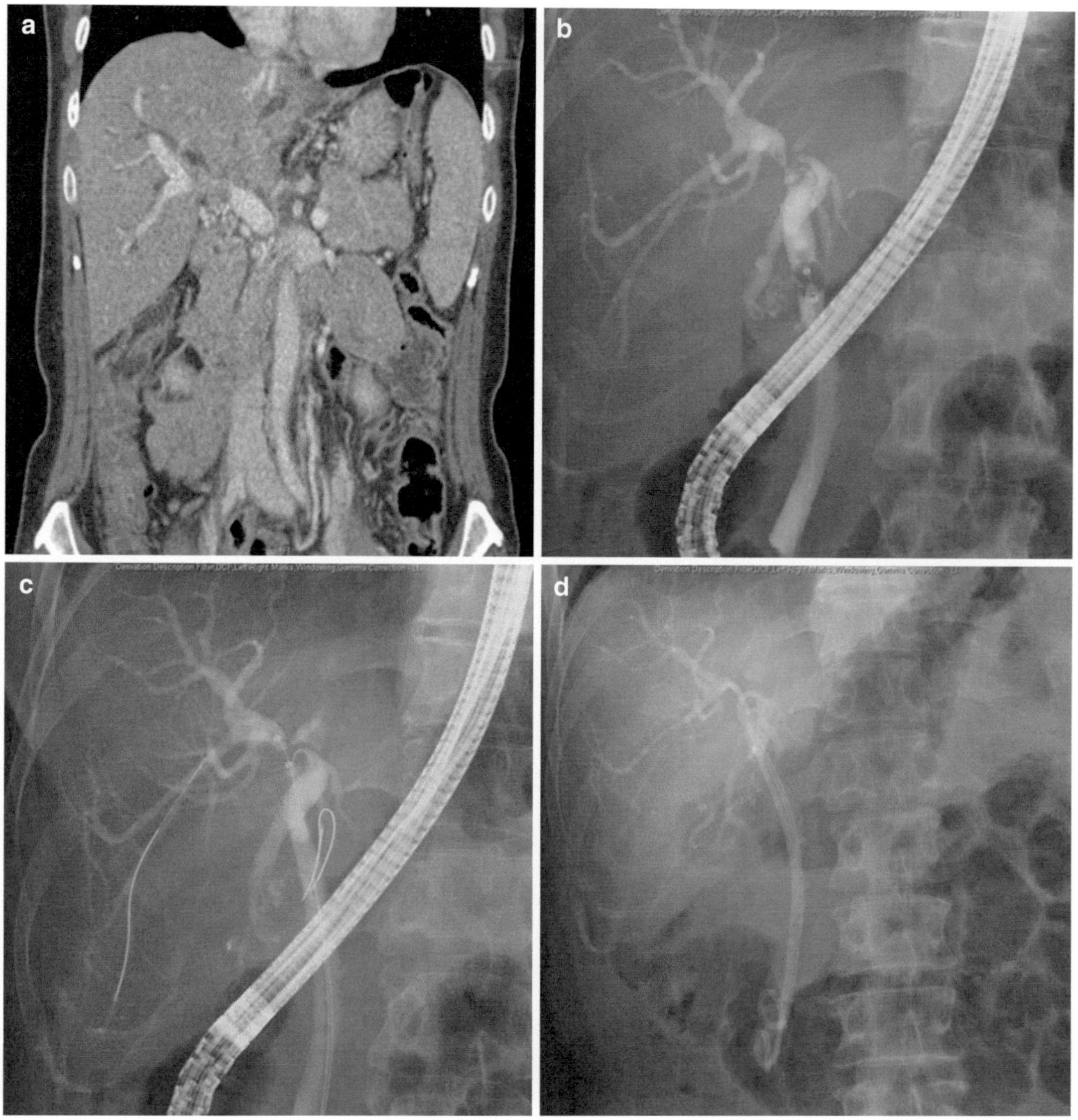

Fig. 7.1 Inserting a plastic stent in patients with Klatskin type IV tumors. A 46-year-old female patient was referred to our hospital because of hyperbilirubinemia. A plastic stent was inserted because the treatment plan was not confirmed. (**a**) A 46-year-old female patient was diagnosed with a Klatskin type IV tumor. Peri-hilar cholangiocarcinoma was revealed by abdominopelvic computed tomography (APCT). Extension to both intrahepatic ducts (IHDs) was noted, and bilateral IHDs were dilated. (**b**) A tight hilar stricture was noted on the cholangiogram. (**c**) Guidewires were passed through the tight stricture to the right and left IHDs. (**d**) Endoscopic retrograde biliary drainage (ERBD) was performed through the right and left IHDs, and complete drainage was achieved

[32]. Therefore, the number of patients who survive longer than the patency of the SEMS, and thus have to undergo a reintervention, has increased. Recurrent biliary obstructions account for 3–45% of cases of bilateral SEMS insertion for malignant hilar obstruction [33]. However, due to the difficulty of endoscopic reintervention for bilateral SEMS, the reported success rate ranges widely, from 44% to 100% [33].

Although various reintervention methods have been used, no optimal method has yet been established. Endoscopic reintervention is less invasive when the SEMS is occluded. If endoscopic reintervention fails, then percutaneous transhepatic drainage should be considered as an alternative. However, external drainage reduces patient quality of life. Therefore, reintervention should always be considered for patients who are expected to have a lengthy survival period [34]. Generally, PSs are used when a SEMS becomes obstructed at an unresectable malignant hilar biliary obstruction [34, 35] (Fig. 7.2). It is not known whether PSs or SEMSs are more useful for reinterventions. One study found that the median time from revisionary stent to recurrent obstruction was significantly longer with a PS. Therefore, when determining the type of stent for a reintervention, a SEMS should be preferred if the patient's life expectancy is expected to be long [34]. However, it should be noted that, when a second stent is inserted into the first stent during a re-intervention, both the PS and SEMS have a

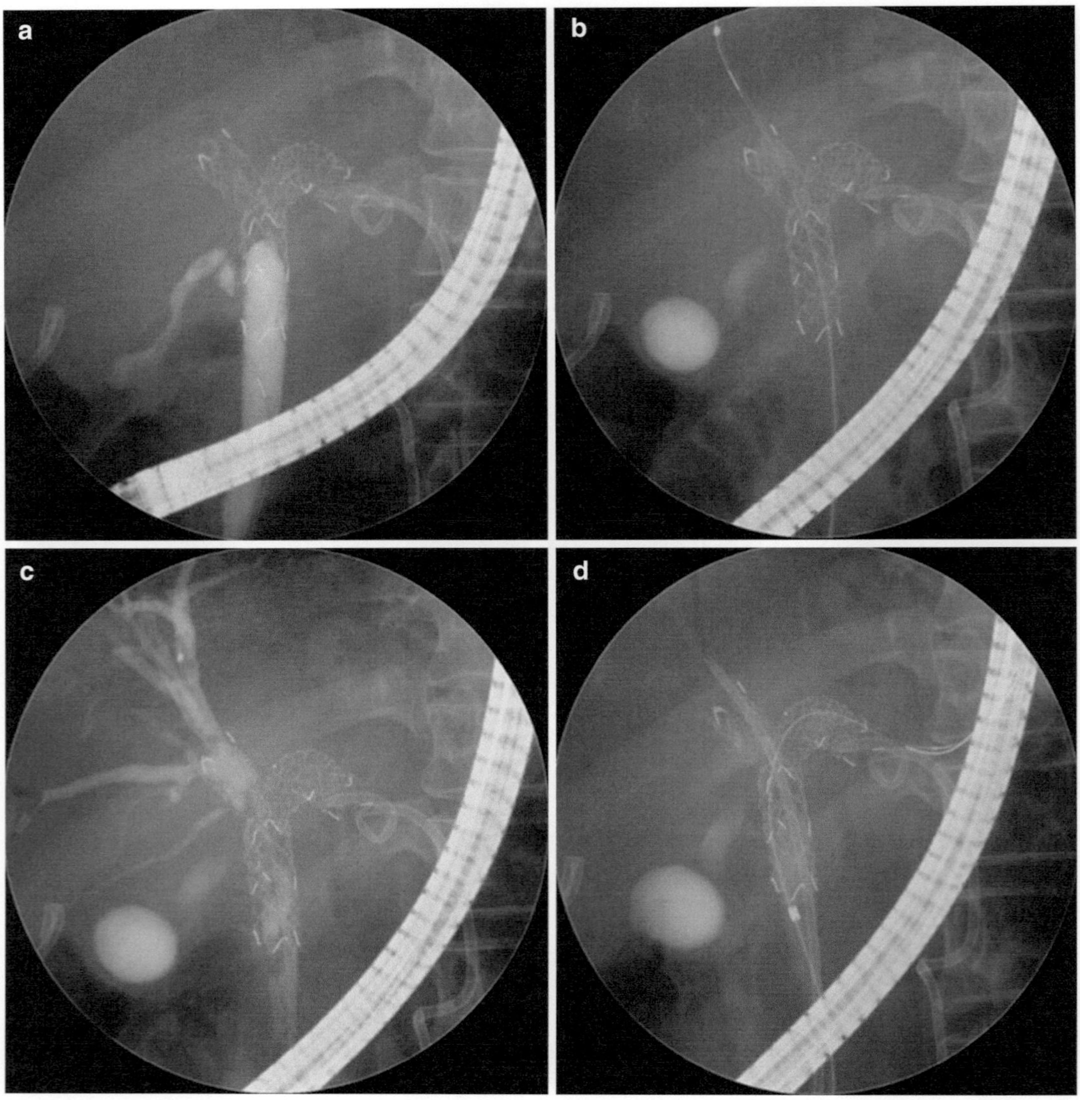

Fig. 7.2 Self-expandable metallic stent (SEMS) occlusion due to tumor ingrowth and revision with plastic stents (PSs). (**a**) The previous SEMS was occluded due to tumor ingrowth. (**b**) A new guidewire was inserted through the previous SEMS into the right IHD. (**c**) A PS was inserted into the right IHD. (**d**) A guidewire was passed through the left IHD and revision via a PS was done

short patency, so that cholangitis and other events can easily occur after the procedure.

SEMSs use should be avoided as the initial procedure for treating advanced malignant hilar tumors because removing the SEMS is difficult, and endoscopic re-intervention may not be effective if the stent does not achieve effective drainage. Therefore, effective drainage should first be attempted by inserting multiple PSs rather than a SEMS during the first procedure. Thereafter, a SEMS may be inserted during a planned ERCP. Replacing the PS several times should also be considered in a planned ERCP, when long-term survival is expected due to a good response to chemotherapy or radiotherapy.

Unilateral Versus Bilateral Stent Placement

Bismuth type III and IV hilar biliary strictures are complex, and there is much debate as to whether unilateral stents are better than bilateral stents in such cases [4]. According to two retrospective studies, bilateral SEMS are more effective in terms of survival or cumulative stent patency than unilateral SEMS [26, 36]. Bilateral maximal biliary drainage can prevent cholangitis and preserve liver function. However, two randomized controlled trials reported no significant differences in drainage success, complications, or mortality rates between bilateral and unilateral SEMS groups [29, 37]. Furthermore, when performing reintervention due to a dysfunctional stent, bilateral stenting is more complicated and difficult than unilateral stenting [29]. Based on these results, DePalma argued that inserting more than one stent for biliary bifurcation tumors should not be performed routinely [37]. A recent retrospective review of the literature suggested that bilateral SEMS may prolong cumulative stent patency only in Bismuth type II patients and may reduce the need for repeated biliary drainage due to stent occlusion [38]. Unilateral drainage is sufficient if the necessary liver volume is drained by unilateral stenting. Bilateral drainage can be considered when the estimated drained liver volume is deemed insufficient by unilateral stenting [23, 36, 38, 39]. According to a study of Bismuth type II–IV high-grade unresectable malignant hilar biliary obstructions, the technical success rates of unilateral and bilateral stenting are equal, but bilateral stenting has a higher clinical success rate and lower re-intervention rate [40]. Therefore, additional well-designed, large-scale trials are needed to determine whether unilateral or bilateral stenting is superior for treating a hilar stricture.

Side-by-Side Versus Stent-in-Stent Placement

Bilateral SEMS can be inserted according to both side-by-side (SBS) and stent-in-stent (SIS) methods. The SIS technique involves inserting the second SEMS into the contralateral hepatic duct through the mesh of the first SEMS. By contrast, the SBS method involves inserting two SEMS parallel to each other into the right hepatic duct (RHD) and left hepatic duct (LHD).

The bilateral SBS technique can be useful when guidewires are inserted into RHD right and LHD. However, the SBS technique has the disadvantage that the stricture and the distal bile duct can be overexpanded. The expansion forces caused by the use of two SEMS can result in severe pain, acute cholecystitis, and portal vein occlusion [1, 41–43].

The bilateral SIS technique is more physiological than the SBS technique, because two SEMS can expand within the diameter of a single stent [9, 10, 44–48]. Therefore, it is advantageous to avoid excessive expansion, particularly for non-dilated bile ducts.

Although transpapillary insertion of bilateral SEMS is technically more difficult than unilateral stenting when using both the SBS and SIS approaches, the 5-Fr delivery system with large-mesh has a high success rate [17]. However, whether the SBS or SIS method is superior remains controversial. According to a retrospective study, no significant difference was observed in technical or functional success rates between the SIS and SBS methods. Cumulative stent patency was longer in the SBS group, but the complication rate was higher [49]. In another retrospective study, no differences were detected in successful drainage, early complications, late complications, or stent patency between SIS and SBS [50]. In another retrospective study, there was no difference in reintervention need, successful reintervention, or procedural length between SBS and SIS groups [51]. Additional prospective comparative studies are therefore required.

The SIS method prevents endoscopic revision of an occluded stent because of the previously positioned wire mesh [9, 45, 52, 53]. Unlike the SIS method, the SBS method is more suitable for reintervention because the meshes do not cross each other. Intervention using the SIS method is easier with greater SEMS diameter, because the SEMS mesh is also larger [34].

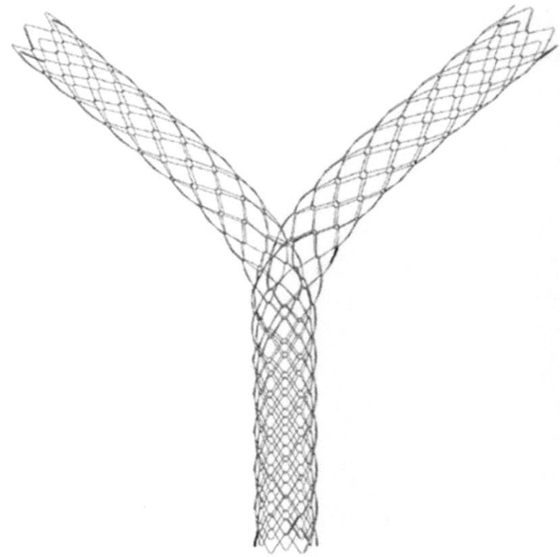

Fig. 7.3 Y-configured metal stent (large-D-cell type; TaeWoong Medical, Seoul, South Korea); unfixed large cell (size: 6 mm) stent with weaved pattern. The large cell size of the LCD TM enabled easy positioning of the second stent

Other Stenting Methods for Overcome Hurdle

The most difficult part of the SIS technique is to insert a second SEMS into the contralateral hepatic duct between the meshes of the first SEMS. To overcome this difficulty, more sophisticated Y-configured SEMS have been developed for hilar biliary strictures (Niti-S large cell D type; TaeWoong Corp., Seoul, South Korea) (Figs. 7.3 and 7.4) [17]. The technical method for inserting a Y-stent is as follows. Patients undergo endoscopic sphincterotomy before stenting. A biliary SEMS is first placed in the RHD or LHD through the hilar obstruction. This process is followed by insertion of a second SEMS using the SIS method, after locating the guidewire through the central mesh of the previously inserted SEMS. A portion of the second stent, including the central mesh, is placed in the common hepatic duct to form the Y-shape (Fig. 7.2) [54]. One study showed that the bilateral SIS technique using large-cell SEMS has a high technical success rate [46]. In addition, the open-cell-SEMS design has a high technical success rate for revision, although it does not prevent tumor ingrowth and bilateral revision remains difficult [45, 46, 52].

A newly designed closed-cell, cross-wire stent is also useful for SIS stenting (Bonastent M-Hilar; Standard SciTech Inc., Seoul, South Korea). This stent consists of proximal and distal parts with hooks and cross-wired structures; the central portion is made up of cross-wired structures alone, which facilitate the SIS technique [44].

It is often difficult to insert the second SEMS using the SBS technique, as the first SEMS is expanded. A small diameter (6-Fr) SEMS has been developed to overcome this problem (Zilver635; Cook Japan, Tokyo, Japan). The small diameter of the SEMS allows for simultaneous, single-step SBS placement, which increases the technical success rate of bilateral SBS stenting [51, 55]. The optimal location of the distal end of the SEMS remains controversial. The distal end of the two SEMS should be located at the same level of the common bile duct (CBD) or duodenum to facilitate subsequent reintervention [20].

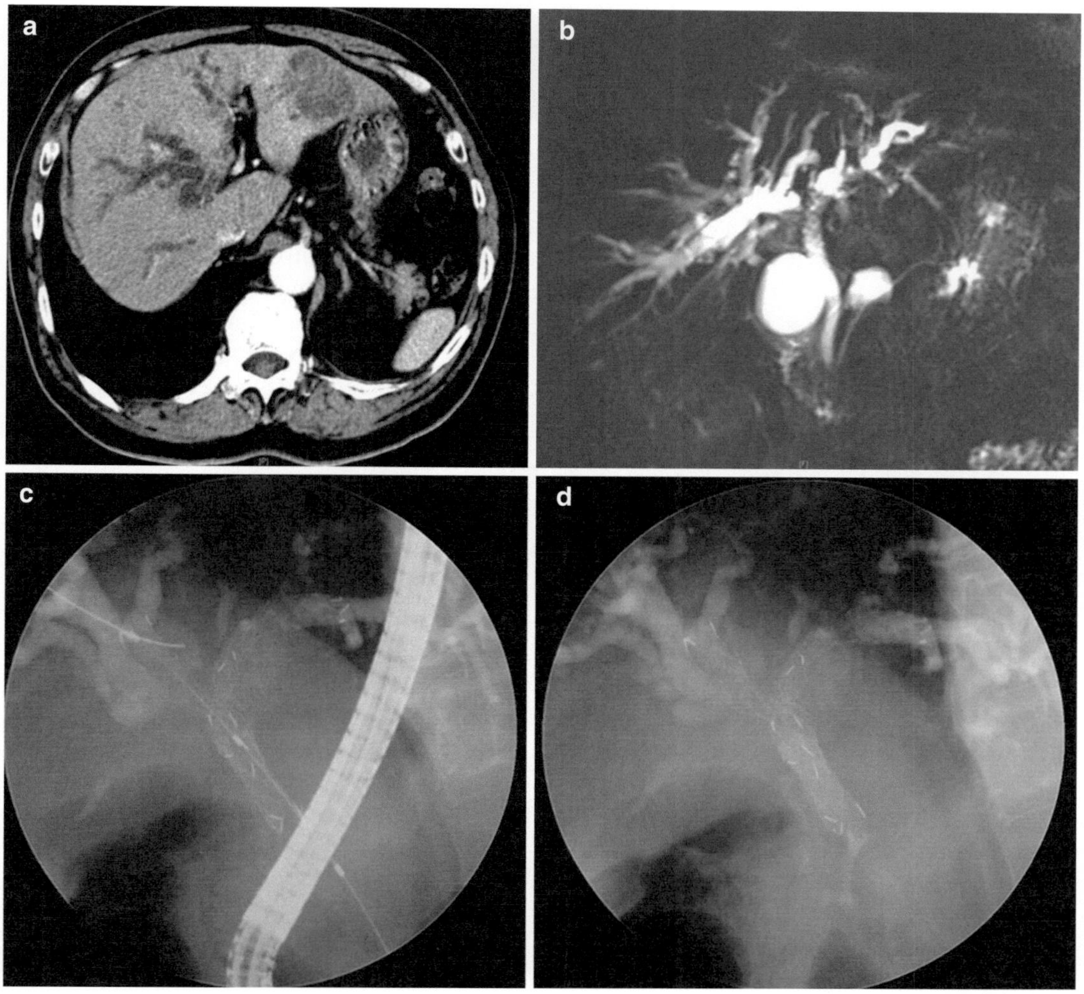

Fig. 7.4 Y-stent fitted during endoscopic retrograde cholangiopancreatography (ERCP) in patients with a Klatskin tumor, Bismuth type IV. (**a**) Bismuth type IV resulting in bilateral IHD dilatation was noted on APCT with infiltrative hilar bile duct cancer. (**b**) A Klatskin tumor type IV resulting in bilateral IHD dilatation was noted on magnetic resonance imaging (MRI) and magnetic resonance cholangiopancreatography (MRCP) images. (**c**) A guidewire and another stent were inserted through the right IHD to insert the Y-stent. (**d**) The Y-stent was inserted successfully through the left and right IHD

Percutaneous Biliary Drainage

Percutaneous transhepatic biliary drainage (PTBD) allows for precise lobar selection, reduces the risk of exposing the biliary tree to duodenal contents, and shows a high success rate with respect to biliary drainage and a low risk of cholangitis [56]. However, PTBD is accompanied by pain and discomfort at the skin puncture site. PTBD is also occasionally accompanied by complications, such as infection and bleeding, so drainage should be internalized in such cases [57]. Percutaneous tract recurrence occurs in 2–5% of patients [58].

Metal stents are superior to PSs in terms of longer patency, lower rate of re-intervention, and lower overall cost [14, 29]. Two methods are used to insert a stent into percutaneous tissue. The "one-stage" procedure is performed without biliary drainage, and the "two-stage" procedure is performed after 5–7 days of biliary drainage [59–61]. Most recent reports prefer the two-stage procedure because of the complex anatomic structure and technical difficulty of malignant hilar obstruction [62–66].

The Asia-Pacific consensus on HC and the European Society of Gastrointestinal Endoscopy failed to conclude definitively whether metal stents should pass the duodenal papilla [30, 67]. If a metal stent is placed above the duodenal papilla, then it has the advantage of preserving duodenal papillary function. However, if the flow of contrast is slow during cholangiography after positioning the stent above the duodenal papilla, then it is necessary to place the stent across the duodenal papilla to increase the therapeutic success rate and reduce post-procedural cholangitis and the re-intervention rate [68].

Percutaneous biliary drainage can be used in Bismuth type III and IV cases and can serve as an alternative if ERCP fails or complete drainage is not achieved by ERCP (Fig. 7.5). The hilar stricture of advanced hilar tumors is tight, tortuous, and involves several branches; this scenario often leads to failure or ineffective stenting. In such cases, the percutaneous approach is favored initially (Figs. 7.6 and 7.7). In addition, revision via a transhepatic route can be performed when occlusion occurs after stenting with ERCP (Fig. 7.8).

Unresectable malignant biliary hilar tumors have been studied in terms of whether unilobar or bilobar drainage is better. When contrast medium is injected into an undrained duct, unilateral drainage increases the possibility of bacterial contamination, which in turn increases the probability that jaundice will not improve [66, 69–71]. Advocates of unilateral drainage emphasize the low complication rate and argue that it is important to not overfill the undrained ducts [24–26, 72]. However, contrast medium can unintentionally fill an undrained lobe behind the hilar stricture. In such cases, additional drainage is needed to control cholangitis. Similarly, bilobar drainage can cause the same problem due to undrained duct contamination [61].

Bismuth II and III cases are associated with an increase in mean survival time and a decrease in the incidence of early cholangitis when two or more stents are inserted [73–75]. The number and type of stents in Bismuth II and III cases are not significantly related to stent patency, but inserting two stents could maintain stent patency rates longer in Bismuth IV cases [76].

The Y stent method (SIS) and T stent method (SIS) can be used to insert bilateral stents. These methods generally involve inserting two stents into the hilum to drain both lobes simultaneously [66]. The T- and Y-configured stents are connected to the CBD via the right-sector ducts, which are both intrahepatic ducts (IHDs), and the LHD. Both types of stents are effective for lowering the bilirubin level after the procedure, but no significant difference was detected in the extent of bilirubin reduction between the two stents types [50]. A "crisscross-configured" method has also been used for trisector drainage. Many studies have suggested that both T-configured and crisscross-configured stents enable effective biliary drainage and show long-term stent patency for a malignant hilar obstruction [60, 61, 77]. However, it remains controversial as to whether the T-configured or crisscross-configured stent is superior; therefore, an additional prospective study is needed.

Stent-in-Stent (T-Configured) and Stent-by-Stent (Y-Configured) Deployment

The advantage of placing a T-configured stent is that bilateral biliary drainage is obtained through single percutaneous transhepatic access. The T- and Y-configured stents both connect one of the ducts in the right sector to the LHD, in a circuit including the CBD [54] (Fig. 7.6).

No significant difference was observed in patency between the two types of stent when used in malignant hilar stricture patients [50]. In other studies, no difference was detected in stent patency between the two types of stent in chemotherapy patients, but patency was longer with the Y- versus T-type stent in patients not undergoing chemotherapy [49]. There are two main reasons why Y-type patency is maintained for longer. First, a Y-type bile duct is drained via two

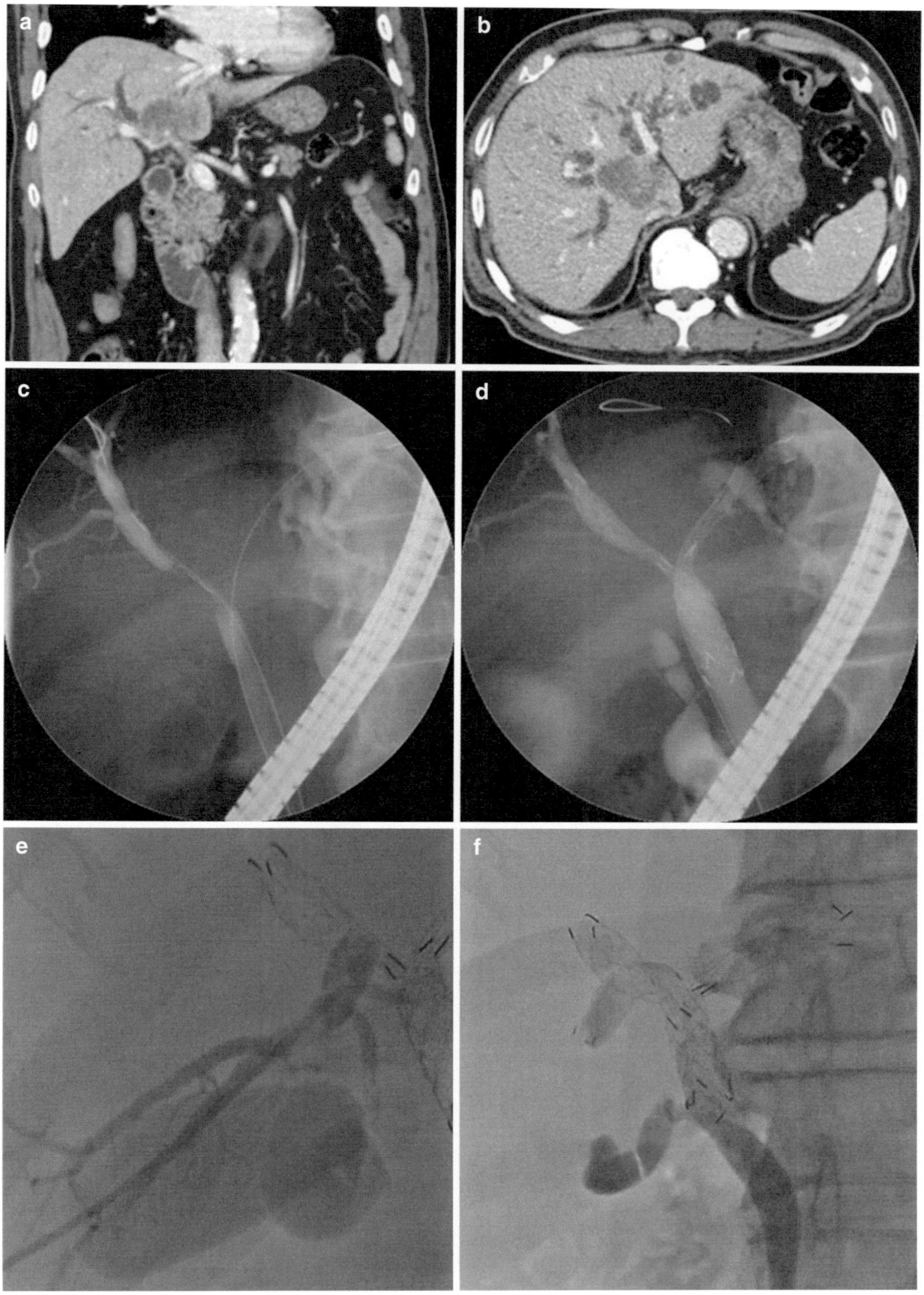

Fig. 7.5 Far-advanced malignant hilar stricture; additional SEMS via percutaneous transhepatic biliary drainage (PTBD). (**a**, **b**) On APCT, intrahepatic cholangiocellular carcinoma (CCC) with hilar invasion was noted. Bilateral IHD dilatation was seen. (**c**) The guidewire was passed through to the left and right IHD during ERCP. (**d**) The Y-stent was inserted during ERCP. (**e**) Additional PTBD via the right IHD was performed to drain another bile duct. (**f**) Additional PTBD using a SEMS was done and successful biliary drainage was achieved

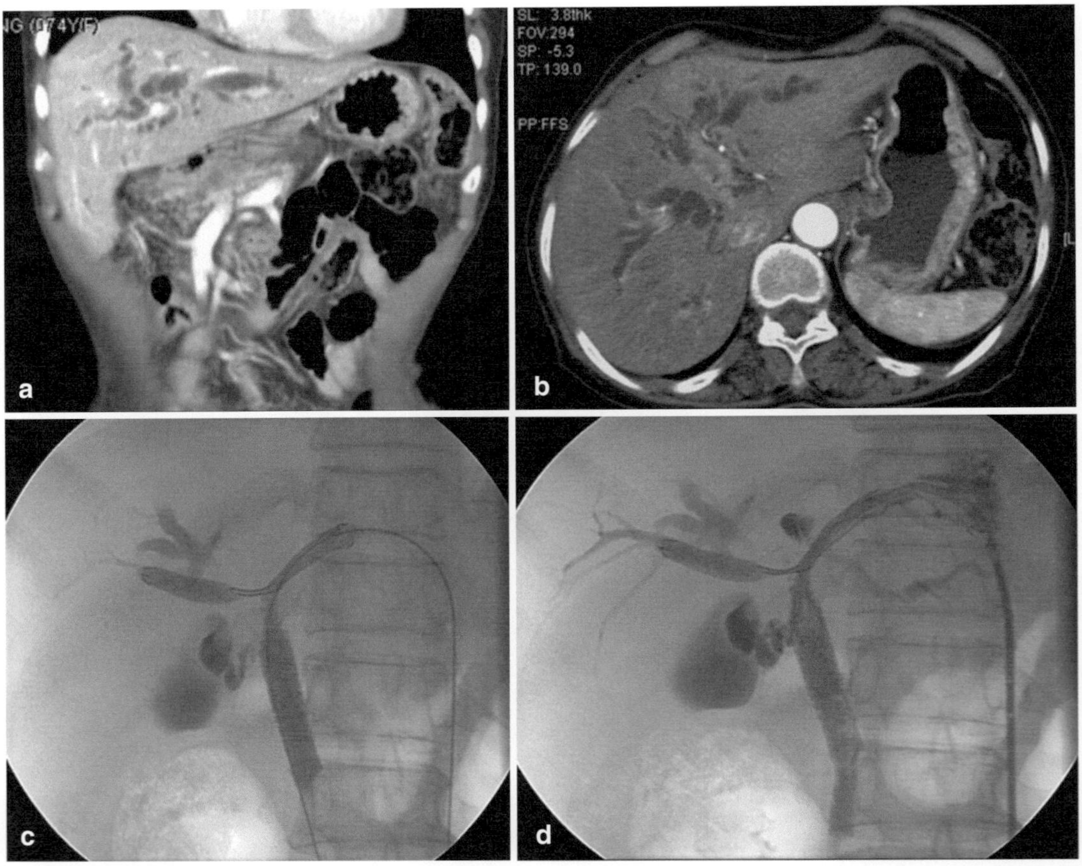

Fig. 7.6 Use of a T-configured stent fitted via the percutaneous method in patients with a Klatskin tumor, Bismuth type IV. (**a**, **b**) Bismuth type IV case with infiltrative hilar bile duct cancer; bilateral IHD dilatation was noted on APCT. (**c**) A 10 × 60 mm stent was inserted from right to left into the main duct via a PTBD catheter. (**d**) A 10 × 80 mm stent was inserted at the left side of the main duct into the common bile duct (CBD) through a previously installed stent mesh

separate channels, unlike the T-type, which forms one channel; thus, bile can be drained to the other side even if one side is closed. Second, because the stent mesh is larger in the T-type stent, patency can be maintained for longer in Y-type stenting because tumor proliferates more readily between the meshes. However, it is difficult to conclude that the Y-type stent is more advantageous simply because of the enhanced maintenance period. A comparison of the advantages of the two types of stents should not only consider maintenance duration but also how effectively bilirubin can be reduced, whether there is a difference in complications and whether re-intervention is easy for an occlusion [78]. The effectiveness of bilirubin reduction after stenting is an important criterion for clinical success. In previous studies, clinical success was considered as a decrease in bilirubin [49, 50, 79]. One study reported successful bilirubin reduction rates of 78.9% and 81.8% for the Y- and T-type stents, respectively, at 1 month after the procedure [50]. Another study reported successful bilirubin reduction rates of 96% and 100% for the Y- and T-types, respectively, at 1 month after the procedure [49]. However, in both of these studies, no significant difference was observed in bilirubin reduction rate between the two stent types. The T-type stent is more effective at reducing bilirubin initially, because

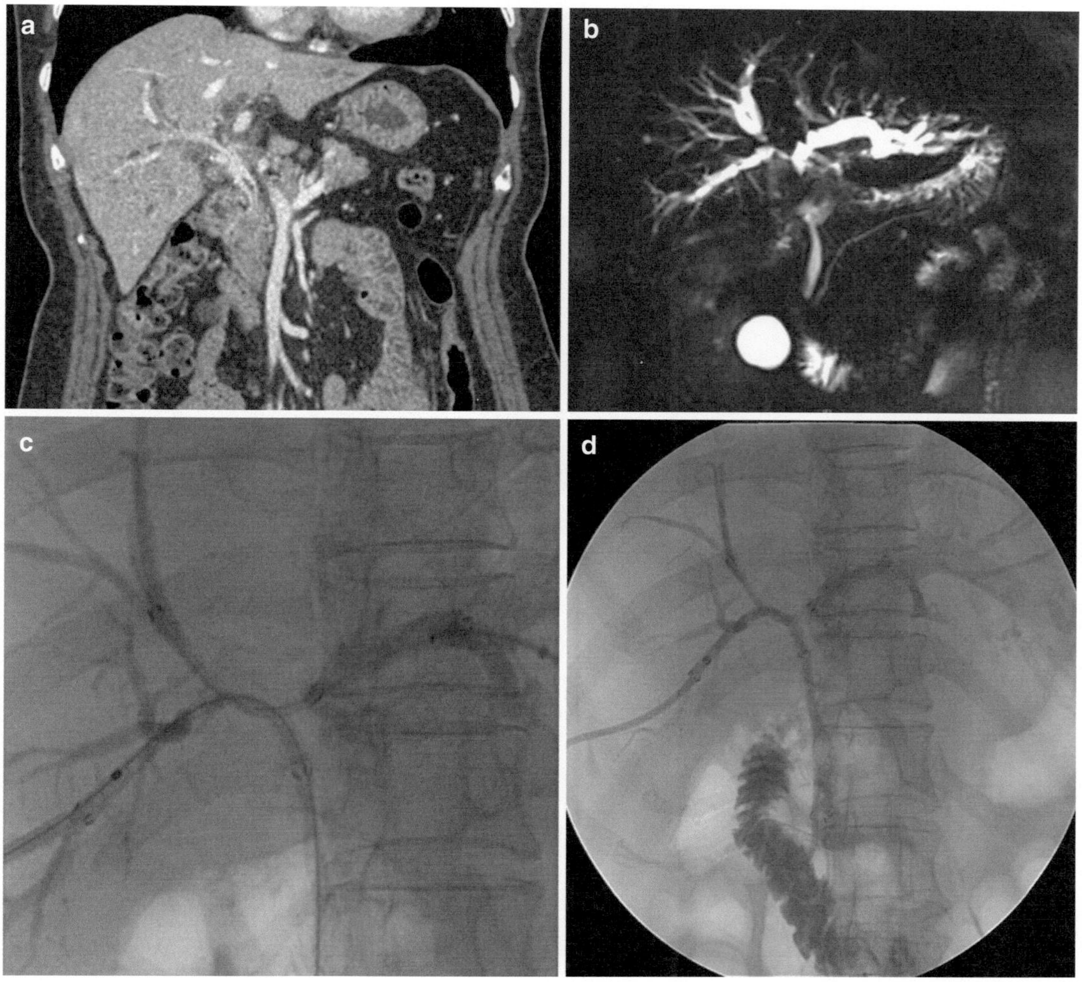

Fig. 7.7 Crisscross-configured stent fitted using the percutaneous method in patients with Klatskin tumor, Bismuth type IIIa. (**a**) A Klatskin type IIIa tumor was noted on APCT. Both IHDs were dilatated. (**b**) On MRI, a Klatskin type IIIa tumor was noted. Both IHDs were dilatated. (**c**, **d**) Left to right anterior (8 mm/6 cm) and right posterior (8 mm/10 cm) stents were inserted into the CBD

the initial lumen of the stent is relatively larger than that of the Y-type stent. On the one hand, the Y-type stent is elongated at the site of tumor narrowing, resulting in a diameter smaller than 16–20 mm, which is the sum of the two stent lumens. On the other hand, in T-type stenting, as the two stents, having an inner diameter of 8–10 mm, overlap with each other, relatively high elasticity and a sufficient diameter can be maintained. However, no significant difference in bilirubin reduction rate was observed between the two stent types at 1 month [78]. This case is because a self-inflating metal stent, when used as a Y-type stent, can retain the stent lumen at 1 month after insertion and a wide lumen diameter of 8–12 mm after expansion. It is thought that a constant lumen can be maintained for several months. In patients who required stenting for more than 1 month, no difference in bilirubin reduction rate was observed between the two stent types [78].

Acute cholangitis and acute cholecystitis are common complications after stenting [80, 81]. Complications may differ somewhat depending on the procedure. The parallel stenting technique, in which the stent is arranged in a Y- or

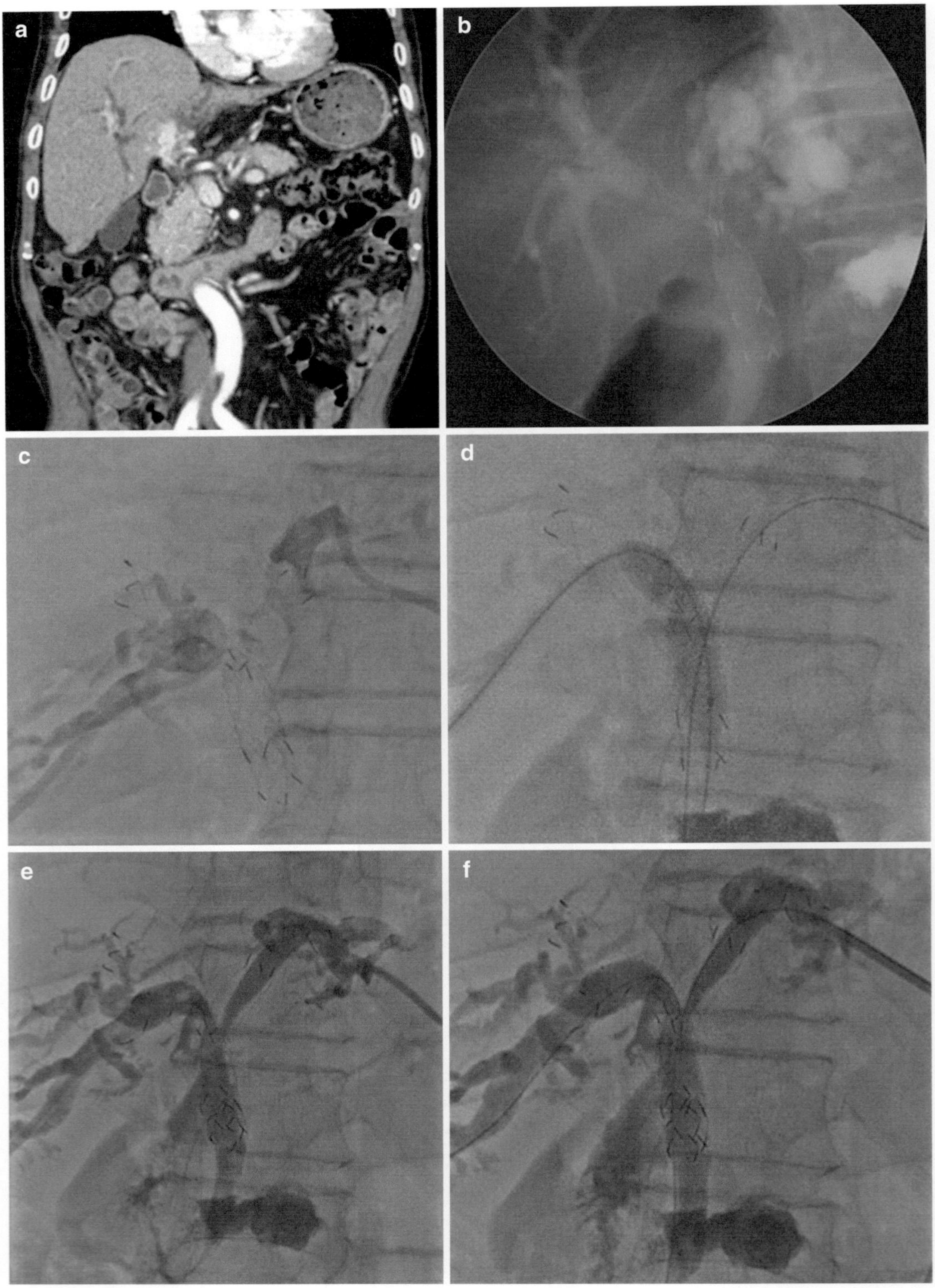

Fig. 7.8 Stent revision by the transhepatic route. (**a**) A Klatskin tumor IV was noted on APCT. (**b**) Y-stent was inserted during ERCP (November 2011). (**c**) Bilateral PTBD was performed after approximately 2 years due to jaundice (February 2014). (**d**) A guidewire was passed through the previous Y-stent during PTBD. (**e**, **f**) Stent revision by the transhepatic route

X-type configuration, is a relatively simple and effective procedure for intrahepatic bile drainage. In some cases, the stent may not be fully deployed at the time of installation, resulting in premature occlusion of the stent due to insufficient bile drainage. In addition, excessive enlargement of the bile duct causes portal vein occlusion and is associated with a high incidence of cholangitis [50, 66, 82]. The T-type is a stent-through-the-wire mesh technique that has the advantage of preventing migration or displacement of the stent, because the two stents overlap partially [64]. However, according to some reports, bile sludge is formed at the site where the stents overlap, which may block the inside of the stent and increase the possibility of early stent occlusion. It is also known that the incidence of tumor proliferation among the meshes in cases of proliferating tumor is higher [49, 66, 83–86].

In the case of stent occlusion, Y-type stenting is performed by puncturing the bile duct of the mesenchyme where one end of the clogged stent is located and reinserting the stent after passing the guidewire through the clogged site. However, when a T-type stent is inserted, the stent cannot be reinserted immediately because its mesh blocks the bile duct. Therefore, it is necessary to perform balloon dilatation through the mesh with a balloon catheter and reinsert the stent through the widened mesh [82, 84]. In other words, the Y-type is relatively advantageous, in terms of ease of reoperation, because the T-type is difficult to reuse if stent occlusion occurs, and a PTBD catheter must be maintained for the entire lifetime in case of failure [43]. In patients with both T- and Y-type stents, bilateral bile duct stents are effective for reducing bilirubin levels following an advanced malignant intrahepatic bile duct obstruction procedure. In particular, no difference in bilirubin reduction rate was observed between the two stent types over a follow-up period of more than 1 month, and there was also no significant difference in retention rate. Therefore, it is necessary to choose the treatment method according to the complications, ease of procedure, and need for re-intervention.

Crisscross-Configured Stent Deployment

Drainage of the right hepatic sector (right anterior duct or right posterior duct) is inevitable in the case of an advanced hilar obstruction that includes the segmental duct, due to the limited drainage volume [61]. A crisscross-configured stent has been developed to overcome this disadvantage (Fig. 7.7) [61]. Hilar tumors that extend beyond the right segmental duct may remain without draining the right segmental duct, even with bilobar drainage. According to a report on the distribution of intrahepatic volume, the right lobe accounts for two-thirds of the total liver volume. Each sector of the right lobe has a similar volume to that of the left hepatic lobe [87]. Therefore, T- and Y-configured stents should be considered as bisectoral drainage methods, particularly for advanced hilar malignancy, rather than bilobar drainage methods. The most effective way to drain three sectors using minimal stenting may be through crisscross-configured stent placement [61].

This method involves three IHDs, to enable "trisector" drainage (right anterior duct [RAD], right posterior duct [RPD], and LHD) [61]. However, the procedure is more complex and requires two or more percutaneous transhepatic approaches, resulting in increased morbidity.

The stent must be located along the biliary ductal anatomy for effective trisector drainage. A RAD-LHD/RPD-CBD pathway is effective if the patient has standard anatomy, with the RPD meeting the RAD and forming the RHD. This case is because the RAD-to-LHD direction is more obtuse and inserting a stent is thus easier. The RAD-LHD/RPD-CBD pathway should be used if the RPD joins the LHD. If the RPD-LHD/RAD-CBD pathway is used, then a transverse stent may become completely separated from a vertical stent, which can lead to failed internal drainage. If this happens, a new stent is needed to connect the two stents.

Although it is unclear whether two stents need to cross in the hepatic hilum, an intersecting stent system has an advantage in terms of system integrity and also secures a large luminal diameter

[61]. Trisectional stents may be used as palliative therapy for longer periods because they can involve the IHDs of the liver to a greater extent than bisectional stents [61].

Endoscopic or Percutaneous Biliary Drainage

Klatskin tumors are classified based on the Bismuth–Corlette classification according to the extent of hepatic duct involvement [19]. MRCP and CT are helpful for classifying HC according to the Bismuth classification and thus for determining the initial treatment method. Endoscopic treatment is preferred to percutaneous drainage for Bismuth types I and II [30]. However, the European Society of Gastrointestinal Endoscopy Guidelines recommend that endoscopic drainage of HC should be performed at high-volume centers with experienced endoscopists and multidisciplinary teams [67]. Other guidelines also recommend a percutaneous approach for Bismuth types III and IV. This scenario is due to the low success rate of endoscopic procedures in Bismuth type III and IV cases and the increased risk of cholangitis following ERCP [30, 88].

However, despite these recommendations, endoscopic biliary drainage is helpful for patients with Bismuth type III or IV, if there is sufficient endoscopic expertise. Endoscopic biliary drainage is less invasive than percutaneous drainage [54].

If endoscopic stenting fails, PTBD should be performed on the same day as ERCP and percutaneous stenting should be maintained for 2–3 days. Furthermore, if endoscopic biliary drainage fails, then immediate conversion to a percutaneous approach is essential because post-procedural cholangitis is common due to residual contrast agent, and the patient's progress may be poor [54].

A malignant hilar stricture is defined as a far-advanced malignant hilar stricture, in which biliary drainage is difficult. Such strictures can be characterized as follows: (1) difficult (tight/long/tortuous), (2) obstructing multiple lobes and segments, and (3) at higher risk of cholangitis on intervention. Planning the treatment strategy for far-advanced malignant hilar strictures requires not only considering the Bismuth type but also consulting with an expert team, including endoscopists and radiologists (Figs. 7.9, 7.10, and 7.11).

Due to recent advances in ERCP technology, biliary drainage of multiple ducts has been tried in some studies. Drainage of more than three biliary ducts involves the LHD, posterior branch of the right hepatic duct (pRHD), and either or both of the anteroinferior branch of the right hepatic duct (aiRHD) and the anterosuperior branch of the right hepatic duct (asRHD) [5]. According to one study, there was no significant difference in complication rates between a group with three or more biliary drainage procedures and one with one or two biliary drainage procedures. Therefore, drainage of multiple ducts with a SEMS can be considered feasible and safe compared to drainage of only one or two ducts. However, to successfully drain multiple ducts, the operator must use appropriate devices, such as guidewires, catheters, and stents. It is also necessary to be familiar with the anatomy of a complicated hepatic duct [89]. In addition, multilateral drainage requires high levels of skill and experience, and use of an endoscopic technique, because re-intervention is difficult. If these conditions are met, then the efficacy of multiple biliary duct drainage may be further enhanced.

Therefore, a percutaneous approach is not always an appropriate alternative in cases where ERCP is considered difficult. Drainage of multiple biliary ducts is feasible and should be tailored to the individual patient, and according to the skills and experience of, and techniques available to, the endoscopist. A palliative endoscopic approach for advanced hilar tumor requires a strategy that preserves as much of the nonatrophied liver as possible during the lifetime of the patient and avoids the potentially lethal complications associated with stent dysfunction [90].

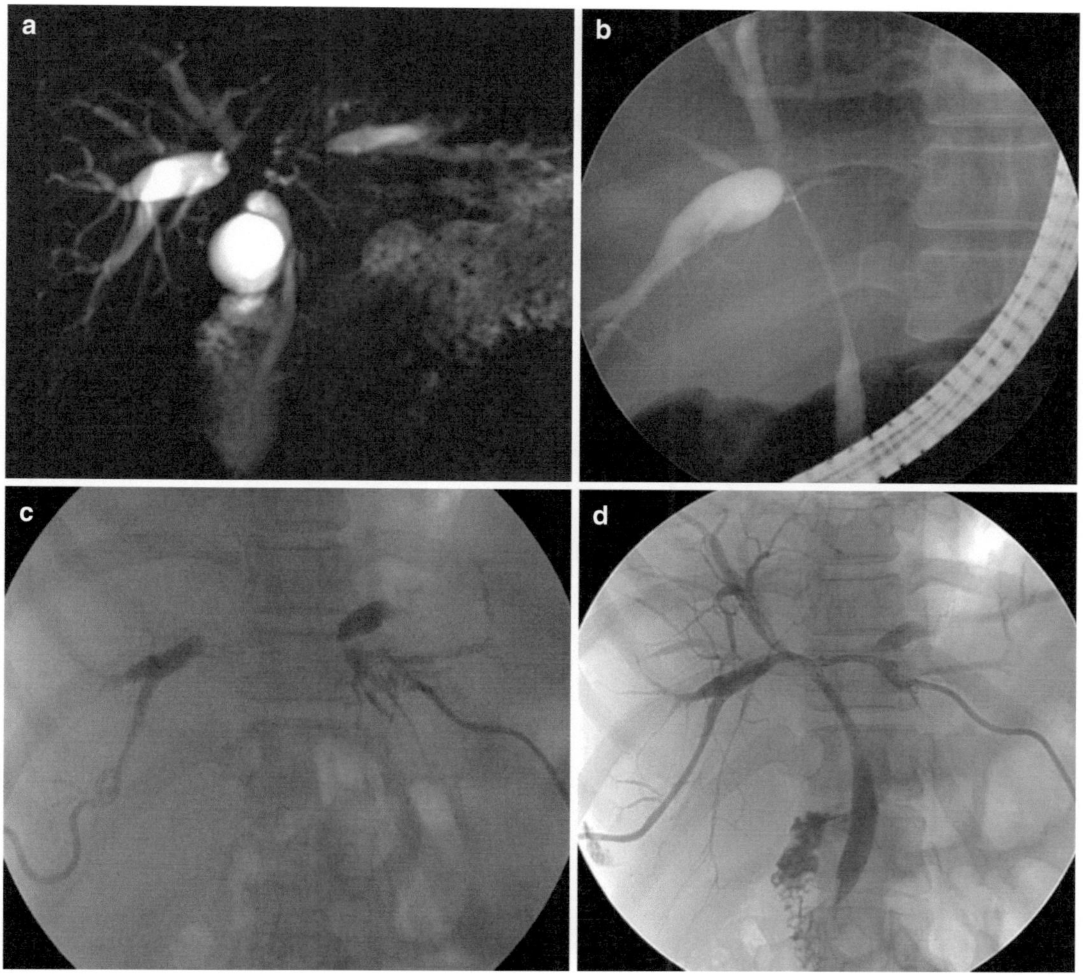

Fig. 7.9 Far-advanced malignant hilar stricture; long and tight stricture. (**a**) A Klatskin type IV tumor was noted on MRI. (**b**) Y-stent insertion failed during ERCP due to failure to inability to pass the guidewire through the stricture. (**c**) A long and tight stricture was seen. (**d**) A crisscross-configured stent was inserted through the right posterior IHD to the CBD and through the left IHD to the right anterior IHD

Summary

In the early 2000s, the success rate of endoscopic biliary drainage of hilar tumors was 55–81% [41, 56]. However, due to the development of stenting devices and endoscopic stenting techniques, the success rate of endoscopic stent insertion is increasing [8, 48, 91]. However, the success rate of endoscopic stenting remains lower for advanced HC than percutaneous stenting [92]. According to a multicenter retrospective study, percutaneous procedures in advanced HC patients showed a significantly higher success rate than endoscopic drainage, and the risk of cholangitis is lower [93].

The most common cause of failure of endoscopic stenting is inability to pass a guidewire along the stricture or to insert the guidewire into the contralateral duct after inserting the initial stenting [54]. Even if the guidewire is successfully positioned, the stent delivery catheter may not pass through the stricture [54]. The percutaneous method is an alternative if endoscopic stenting fails (Figs. 7.7, 7.8, and 7.9). According

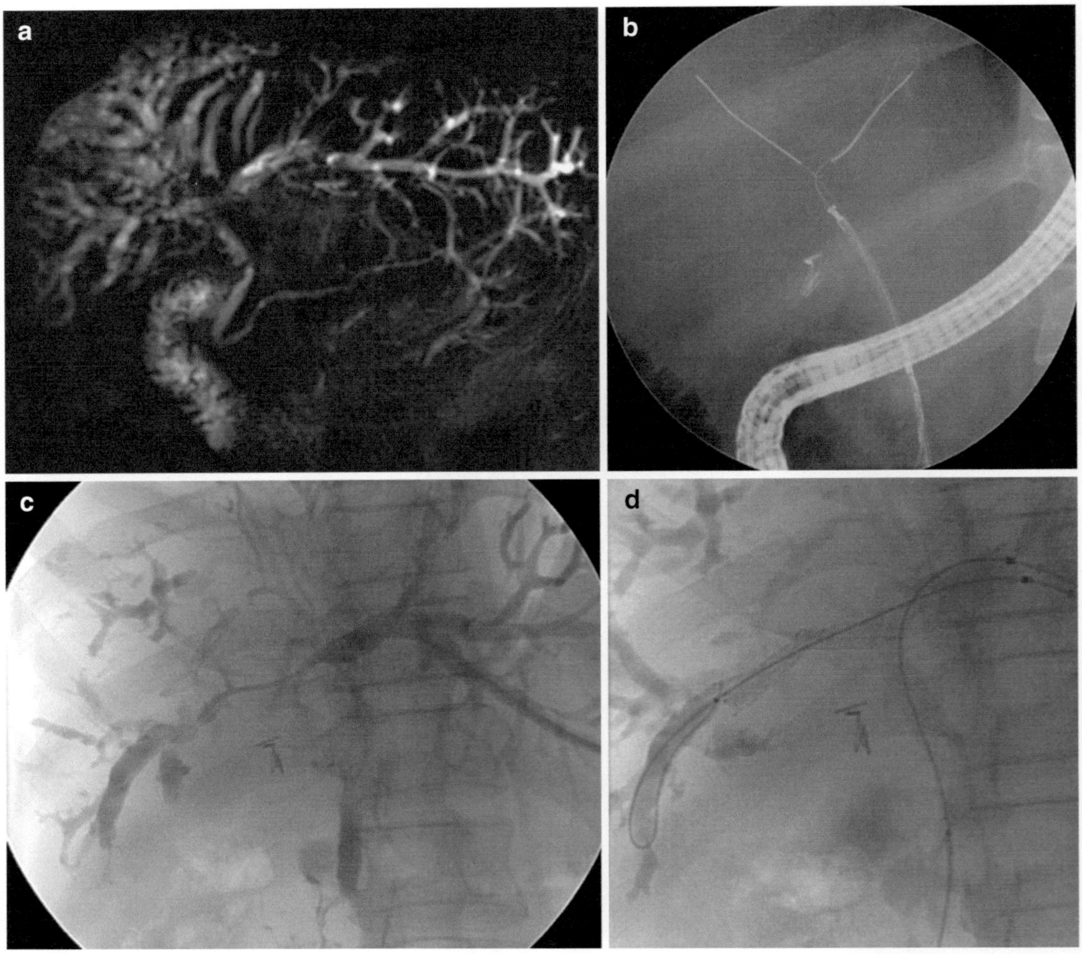

Fig. 7.10 Far-advanced malignant hilar stricture; failed insertion of the catheter. (**a**) A Klatskin type IV tumor was noted on MRI. (**b**) Y-stent insertion failed during ERCP due to inability to pass the stent through the stricture. (**c**) PTBD was achieved through the left IHD. (**d**) A T-stent was inserted during PTBD

to a radiologic study on passing a guidewire through a stricture, acute angulation between the left IHD and CBD is an independent predictor of failure to pass a guidewire [54]. The angle between small IHDs and CBDs makes it difficult to locate an entrance point for the guidewire, which renders the guidewire and catheter difficult to engage [54]. Obstruction is more complex in HCs of Bismuth types III and IV, because the obstructed site is narrower, longer, serpentine, and contains more mesenchyme [54]. Percutaneous biliary stenting can accurately distinguish the bile duct for drainage, whereas endoscopic biliary drainage only occurs in a retrograde direction, making manipulation of instruments more difficult [54].

Evaluating bile ducts according to their radiological characteristics is difficult because radiographs are an indirect measurement modality. A direct cholangiogram during ERCP or PTBD is more accurate than preoperative radiological imaging [94]. Determination of whether or not the catheter can be passed through the guidewire can be achieved most accurately by ERCP [54].

According to a prospective study of endoscopic stenting for preoperative biliary drainage, a significant factor in stenting failure is a proxi-

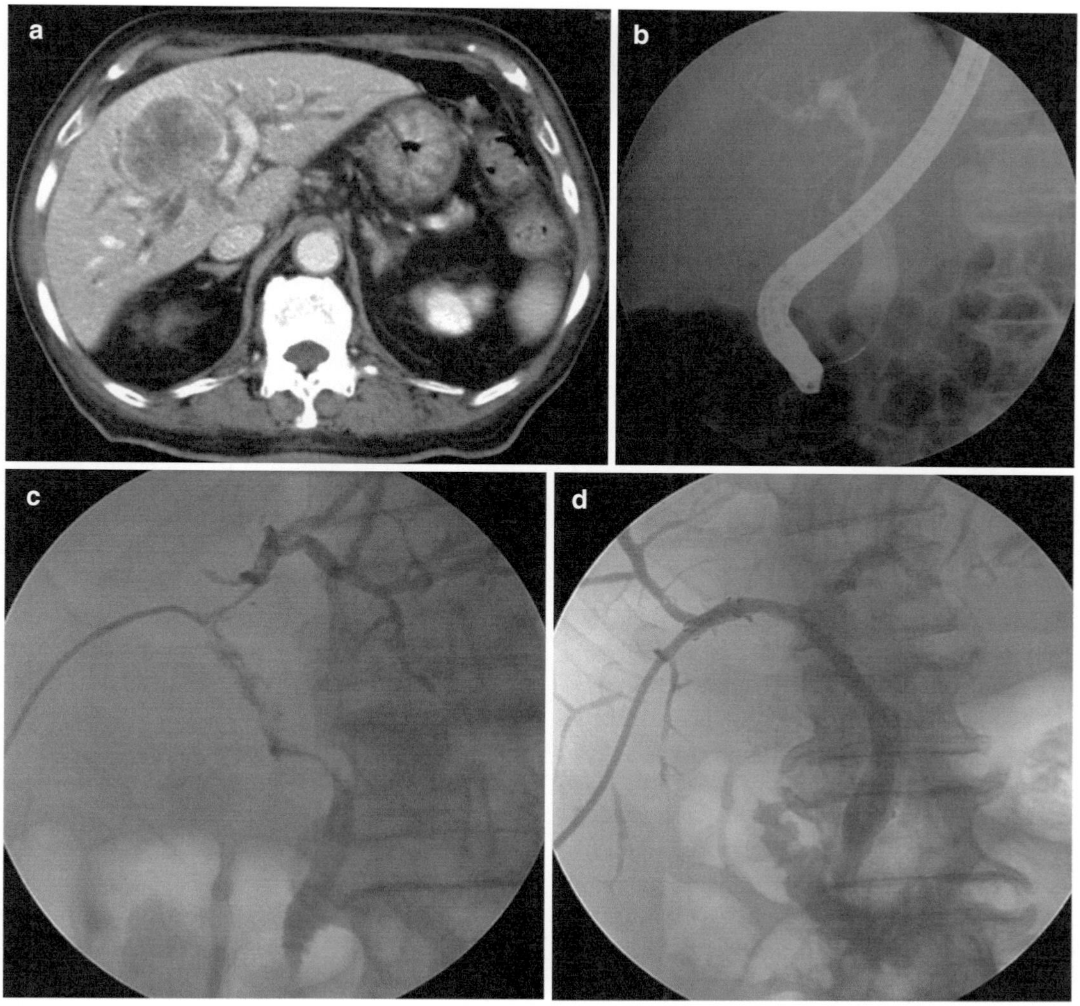

Fig. 7.11 Far-advanced malignant hilar stricture; failed bilateral guidewire insertion. (**a**) A CCC with hilar invasion was noted on APCT. (**b**) Y stent insertion failed due to inability to pass the guidewire bilaterally. (**c**) PTBD was achieving through the right IHD. (**d**) A T-stent was inserted during PTBD

mal biliary obstruction (Bismuth type III or IV) and total bilirubin level (>8.8 mg/dl) [95]. Complications of percutaneous and endoscopic approaches differ by study [54, 96] and may be reduced when performed by a skilled radiologist using certain techniques and tools [54].

The advantages of a percutaneous approach are as follows: [30, 61, 63, 66] (1) easier manipulation of the guidewire and catheter, (2) the possibility of precise selection of lobes or segments for drainage, (3) the availability of a variety of stent designs (T-configured, single- and dual-access, and crisscross-configured), and (4) the possibility of stent patency evaluation before removing the external drainage catheter. Therefore, even though there is controversy regarding unilateral versus bilateral drainage in cases of HC, clinicians should perform percutaneous drainage before bilateral endoscopic stenting for advanced HC without hepatic atrophy. Even if the endoscopic approach fails, “rendezvous” percutaneous and endoscopic procedures or percutaneous drainage will resolve obstructive cholestasis in hilar carcinoma [54]. However, the percutaneous approach also has some disadvantages: (1) pain at the puncture site, (2) a two-step process necessitating a prolonged hospital stay, (3) potential for vascular injury or bile leak, and (4) outcome dependent on operator skill.

In conclusion, malignant hilar stricture requires a highly tailored treatment approach that should emphasize both clinical success and patient safety. The use of unilateral or bilateral stenting should be determined based on drainage volume and liver function. Excessive multi-stenting, particularly to an atrophied area, should be avoided to reduce the risk of cholangitis. Securing a larger drainage volume from the normal liver is beneficial. Effective biliary decompression is not merely a technical question of how many stents can be inserted; the ultimate goal is to achieve a drainage configuration that optimizes function. Thus, inserting a PS is recommended for initial biliary drainage. Insertion of a SEMS should be considered after confirming good biliary drainage with a removable stent. The second stent has shorter patency, regardless of the stent type.

The first-line stent insertion method for patients with advanced and difficult Bismuth types (III and IV) should be the percutaneous approach, due to its high success rate and good clinical outcomes. Furthermore, acute angulation between the left IHD and CBD increases the likelihood of endoscopic stent failure. If the endoscopic approach fails, then subsequent percutaneous drainage must be performed to prevent cholangitis, which will in turn reduce morbidity and mortality [54]. If complete biliary drainage is not achieved through ERCP, percutaneous methods should be considered. In addition, biliary drainage, particularly for advanced malignant hilar lesions, should be performed at institutions with expert operators and fully equipped units.

References

1. Cheng JL, Bruno MJ, Bergman JJ, Rauws EA, Tytgat GN, Huibregtse K. Endoscopic palliation of patients with biliary obstruction caused by nonresectable hilar cholangiocarcinoma: efficacy of self-expandable metallic wallstents. Gastrointest Endosc. 2002;56:33–9.
2. Juttijudata P, Chiemchalsri C, Palavatana C, Churnratanakul S. Causes of cholestasis in Thailand: a study of 276 consecutive patients. Am J Surg. 1984;147:360–6.
3. De Groen PC, Gores GJ, Larusso NF, Gunderson LL, Nagorney DM. Biliary tract cancers. N Engl J Med. 1999;341:1368–78.
4. Bismuth H, Castaing D, Traynor O. Resection or palliation: priority of surgery in the treatment of hilar cancer. World J Surg. 1988;12:39–47.
5. Uchida D, Kato H, Muro S, et al. Efficacy of endoscopic over 3-branched partial stent-in-stent drainage using self-expandable metallic stents in patients with unresectable hilar biliary carcinoma. J Clin Gastroenterol. 2015;49(6):529–36.
6. Deviere J, Baize M, de Toeuf J, Cremer M. Long-term follow-up of patients with hilar malignant stricture treated by endoscopic internal biliary drainage. Gastrointest Endosc. 1988;34:95–101.
7. Martin RC 2nd, Vitale GC, Reed DN, Larson GM, Edwards MJ, McMasters KM. Cost comparison of endoscopic stenting vs surgical treatment for unresectable cholangiocarcinoma. Surg Endosc. 2002;16:667–70.
8. Peters RA, Williams SG, Lombard M, Karani J, Westaby D. The management of high-grade hilar strictures by endoscopic insertion of self-expanding metal endoprostheses. Endoscopy. 1997;29:10–6.
9. Chahal P, Baron TH. Expandable metal stents for endoscopic bilateral stent-within-stent placement for malignant hilar biliary obstruction. Gastrointest Endosc. 2010;71:195–9.
10. Park DH, Lee SS, Moon JH, et al. Newly designed stent for endoscopic bilateral stent-in-stent placement of metallic stents in patients with malignant hilar biliary strictures: multicenter prospective feasibility study (with videos). Gastrointest Endosc. 2009;69:1357–60.
11. Stoker J, Lameris JS, van Blankenstein M. Percutaneous metallic self-expandable endoprostheses in malignant hilar biliary obstruction. Gastrointest Endosc. 1993;39:43–9.
12. Sawas T, Al Halabi S, Parsi MA, Vargo JJ. Self-expandable metal stents versus plastic stents for malignant biliary obstruction: a meta-analysis. Gastrointest Endosc. 2015;82:256–67 e7.
13. Perdue DG, Freeman ML, DiSario JA, et al. Plastic versus self-expanding metallic stents for malignant hilar biliary obstruction: a prospective multicenter observational cohort study. J Clin Gastroenterol. 2008;42:1040–6.
14. Sangchan A, Kongkasame W, Pugkhem A, Jenwitheesuk K, Mairiang P. Efficacy of metal and plastic stents in unresectable complex hilar cholangiocarcinoma: a randomized controlled trial. Gastrointest Endosc. 2012;76:93–9.
15. Wagner HJ, Knyrim K, Vakil N, Klose KJ. Plastic endoprostheses versus metal stents in the palliative treatment of malignant hilar biliary obstruction.

A prospective and randomized trial. Endoscopy. 1993;25:213–8.
16. Soehendra N, Reynders-Frederix V. Palliative bile duct drainage – a new endoscopic method of introducing a transpapillary drain. Endoscopy. 1980;12:8–11.
17. Itoi T, Sofuni A, Itokawa F, Tonozuka R, Ishii K. Current status and issues regarding biliary stenting in unresectable biliary obstruction. Dig Endosc. 2013;25 Suppl 2:63–70.
18. Itoi T, Kasuya K, Abe Y, Isayama H. Endoscopic placement of a new short-term biodegradable pancreatic and biliary stent in an animal model: a preliminary feasibility study (with videos). J Hepatobiliary Pancreat Sci. 2011;18:463–7.
19. Bismuth H. Surgical anatomy and anatomical surgery of the liver. World J Surg. 1982;6:3–9.
20. Fukasawa M, Takano S, Shindo H, Takahashi E, Sato T, Enomoto N. Endoscopic biliary stenting for unresectable malignant hilar obstruction. Clin J Gastroenterol. 2017;10:485–90.
21. Dowsett J, Vaira D, Hatfield A, et al. Endoscopic biliary therapy using the combined percutaneous and endoscopic technique. Gastroenterology. 1989;96:1180–6.
22. Vienne A, Hobeika E, Gouya H, et al. Prediction of drainage effectiveness during endoscopic stenting of malignant hilar strictures: the role of liver volume assessment. Gastrointest Endosc. 2010;72:728–35.
23. Takahashi E, Fukasawa M, Sato T, et al. Biliary drainage strategy of unresectable malignant hilar strictures by computed tomography volumetry. World J Gastroenterol: WJG. 2015;21:4946.
24. Rerknimitr R, Kladcharoen N, Mahachai V, Kullavanijaya P. Result of endoscopic biliary drainage in hilar cholangiocarcinoma. J Clin Gastroenterol. 2004;38:518–23.
25. De Palma GD, Galloro G, Siciliano S, Iovino P, Catanzano C. Unilateral versus bilateral endoscopic hepatic duct drainage in patients with malignant hilar biliary obstruction: results of a prospective, randomized, and controlled study. Gastrointest Endosc. 2001;53:547–53.
26. Chang W-H, Kortan P, Haber GB. Outcome in patients with bifurcation tumors who undergo unilateral versus bilateral hepatic duct drainage. Gastrointest Endosc. 1998;47:354–62.
27. Ducreux M, Liguory C, Lefebvre J, et al. Management of malignant hilar biliary obstruction by endoscopy results and prognostic factors. Dig Dis Sci. 1992;37:778–83.
28. Freeman ML, Overby C. Selective MRCP and CT-targeted drainage of malignant hilar biliary obstruction with self-expanding metallic stents. Gastrointest Endosc. 2003;58:41–9.
29. Mukai T, Yasuda I, Nakashima M, et al. Metallic stents are more efficacious than plastic stents in unresectable malignant hilar biliary strictures: a randomized controlled trial. J Hepatobiliary Pancreat Sci. 2013;20:214–22.
30. Rerknimitr R, Angsuwatcharakon P, Ratanachu-ek T, et al. Asia-Pacific consensus recommendations for endoscopic and interventional management of hilar cholangiocarcinoma. J Gastroenterol Hepatol. 2013;28:593–607.
31. Kato H, Tsutsumi K, Kawamoto H, Okada H. Current status of endoscopic biliary drainage for unresectable malignant hilar biliary strictures. World J Gastrointest Endosc. 2015;7:1032.
32. Valle J, Wasan H, Palmer DH, et al. Cisplatin plus gemcitabine versus gemcitabine for biliary tract cancer. N Engl J Med. 2010;362:1273–81.
33. Lee TH, Moon JH, Park SH. Bilateral metallic stenting in malignant hilar obstruction. Clin Endosc. 2014;47:440–6.
34. Inoue T, Naitoh I, Okumura F, et al. Reintervention for stent occlusion after bilateral self-expandable metallic stent placement for malignant hilar biliary obstruction. Dig Endosc. 2016;28:731–7.
35. Okabe Y, Ishida Y, Ushijima T, Sugiyama G, Sata M. Technique of reintervention for stent dysfunction in patients with malignant hilar biliary stricture. Dig Endosc. 2013;25(Suppl 2):90–3.
36. Naitoh I, Ohara H, Nakazawa T, et al. Unilateral versus bilateral endoscopic metal stenting for malignant hilar biliary obstruction. J Gastroenterol Hepatol. 2009;24:552–7.
37. De Palma GD, Pezzullo A, Rega M, et al. Unilateral placement of metallic stents for malignant hilar obstruction: a prospective study. Gastrointest Endosc. 2003;58:50–3.
38. Liberato MJA, Canena JMT. Endoscopic stenting for hilar cholangiocarcinoma: efficacy of unilateral and bilateral placement of plastic and metal stents in a retrospective review of 480 patients. BMC Gastroenterol. 2012;12:103.
39. Iwano H, Ryozawa S, Ishigaki N, et al. Unilateral versus bilateral drainage using self-expandable metallic stent for unresectable hilar biliary obstruction. Dig Endosc. 2011;23:43–8.
40. Lee TH, Kim TH, Moon JH, et al. Bilateral versus unilateral placement of metal stents for inoperable high-grade malignant hilar biliary strictures: a multicenter, prospective, randomized study (with video). Gastrointest Endosc. 2017;86:817–27.
41. Dumas R, Demuth N, Buckley M, et al. Endoscopic bilateral metal stent placement for malignant hilar stenoses: identification of optimal technique. Gastrointest Endosc. 2000;51:334–8.
42. Chennat J, Waxman I. Initial performance profile of a new 6F self-expanding metal stent for palliation of malignant hilar biliary obstruction. Gastrointest Endosc. 2010;72:632–6.
43. Lee TH, Park do H, Lee SS, et al. Technical feasibility and revision efficacy of the sequential deployment of endoscopic bilateral side-by-side metal stents for malignant hilar biliary strictures: a multicenter prospective study. Dig Dis Sci. 2013;58:547–55.
44. Kawamoto H, Tsutsumi K, Fujii M, et al. Multiple stenting in a patient with a high-grade malignant

hilar biliary stricture: endoscopic four-branched partial stent-in-stent deployment of metallic stents. Endoscopy. 2007;39(Suppl 1):E167–8.
45. Kim JY, Kang DH, Kim HW, et al. Usefulness of slimmer and open-cell-design stents for endoscopic bilateral stenting and endoscopic revision in patients with hilar cholangiocarcinoma (with video). Gastrointest Endosc. 2009;70:1109–15.
46. Kogure H, Isayama H, Nakai Y, et al. Newly designed large cell Niti-S stent for malignant hilar biliary obstruction: a pilot study. Surg Endosc. 2011;25:463–7.
47. Hwang JC, Kim JH, Lim SG, Kim SS, Yoo BM, Cho SW. Y-shaped endoscopic bilateral metal stent placement for malignant hilar biliary obstruction: prospective long-term study. Scand J Gastroenterol. 2011;46:326–32.
48. Lee T, Moon J, Kim J, et al. Primary and revision efficacy of cross-wired metallic stents for endoscopic bilateral stent-in-stent placement in malignant hilar biliary strictures. Endoscopy. 2013;45:106–13.
49. Naitoh I, Hayashi K, Nakazawa T, et al. Side-by-side versus stent-in-stent deployment in bilateral endoscopic metal stenting for malignant hilar biliary obstruction. Dig Dis Sci. 2012;57:3279–85.
50. Kim KM, Lee KH, Chung YH, et al. A comparison of bilateral stenting methods for malignant hilar biliary obstruction. Hepato-Gastroenterology. 2012;59:341–6.
51. Law R, Baron TH. Bilateral metal stents for hilar biliary obstruction using a 6Fr delivery system: outcomes following bilateral and side-by-side stent deployment. Dig Dis Sci. 2013;58:2667–72.
52. Lee JH, Kang DH, Kim JY, et al. Endoscopic bilateral metal stent placement for advanced hilar cholangiocarcinoma: a pilot study of a newly designed Y stent. Gastrointest Endosc. 2007;66:364–9.
53. Kawamoto H, Tsutsumi K, Fujii M, et al. Endoscopic 3-branched partial stent-in-stent deployment of metallic stents in high-grade malignant hilar biliary stricture (with videos). Gastrointest Endosc. 2007;66:1030–7.
54. Jang SI, Hwang JH, Lee KH, et al. Percutaneous biliary approach as a successful rescue procedure after failed endoscopic therapy for drainage in advanced hilar tumors. J Gastroenterol Hepatol. 2017;32:932–8.
55. Kawakubo K, Kawakami H, Kuwatani M, et al. Single-step simultaneous side-by-side placement of a self-expandable metallic stent with a 6-Fr delivery system for unresectable malignant hilar biliary obstruction: a feasibility study. J Hepatobiliary Pancreat Sci. 2015;22:151–5.
56. Mansfield SD, Barakat O, Charnley RM, et al. Management of hilar cholangiocarcinoma in the North of England: pathology, treatment, and outcome. World J Gastroenterol. 2005;11:7625–30.
57. Goenka MK, Goenka U. Palliation: hilar cholangiocarcinoma. World J Hepatol. 2014;6:559.
58. Kang MJ, Choi Y-S, Jang J-Y, Han IW, Kim S-W. Catheter tract recurrence after percutaneous biliary drainage for hilar cholangiocarcinoma. World J Surg. 2013;37:437–42.
59. Yoshida H, Tajiri T, Mamada Y, et al. One-step insertion of an expandable metallic stent for unresectable common bile duct carcinoma. J Nippon Med Sch. 2003;70:179–82.
60. Gwon DI, Ko G-Y, Kim JH, et al. Percutaneous bilateral metallic stent placement using a stentinstent deployment technique in patients with malignant hilar biliary obstruction. Am J Roentgenol. 2013;200:909–14.
61. Bae J-I, Park AW, Choi SJ, et al. Crisscross-configured dual stent placement for trisectoral drainage in patients with advanced biliary hilar malignancies. J Vasc Interv Radiol. 2008;19:1614–9.
62. Brountzos EN, Ptochis N, Panagiotou I, Malagari K, Tzavara C, Kelekis D. A survival analysis of patients with malignant biliary strictures treated by percutaneous metallic stenting. Cardiovasc Intervent Radiol. 2007;30:66–73.
63. Gwon DI, Ko GY, Kim JH, et al. Percutaneous bilateral metallic stent placement using a stentin-stent deployment technique in patients with malignant hilar biliary obstruction. AJR Am J Roentgenol. 2013;200:909–14.
64. Gwon DI, Ko GY, Yoon HK, et al. Safety and efficacy of percutaneous Y-configured covered stent placement for malignant hilar biliary obstruction: a prospective, pilot study. J Vasc Interv Radiol. 2012;23:528–34.
65. Gwon DI, Ko G-Y, Sung K-B, et al. Percutaneous biliary metallic stent placement in patients with unilobar portal vein occlusion caused by advanced hilar malignancy: outcome of unilateral versus bilateral stenting. Am J Roentgenol. 2011;197:795–801.
66. Kim CW, Park AW, Won JW, Kim S, Lee JW, Lee SH. T-configured dual stent placement in malignant biliary hilar duct obstructions with a newly designed stent. J Vasc Interv Radiol. 2004;15:713–7.
67. Dumonceau JM, Tringali A, Blero D, et al. Biliary stenting: indications, choice of stents and results: European Society of Gastrointestinal Endoscopy (ESGE) clinical guideline. Endoscopy. 2012;44:277–98.
68. Li M, Bai M, Qi X, et al. Percutaneous transhepatic biliary metal stent for malignant hilar obstruction: results and predictive factors for efficacy in 159 patients from a single center. Cardiovasc Intervent Radiol. 2015;38(3):709–21.
69. LaBerge JM, Doherty M, Gordon RL, Ring EJ. Hilar malignancy: treatment with an expandable metallic transhepatic biliary stent. Radiology. 1990;177:793–7.
70. Lee M, Dawson S, Mueller P, et al. Percutaneous management of hilar biliary malignancies with metallic endoprostheses: results, technical problems, and causes of failure. Radiographics. 1993;13:1249–63.
71. Inal M, Akgul E, Aksungur E, Seydaoglu G. Percutaneous placement of biliary metallic stents in patients with malignant hilar obstruction: unilobar versus bilobar drainage. J Vasc Interv Radiol. 2003;14:1409–16.
72. Cowling MG, Adam AN. Internal stenting in malignant biliary obstruction. World J Surg. 2001;25:355–8.

73. Kim KR, Kim JH, Park WK, et al. The effect of percutaneous bilateral metalic stent for hilar cholangiocarcinoma. Yeungnam Univ J Med. 2005;22:211–20.
74. Bulajic M, Panic N, Radunovic M, et al. Clinical outcome in patients with hilar malignant strictures type II Bismuth-Corlette treated by minimally invasive unilateral versus bilateral endoscopic biliary drainage. Hepatobiliary Pancreat Dis Int. 2012;11:209–14.
75. Devière J, Baize M, de Toeuf J, Cremer M. Long-term follow-up of patients with hilar malignant stricture treated by endoscopic internal biliary drainage. Gastrointest Endosc. 1988;34:95–101.
76. Inal M, Akgül E, Aksungur E, Seydaoğlu G. Percutaneous placement of biliary metallic stents in patients with malignant hilar obstruction: unilobar versus bilobar drainage. J Vasc Interv Radiol. 2003;14:1409–16.
77. Karnabatidis D, Spiliopoulos S, Katsakiori P, Romanos O, Katsanos K, Siablis D. Percutaneous trans-hepatic bilateral biliary stenting in Bismuth IV malignant obstruction. World J Hepatol. 2013;5:114.
78. Koh E, Jin GY, Hwang SB, et al. A comparison of Y-type and T-type metallic bilateral biliary stents in patients with malignant hilar biliary obstruction. J Korean Soc Radiol. 2013;68(4):297–303.
79. Hong HP, Kim SK, Seo T-S. Percutaneous metallic stents in patients with obstructive jaundice due to hepatocellular carcinoma. J Vasc Interv Radiol. 2008;19:748–54.
80. Sol YL, Kim CW, Jeon UB, et al. Early infectious complications of percutaneous metallic stent insertion for malignant biliary obstruction. Am J Roentgenol. 2010;194:261–5.
81. Stoker J, Lameris JS. Complications of percutaneously inserted biliary Wallstents. J Vasc Interv Radiol. 1993;4:767–72.
82. Jeon YS, Kim JH. T-configured dual stent placement in malignant biliary hilar obstruction: technique and clinical application. J Korean Soc Radiol. 2010;62:211–8.
83. Han Y-M, Jin G-Y, Lee S-O, Kwak H-S, Chung G-H. Flared polyurethane-covered self-expandable nitinol stent for malignant biliary obstruction. J Vasc Interv Radiol. 2003;14:1291–301.
84. Eum JS, Kang DH, Choi CW. A preliminary study on the usefullness of a zilver stent for bilateral stenting in patients withadvanced hilar cholangiocarcinoma. Korean J Gastrointest Endosc. 2008;36:354–60.
85. Kogure H, Isayama H, Kawakubo K, et al. Endoscopic bilateral metallic stenting for malignant hilar obstruction using newly designed stents. J Hepatobiliary Pancreat Sci. 2011;18:653–7.
86. Gwon DI, Ko GY, Yoon HK, et al. Prospective evaluation of a newly designed T-configured stent graft system for palliative treatment of advanced hilar malignant biliary obstructions. J Vasc Interv Radiol. 2010;21:1410–8.
87. Abdalla EK, Denys A, Chevalier P, Nemr RA, Vauthey J-N. Total and segmental liver volume variations: implications for liver surgery. Surgery. 2004;135:404–10.
88. Khan SA, Davidson BR, Goldin RD, et al. Guidelines for the diagnosis and treatment of cholangiocarcinoma: an update. Gut. 2012;61:1657–69.
89. Ohkubo M, Nagino M, Kamiya J, et al. Surgical anatomy of the bile ducts at the hepatic hilum as applied to living donor liver transplantation. Ann Surg. 2004;239:82.
90. Kawakami H, Itoi T, Kuwatani M, Kawakubo K, Kubota Y, Sakamoto N. Technical tips and troubleshooting of endoscopic biliary drainage for unresectable malignant hilar biliary obstruction. J Hepatobiliary Pancreat Sci. 2015;22:E12–21.
91. Hara T, Yamaguchi T, Sudo K, et al. Expansion of metallic mesh stent hole using a Soehendra stent retriever in multiple stenting of biliary hilar obstruction. Endoscopy. 2008;40(Suppl 2):E147–8.
92. Walter T, Ho CS, Horgan AM, et al. Endoscopic or percutaneous biliary drainage for Klatskin tumors? J Vasc Interv Radiol. 2013;24:113–21.
93. Paik WH, Park YS, Hwang JH, et al. Palliative treatment with self-expandable metallic stents in patients with advanced type III or IV hilar cholangiocarcinoma: a percutaneous versus endoscopic approach. Gastrointest Endosc. 2009;69:55–62.
94. Lee SS, Kim MH, Lee SK, et al. MR cholangiography versus cholangioscopy for evaluation of longitudinal extension of hilar cholangiocarcinoma. Gastrointest Endosc. 2002;56:25–32.
95. Wiggers JK, Groot Koerkamp B, Coelen RJ, et al. Preoperative biliary drainage in perihilar cholangiocarcinoma: identifying patients who require percutaneous drainage after failed endoscopic drainage. Endoscopy. 2015;47:1124–31.
96. Born P, Rosch T, Bruhl K, et al. Long-term outcome in patients with advanced hilar bile duct tumors undergoing palliative endoscopic or percutaneous drainage. Z Gastroenterol. 2000;38:483–9.

Palliative Therapy for Malignant Biliary Obstruction

8

Woo Hyun Paik, Dongwook Oh, and Do Hyun Park

Part I

Dongwook Oh and Do Hyun Park

Introduction

Malignant biliary obstruction results from various tumors such as pancreatic cancer, cholangiocarcinoma, and gallbladder cancer. Malignant biliary obstruction could contribute to poor clinical outcomes including cholangitis, delay in treatment, decreased quality of life, and increased mortality [1]. Palliative treatment with biliary stent placement is crucial to alleviate symptoms and potentially prevent adverse events [2].

Palliative biliary drainage can be performed by two methods: endoscopic stenting and percutaneous drainage. Currently, endoscopic biliary drainage is preferred because of minimal invasiveness, less mortality, shorter hospitalization period, and recent progress in endoscopic devices [3]. Current guidelines recommend endoscopic biliary drainage rather than percutaneous approach in terms of quality of life, adverse events, shorter hospitalization, and lower total costs [4]. Therefore, transpapillary stent placement with endoscopic retrograde cholangiopancreatography (ERCP) has become the standard of care for malignant biliary obstruction. However, the presence of duodenal obstruction that can occur in later stages of malignancy or surgically altered anatomy often preclude accessing bile duct with ERCP [5]. With recent advance endoscopic ultrasound (EUS), transmural stent placement under EUS guidance has emerged as an alternative procedure to percutaneous biliary drainage after failed ERCP [6]. Here, we review both established and emerging areas of EUS and ERCP in the management of palliative malignant biliary obstruction.

Choice of Biliary Stent for Endoscopic Drainage

Currently, two types of biliary stents are available for biliary drainage: plastic stents (PSs) and self-expandable metal stents (SEMSs) (Fig. 8.1). SEMSs can be either uncovered or covered with material to prevent tumor ingrowth [7]. Several factors could affect the choice of biliary stent such as life expectancy, presence of distant metastasis, cause/site/length of malignant stricture, diameter of bile duct, site of the cystic duct,

W. H. Paik
Department of Internal Medicine, Seoul National University Hospital, Seoul National University College of Medicine, Seoul, South Korea

D. Oh · D. H. Park (✉)
Division of Gastroenterology, Department of Internal Medicine, Asan Medical Center, University of Ulsan College of Medicine, Seoul, South Korea
e-mail: dhpark@amc.seoul.kr

D. K. Lee (ed.), *Advanced ERCP for Complicated and Refractory Biliary and Pancreatic Diseases*,
https://doi.org/10.1007/978-981-13-0608-2_8

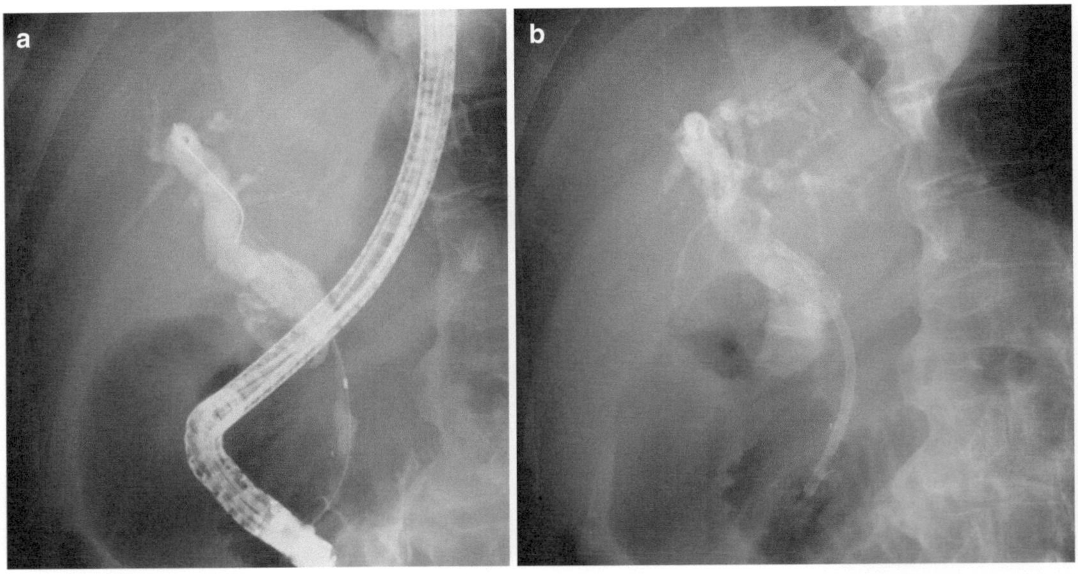

Fig. 8.1 A 63-year-old man with pancreatic adenocarcinoma developed biliary obstruction due to common bile duct invasion. (**a**) There is a common bile duct stricture with dilatation of proximal bile duct. (**b**) A plastic biliary stent is inserted with satisfactory position

tumor involvement of the pancreatic duct, or future treatment [3]. Theoretically, SEMSs have a larger lumen (6–10 mm) compared with PSs (5–10 Fr), and SEMS may have several advantages over a PS, such as prolonged stent patency, fewer repeat interventions, and decreased hospital stays [8].

For the management of distal biliary obstruction, current guidelines recommend the placement of SEMS rather than that of PS for palliative drainage [4, 9]. Although the technical success rates for SEMSs and PSs were similar, SEMSs showed longer stent patency, lower adverse event rates, and fewer re-interventions as compared with PSs [10]. Different types of SEMS including covered SEMSs (CSEMSs) and uncovered SEMSs (USEMSs) can be used in palliative cases. USEMSs have a mesh design that allows them to embed in the biliary duct wall, but it also makes them susceptible to tissue ingrowth, which can lead to occlusion in as many as 20% of patients. CSEMSs were designed to prevent tissue ingrowth, but because of this they are known to have increased rates of migration (Fig. 8.2) [11]. Several studies have demonstrated the trade-off between tissue ingrowth in USEMS and migration in CSEMS. Due to the downside of each USEMS and CSEMS, there was no advantage of CSEMS, compared with UCSEMS, in terms of the proportion of stent dysfunction, overall adverse events, or patent survival (Table 8.1) [12, 13].

The types of stents used for drainage in hilar biliary stricture include PSs and SEMSs. In patients with malignant hilar biliary strictures, CSEMSs are not indicated because they would block the contralateral hepatic duct and intrahepatic side branches and potentially cause cholangitis [11]. The median patency of PS is 1.4–3 months, whereas a larger diameter SEMS provides a longer patency at 6–10 months [14]. Several studies demonstrated that USEMS placement for palliative treatment of hilar biliary obstruction seems to be superior to PS placement in terms of stent patency, adverse events, and reintervention [15–17]. USEMSs seem to be better stents for palliative endoscopic drainage as compared to PSs. Based on these results, therefore, SEMS placement is recommended in patients with a predicted survival of longer than 3 months for palliation with respect to clinical outcomes in Asia-Pacific consensus [14].

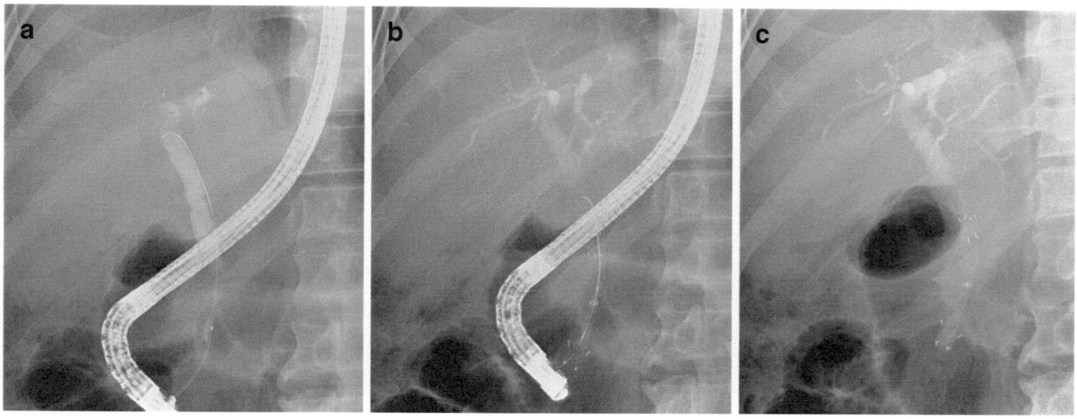

Fig. 8.2 A 53-year-old man was diagnosed with pancreatic adenocarcinoma (**a**) ERCP shows a distal common bile duct stricture. (**b**) A single fully covered self-expandable metal stent was inserted. (**c**) Final image after deployment of the stent

Stent dysfunction is inevitable regardless of stent types. For plastic stents, the development of biofilm and bacterial colonization is the most important factor [18]. SEMSs have been developed to overcome the limitations of plastic stents such as early occlusion due to small caliber of plastic stents, but SEMSs can still occlude [19]. For USEMS, tissue ingrowth through the mesh interstices at the level of the tumor remains the most likely source of occlusion. The occlusion or dysfunction of fully CSEMS may occur due to stent migration, overgrowth of tissue at the ends of the stent, cholecystitis due to covering of cystic duct by CSEMS or accompanying tumor invasion of cystic duct, or food debris [1]. Therefore, clinicians should know the characteristics of each stent and be able to choose the best stent for the situation.

The diagnosis of stent dysfunction has not been standardized. It is usually based on the combination of clinical criteria and liver function tests, complemented with transabdominal ultrasound in some cases. Recent studies have mostly used paraclinical tests, as in the study by Schmidt et al. who defined stent dysfunction as the presence of two of the three following criteria: (a) ultrasound showing new dilatation of intrahepatic or extrahepatic bile ducts, (b) bilirubin ≥2 mg/dL (34.2 μmol/L) with an increase ≥1 mg/dL (17.1 μmol/L) compared to the value after initial successful drainage or elevation of alkaline phosphatases/gamma-glutamyl transferase to more than twice the upper limit of normal values with an increase of at least 30 U/L, and (c) signs of cholangitis (fever and leukocyte count >10,000 μL^{-1} or C-reactive protein (CRP) >20 mg/dL) [4, 20]. According to ESGE guidelines, when stent dysfunction occurred in patients with plastic stents, a plastic stent should be replaced by a SEMS. In cases of SEMSs, a plastic stent or a new SEMS should be inserted within the original SEMS [4].

Necessity of Endoscopic Sphincterotomy for Biliary Stent Placement

Endoscopic sphincterotomy (EST) has been performed as a way to prevent pancreatitis after stent placement by reducing tension at the pancreatic duct orifice [21]. In addition, EST has been considered to ease the deployment of stent. However, EST has flaws such as bleeding and stent migration [22]. In a meta-analysis by Cui et al., EST before stent placement was associated with a lower rate of pancreatitis (OR, 0.34; 95% CI, 0.12–0.93), but a higher rate of bleeding (OR, 9.70; 95% CI, 1.21–77.75) [23]. A recent study by Hayashi et al. revealed that EST in patients with nonresectable pancreatic cancer has no benefit for preventing pancreatitis [24].

Table 8.1 Meta-analyses comparison of covered and uncovered self-expandable metal stents for distal biliary obstruction

Author, year	Included studies	Number of patients (USEMS/CSEMS)	Stent patency	Overall adverse events	Tumor in growth	Tumor over growth	Stent migration	Cholecystitis	Pancreatitis
Saleem et al., 2011 [12]	5 RCTs	781 (386/395)	WMD 60.56 days (95% CI 25.96–95.17), higher in CSEMS	NA	RR 0.23 (95% CI 0.08–0.67), lower in CSEMS	RR 2.03 (95% CI 1.08–3.78), higher in CSEMS	RR 8.11 (95% CI 1.47–44.75), higher in CSEMS	RR 1.27 (95% CI 0.41–3.92), no difference in both groups	RR 1.27 (95% CI 0.25–6.39), no difference in both groups
Almadi et al., 2013 [13]	9 RCTs	1061 (522/539)	6 months: OR 1.82 (95% CI 0.63–5.25) 12 months: OR 1.25 (95% CI 0.65–2.39), no difference in both groups	NA	OR 0.19 (95% CI 0.07–0.55), lower in CSEMS	OR 1.88 (9% CI 1.02–3.45), higher in CSEMS	OR 7.13 (95% CI 0.44–25.9), higher in CSEMS	NA	OR 1.07 (95% CI 0.44–2.59), no difference in both groups
Yang et al., 2013 [88]	5 RCTs	781 (386/395)	HR 0.73, (95% CI 0.41–1.32), no difference in both groups	NA	RR 0.21 (95% CI 0.06–0.69), lower in CSEMS	RR 2.03 (95% CI 1.08–3.78), higher in CSEMS	RR 8.11 (95% CI 1.47–44.76), higher in CSEMS		
Chen et al., 2016 [89]	6 RCTs, 2 retrospective	1067 (533/524)		HR 0.87 (95% CI 0.58–1.30), no difference in both groups	OR 0.74 (0.57–0.97), lower in CSEMS	NA	NA	NA	NA
Li et al., 2016 [90]	14 RCTs	1417 (700/717)	HR 0.93 (95% CI 0.19–4.53), no difference in both groups	RR 1.26 (95% CI 0.94–1.68), no difference in both groups	RR 0.25 (95% CI 0.12–0.52), lower in CSEMS	RR 1.76 (95% CI 1.03–3.02), higher in CSEMS	RR 9.33 (95% CI 2.54–34.24), higher in CSEMS	NA	NA

USEMS uncovered self-expandable metal stent, *CSEMS* covered self-expandable metal stent, *RCT* randomized controlled trial, *WMD* weighted mean difference, *NA* not available

However, in patients with hilar obstruction, limited data are available on the outcome of ES before stent placement. In a retrospective study by Tarnasky et al., post-procedure pancreatitis after stent placement was frequently observed in patients with proximal CBD obstruction without EST (four of 24 patients) compared to those with distal or no stricture (0 of 59 patients) [25]. In a randomized controlled study by Zhou et al., patients with proximal bile duct obstruction showed a higher incidence of PEP among patients who did not undergo EST [26]. Therefore, prospective studies are warranted to compare the outcomes of EST before stent placement.

Position of Distal End of Stent: Transpapillary vs. Suprapapillary Stent Placement

It has been postulated that stent insertion where the distal tip remains above the papilla could prevent the reflux of bacteria and undigested materials into the biliary system and the stent and thus contribute to prolonged patency [11]. In a randomized trial by Pedersen et al., there was no difference in stent patency in terms of plastic stent placement [27]. In cases with SEMS placement, transpapillary stent placement was the most significant factor for cholangitis after SEMS placement [28]. Thus, further prospective comparative studies are mandatory.

Optimal Endoscopic Drainage of Malignant Hilar Stricture

Endoscopic drainage for malignant hilar stricture remains challenging with no definite consensus on the optimal approach. There has been considerable debate with respect to optimal type of stent, drainage area (unilateral or bilateral drainage), and bilateral metal stenting method [stent-in-stent (SIS) or side-by-side (SBS)]. Currently, there was no clear consensus on the best endoscopic drainage method for performing unilateral or bilateral stenting in patients with hilar obstruction. Although unilateral drainage is technically easier than bilateral drainage, bilateral drainage is more physiological and has superiority in drainage liver volume compared with unilateral stenting [7]. Before biliary drainage, appropriate pre-ERCP mapping of the site of obstruction is important. At least, a unilateral drainage procedure should be performed if only one side is opacified. In experienced centers, if the endoscopist has confidence in its success or if both sides have been injected with contrast, bilateral biliary drainage should be performed [11].

With recent advancement of dedicated SEMS for hilar drainage, bilateral SEMS placement demonstrated the relatively high success rate, regardless of bilateral stenting method. Currently, there was no consensus for the optimal method performing bilateral SEMS deployment. SBS method has become easier with the availability of small-diameter delivery catheters that can be passed simultaneously in a standard therapeutic channel duodenoscope and permit simultaneous SEMS deployment [4, 29]. On the one hand, a concern in the SBS method is overexpansion of the stricture and distal bile duct by two SEMSs. The excessive expansion force of two SEMSs can cause severe pain, acute cholecystitis, and occlusion of the portal vein [30]. On the other hand, SIS method is suitable for nondilated bile ducts due to avoiding excessive expansion of the bile duct. Recent meta-analysis showed similar results between SIS and SBS methods in terms of technical success, successful drainage, adverse events, and stent patency [31]. Therefore, further well-designed large-scale studies comparing these methods are warranted.

Endoscopic Biliary Stenting in Patients with Duodenal Obstruction

Patients with periampullary cancer are often diagnosed at the advanced stage and are not suitable for surgical treatment. In these patients, malignant duodenal obstruction frequently develops concomitant biliary obstruction and require biliary intervention as their malignancies progresses [32]. In the past, the standard treatment for duodenal obstruction was bypass gastrojejunostomy. As the development of endoscopically placed SEMS, endoscopic duodenal stenting has been increasingly used for palliative treatment.

Combined biliary obstruction and duodenal obstruction is categorized according to the location and sequences. Type 1 strictures occur in the first part of the duodenum without involvement of the papilla. Type 2 strictures affect the second part of the duodenum with involvement of the ampullary region. Type 3 strictures occur in the third part of the duodenum distal to and without involvement of the major papilla [33]. Of the three types of malignant biliary-duodenal obstruction, technical difficulty to achieve successful combined biliary and duodenal palliation is least in patients with type 3 duodenal stenosis, while type 1 is intermediate and type 2 is the most technically difficult [34].

In patients with type 1 duodenal obstruction, biliary stent placement could be achieved by passage of a side-viewing duodenoscope through the duodenal obstruction. However, it may be difficult and have a risk of duodenal perforation [35]. Duodenal stricture can be dilated using a balloon before biliary stent placement. However, bleeding or luminal edema resulting from duodenal dilation can interfere with biliary stent placement [36]. If the duodenoscope cannot be passed through the stricture despite balloon dilation, a duodenal stent is placed across the stricture. It is important that the duodenal stent be placed with the distal end positioned proximal to the level of the major papilla to allow the bile duct to be accessed [34]. If the duodenoscope cannot be passed through the duodenal stent lumen because of inadequate stent expansion, then balloon dilation of the duodenal stent may be needed.

Biliary stenting is challenging in patient with type 2 duodenal obstruction. In type 2 duodenal obstruction, duodenal obstruction is often preceded by or simultaneous with biliary obstruction [37]. Because major papilla can be compromised by covered SEMS in type 2 duodenal obstruction, uncovered duodenal SEMS may be preferred. Identification or cannulation of duodenal papilla is often difficult because the major papilla is not endoscopically identifiable due to extensive tumor infiltration. Although successful cannulation of the papilla through the mesh of a duodenal stent is difficult, biliary stent placement may be achieved after duodenal stent placement [36]. In previous studies, various methods such as removal of stent wires with forceps, argon plasma coagulation to melt stent struts, and balloon dilatation of the stent interstices for facilitating biliary access have been performed, but are not always successful and require a very technically demanding and lengthy procedure [33, 38].

For biliary stent placement in type 3 duodenal obstruction, biliary drainage is easier than type 1 or type 2 obstruction. The tumor encases the bile duct causing biliary obstruction and extends inferiorly causing duodenal obstruction below the level of the major papilla [34]. Duodenoscope can be reached to the major papilla, and it is not necessary to pass the duodenoscope beyond the duodenal obstruction. When the proximal level of the duodenal obstruction is close to the major papilla, it is better to avoid placing the duodenal stent across the papilla so that biliary access is preserved both at the time of the initial biliary stenting and reintervention for stent occlusion.

A recent study revealed that endoscopic biliary cannulation was difficult (13/38, 34.2%) in patients with biliary obstruction and a papilla obscured by a preexisting duodenal stent [39]. In a more recent study that included 71 cases with combined duodenal and biliary obstruction who underwent ERCP through a previously placed enteral stent, the technical success rate in patients with type 2 duodenal obstruction (16/21, 76%) was lower than in patients with type 1 (40/46, 87%) or type 3 (4/4, 100%) obstruction [40]. If the biliary drainage cannot be accessed through a transpapillary approach after duodenal stent placement, then biliary access can be achieved using a percutaneous or EUS approach.

Part II

Woo Hyun Paik and Do Hyun Park

EUS-Guided Biliary Drainage for Malignant Biliary Obstruction

EUS-guided biliary drainage (EUS-BD) has been introduced as an alternative treatment option to percutaneous transhepatic biliary drainage (PTBD) after failed ERCP [41, 42]. EUS-BD may be advantageous over ERCP or PTBD as follows: (1) ERCP is impossible when the papilla is not accessible with endoscopy; however, EUS-BD is possible even in surgically altered anatomy or inaccessible papilla. (2) One of the most common and serious adverse events of ERCP is procedure-related acute pancreatitis. In EUS-BD, traumatic papillary manipulation that can lead to acute pancreatitis could be prevented. (3) The stent patency might be longer in EUS-BD than in ERCP because the stents are not needed to be deployed across the stricture site [6, 43]. EUS-BD shows similar efficacy compared to PTBD when performed by expertise and may be more comfortable and physiologic to the patients than PTBD because EUS-BD is an internal drainage [43]. However, EUS-BD remains limited because of the complexity of this procedure and lack of dedicated device for EUS-BD.

Types of EUS-BD

EUS-BD implies three different approaches to the bile duct: rendezvous technique, antegrade stenting, and transmural stenting (Fig. 8.3) [42]. The accessibility to the papilla should be considered first. If the papilla is accessible with endoscopy, rendezvous technique may be preferred. EUS-guided rendezvous technique is available when the ampulla is endoscopically accessible and ERCP with selective cannulation of the bile duct fails. However, in rendezvous technique, negotiating guidewire to pass through the ampulla is sometimes difficult. When the guidewire traverses through the papilla with transgastric intrahepatic approach, antegrade stenting may be available. Antegrade stenting is useful especially when the papilla is inaccessible with endoscopy. When all these approaches fail, transmural stenting should be considered, and the transmural stenting usually has two methods: hepaticogastrostomy and choledochoduodenostomy. EUS-guided choledochoduodenostomy (EUS-CDS) may be technically easier than EUS-guided hepaticogastrostomy (EUS-HGS). EUS-HGS has many more types of adverse events than EUS-CDS, and it has potential risk of life-threatening adverse events including peritoneal stent migration, mediastinitis, and pneumomediastinum [44]. EUS-CDS may be more vulnerable to bile leak than EUS-HGS. In cases of surgically altered anatomy or duodenal obstruction, hepaticogastrostomy may be considered first. In patients with acute cholecystitis and high risk of surgery, EUS-guided gallbladder drainage (EUS-GBD) may be considered. In addition, EUS-GBD can be a possible alternative route for decompression of the bile duct when ERCP fails and biliary ducts are not dilated enough [45].

Indication of EUS-BD

The first indication of EUS-BD is when selective deep cannulation of the bile duct with ERCP fails. EUS-BD has the advantage that it can be performed directly by the same operator if ERCP fails. EUS-BD can be considered initially when

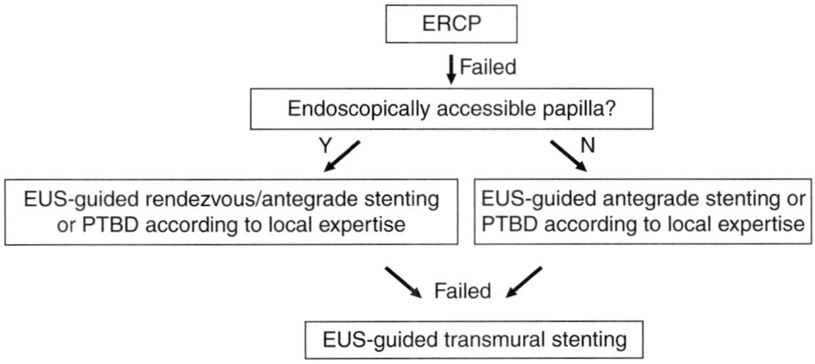

Fig. 8.3 Treatment algorithm for malignant biliary obstruction

surgically altered anatomy or duodenal obstruction is accompanied. Recently, primary palliation of cholestasis with EUS-BD instead of ERCP in malignant biliary obstruction has been introduced, and the indication of EUS-BD is expected to expand gradually [6]. Regarding the level of biliary obstruction, distal biliary obstruction may be easily resolved by EUS-BD. In terms of hilar biliary obstruction, drainage of the left intrahepatic duct is more appropriate with EUS-BD. Drainage of right intrahepatics is challenging with EUS-BD; however, several techniques such as bridging method (insertion of uncovered metal stent between the right and left intrahepatics to across the hilum and then insertion of covered metal stent as EUS-HGS) or hepaticoduodenostomy have been introduced [46, 47]. EUS-BD is contraindicated when bleeding tendency or uncorrected coagulopathy is present.

Preparation Prior to EUS-BD

Antibiotic prophylaxis is required before EUS-BD. There is no consensus about fasting time in EUS-BD; however, we recommend fasting time as minimal 4–6 h before the procedure. EUS-BD can be performed under conscious sedation or general anesthesia. If there is gastric outlet obstruction, then longer fasting time would be required to prevent peritonitis by remnant food. CO_2 insufflation during the procedure is recommended to reduce the risk of pneumoperitoneum [48]. Puncture of the bile duct can be performed with conventional 19-G EUS-guided fine needle aspiration needle. Recently, novel needle for EUS-BD (EUS access needle, Cook Medical, Bloomington, USA) has been developed, and it has blunt needle tip that can prevent shearing the coating off guidewires.

EUS-BD is performed under a real-time imaging with curvilinear array echoendoscope and fluoroscopy. Selection of a guidewire is important in EUS-BD, and a 0.025-in. VisiGlide guidewire (Olympus America, San Jose, USA) is preferred in EUS-BD because of its adequate stiffness and improved negotiation capability. Sometimes, 0.035-in. guidewires (Jagwire, Boston Scientific, Natick, USA; Tracer, Cook Medical) may be useful. Diluted contrast is used in EUS-BD to facilitate the visualization of the guidewires. When guidewire negotiation is difficult, 4 Fr cannula can be used to advance a guidewire through the fistula and into the intrahepatics.

Fistula dilation can be performed with 4 Fr cannula, 6 and 7 Fr bougie catheter, 4-mm balloon catheter (Hurricane RX, Boston Scientific), needle knife, and 6 Fr cystotome (Cook Medical). The use of a needle knife for fistula dilation is not recommended for the risk of adverse events including pneumoperitoneum and bleeding [49].

In EUS-BD, fully covered or partially covered metal stents are superior to plastic stents in terms of bile leak. To prevent stent migration, several types of metal stents with flared end, uncovered portion at the bile duct side, flaps, or flanges have been developed. In addition, the use of a lumen-apposing self-expandable metal stent for EUS-CDS or EUS-guided gallbladder drainage has been reported. In EUS-HGS, longer stents are favored to prevent proximal and distal migration. Recently, a novel dedicated device for one-step EUS-BD without additional fistula dilation has been introduced, which may result in shortened procedural time with less procedure-related adverse events [50].

EUS-BD Protocol

Rendezvous Technique

The extra- or intrahepatics are accessed with EUS needle. The extrahepatic approach may be preferred because intrahepatic approach requires more difficult guidewire manipulation that has to pass through the stricture site and the papilla. The extrahepatic bile duct can be assessed by two methods: push and pull. Although pull methods have more unstable scope position than push methods, negotiation of guidewire across the papilla is easier with pull methods. The intrahepatics can be approached via B2 or B3 duct. Because B2 duct is less angulated than B3, B2 is preferred over B3. After puncturing the bile duct, a small amount of bile juice is aspirated to confirm the bile duct access. Contrast is injected to obtain cholangiography, and then a guidewire negotiates a stricture site and pass through the papilla in an antegrade manner. Guidewire manipulation is the most difficult step in rendezvous technique. Coiling of the guidewire inside the duodenum is necessary to prevent loss of guidewire during withdrawal of the needle and the echoendoscope. After removal of the EUS needle and echoendoscope, conventional duodenoscope is intubated into the duodenum. Usually, selective deep cannulation of the bile duct is possible following the existing guidewire; however, when this method fails, the loops of guidewire is caught with a biopsy forceps or snare, and then the guidewire is pulled through the working channel, and the catheter or sphincterotome is inserted along the guidewire. The rendezvous technique may be the safest way in EUS-BD; however, this technique is cumbersome and time consuming.

Antegrade Stenting

The initial steps of antegrade stenting are similar to those of rendezvous technique. With a 19-G EUS needle, the intrahepatics are punctured and cholangiogram is obtained. The intrahepatics B2 may be preferred than B3 because B2 is usually more straightened. After guidewire manipulation passes across the stricture site and the papilla, a couple of loops of guidewire are placed inside the duodenum, and then the needle and the echoendoscope are withdrawn. A 4-mm balloon catheter is useful for dilatation of the papilla and stricture site to facilitate advancement of the stent delivery system. Lastly, the biliary metal stents are placed along the guidewire in an antegrade manner. To prevent the bile leak at the puncture site, 5 Fr nasobiliary drainage may be placed temporally. Usually, an uncovered metal stent is placed in EUS-guided antegrade transpapillary stenting. Therefore, stent dysfunction related to tumor ingrowth may occur. EUS-guided HGS with transmural stenting may be performed in the same session of EUS-guided antegrade stenting because of possible stent revision via fistula tract maintained by HGS stenting.

Transmural Drainage

As previously mentioned, EUS-CDS and EUS-HGS are two main methods in EUS-guided transmural drainage. Sometimes, EUS-guided choledochoantrostomy or hepaticoduodenostomy could be available. The basic steps of EUS-guided transmural drainage are as follows: accessing the biliary system with EUS needle, injection of contrast media for cholangiography, guidewire manipulation, fistula dilatation, and stent deployment.

When performing EUS-CDS, long scope position is preferred because it guides the direction of needle toward hilum of the liver and facilitates guidewire manipulation. Because the common bile duct runs parallel to the portal vein, it is easy to identify the common bile duct on EUS. Before puncturing the bile duct, color Doppler imaging can be used to identify the intervening vasculature. After confirming access of the common bile duct by aspiration of bile juice, radiocontrast is administered to obtain cholangiography. Then, a guidewire is manipulated to be placed into the intrahepatics, and EUS needle is removed gently. During guidewire negotiation, excessive manipulation may cause shearing of guidewire coating. Fistula tract is dilated to facilitate the advancement of stent delivery system. Mechanical dilation is preferred over cautery dilation due to safety issue. A 4-mm hurricane balloon catheter is preferred over sequential dilatation with a 4 Fr cannula and bougie catheter because sequential dilatation lengthens procedural time and may cause separation between the bile duct and the duodenum. In EUS-CDS, the length of metal stent is mainly 5–6 cm. After inserting stent delivery system, stent deployment should be performed under EUS and fluoroscopic guidance rather than endoscopic view. It is important to attach the tip of echoendoscope to the duodenum to prevent stent migration or displacement of echoendoscope. Finally, flows of bile juice from the stent placed in the duodenum can be seen by endoscopic view (Fig. 8.4).

For successful EUS-HGS, the puncture site should be selected carefully. At the optimal access point, the intrahepatics runs from the upper left to the lower right on EUS imaging, and the diameter of the intrahepatics is more than 5 mm and the length is more than 1 cm [51]. B3 is preferred over B2 to prevent puncturing from the esophagus. B3 puncture is usually achieved in the lesser curvatures of stomach body; thus, during deployment, the tip of the stent in the stomach can be verified, and stent migration can be prevented. A guidewire negotiates toward the liver hilum. When the guidewire is advanced into the peripheral biliary tract, liver impaction method that withdraws the EUS needle into the hepatic parenchyma can prevent guidewire kinking with the EUS needle [52]. Fistula dilation is performed the same way as EUS-CDS. In terms of stent deployment, the front one-half of a metal stent is deployed under EUS and fluoroscopic guidance, and then the remaining is deployed inside the working channel to stabilize the position of the echoendoscope. Finally, the scope is pulled out gently, and this stent deployment technique may secure the stable position of the metal stent and shorten the distance between the liver parenchyma and the stomach (Fig. 8.5) [53]. To prevent stent migration by shortening of the stent, a long stent of 10 cm or more and over 3 cm of gastric ends is recommended in EUS-HGS.

EUS-guided gallbladder drainage (EUS-GBD) is useful in patients with acute cholecystitis caused by malignant cystic duct obstruction who are not suitable for surgery [54]. In addition, EUS-GBD could be a potential alternative treatment for decompression of the biliary obstruction when ERCP fails and the bile duct is not dilated [45].

When Duodenal Obstruction Is Accompanied

The duodenal obstruction is often accompanied in malignant biliary obstruction, and ERCP and stent placement are challenging in these cases. When the ampulla of Vater is inaccessible with endoscopy or ERCP fails because of the duodenal obstruction, EUS-BD may be a good rescue method for the palliation of malignant biliary obstruction. If the patient has obstructive symptoms related to duodenal obstruction, duodenal stenting may be preceded before EUS-BD. And then, EUS-BD with transmural approach is preferred to rendezvous technique or antegrade approach. Rendezvous technique is not available in patients with type 1 duodenal obstruction. Antegrade stenting may be very difficult in patients with type 2 duodenal obstruction since negotiation of guidewire passing through the ampulla of Vater invaded by tumors may be challenging. Comparing EUS-CDS and EUS-HGS in patients with duodenal obstruction, EUS-HGS might be preferred to EUS-CDS, where EUS-CDS has more chances to occur duodenobiliary reflux and food impaction as sump syndrome because of the accompanying duodenal obstruction [55].

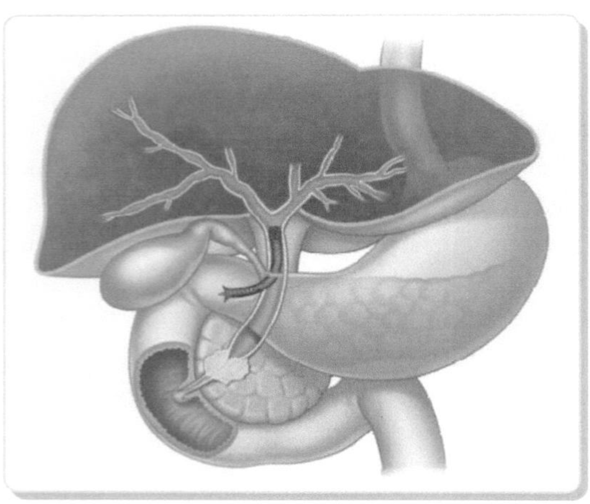

Fig. 8.4 EUS-guided choledochoduodenostomy

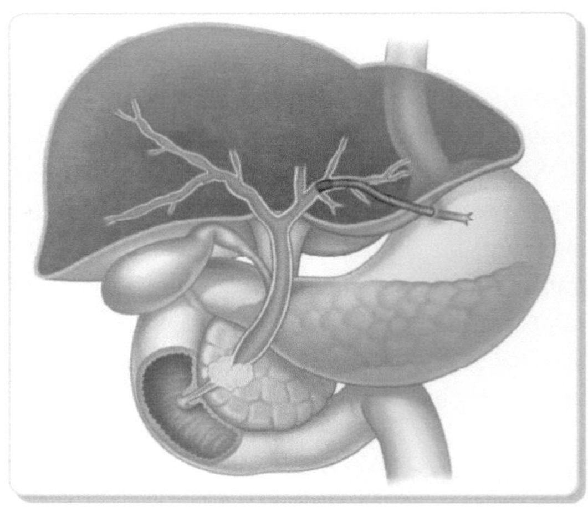

Fig. 8.5 EUS-guided hepaticogastrostomy

Part III

Woo Hyun Paik, Dongwook Oh, and
Do Hyun Park

Palliative Local Ablation Therapy for Malignant Biliary Tract Cancers

Complete radical resection is the only way to achieve potential cure in malignant biliary tract cancers. However, patients with malignant biliary tract cancers usually present at an advanced stage, with more than 50% being unresectable at the initial diagnosis [56]. Therefore, the two alternative treatment modalities, photodynamic therapy (PDT) and radiofrequency ablation (RFA), have been developed to improve survival or stent patency in malignant biliary obstruction.

Photodynamic Therapy (PDT)

Basics of PDT

Cholangiocarcinoma is characterized by a relatively slow growth rate and a low propensity for metastasis than other tumors [56]. Hematogenous spread of cholangiocarcinoma is rare; therefore, a local ablative therapy may play an important role. Painless jaundice by biliary obstruction is usually accompanied in these patients, and successful palliation of biliary obstruction remains the main goal for reducing morbidity and mortality in patients with unresectable cholangiocarcinoma [57].

PDT is based on the relatively specific accumulation of photosensitizers in malignant cells. After intravenous administration of a photosensitizing agent, it is activated by irradiating light of a specific wavelength to cause ischemic necrosis proportional to tissue oxygenation [57]. The mechanisms of tissue necrosis by PDT are as follows: (1) direct cytotoxic effects on tumor cells, (2) ischemic necrosis due to the sensitivity of tumor microvessels to PDT, and (3) induction of inflammatory reaction that leads to the development of systemic immunity [58]. Photoradiation is usually performed by ERCP (Fig. 8.6) and sometimes by percutaneous approach. The laser fiber for photoactivation is a 3 m length having a 3–4 cm cylindrical diffuse with radiopaque markers on both sides of the diffuser. After advancing a catheter across the biliary stricture, the cylindrical diffuser is inserted into a catheter at the level of the malignant stricture to be treated. The catheter has a transparent shaft to allow a light delivery from laser fiber inside the catheter while preventing the loaded laser fiber from breaking. When the length of the tumor exceeds the maximal diffuse length, overlap of treated fields was avoided by a stepwise pullback of the fiber under fluoroscopic guidance. Because the laser fiber is stiff and vulnerable, care should be taken not to be broken during the procedure. After PDT, usually plastic biliary stents are placed across the treated site. PDT imparts prolonged photosensitivity and requires patients to avoid sunlight for at least 4 weeks. The PDT is recommended to be repeated every 3 months because mean thickness of the tumor increases at 4 months after PDT [59].

Indication of PDT

PDT with biliary stenting has been used for palliative local treatment for unresectable biliary cancers. Cholangiocarcinoma can be classified into three categories according to the macroscopic growth pattern: periductal infiltrating type, mass-forming type, and intraductal growth type [60]. The tumoricidal effect of PDT is limited to the superficial 4–4.5 mm depth of the tumor wall; therefore, mass-forming type and large intraductal papillary growing type may be less effective in PDT. Because the depth of energy transfer through the PDT is limited, the effect of PDT may be achieved through temporary improvement of cholestasis by recanalization of the bile duct wall rather than complete tumor ablation [61]. Therefore, the appropriate indication of PDT may be (1) periductal infiltrating type without hematogenous metastasis regardless of nodal metastasis, (2) superficial intraductal

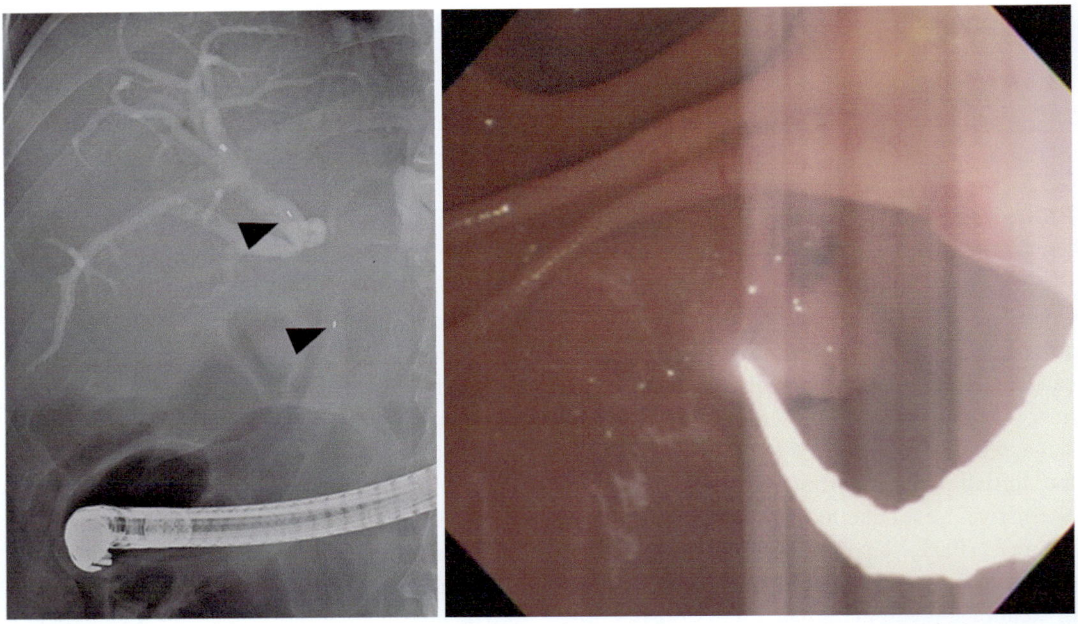

Fig. 8.6 Photodynamtic therapy in hilar cholangiocarcinoma. The radiopaque markers are located at the stricture site (black arrowheads) under fluoroscopic guidance with ERCP, and light is emitted from the laser fiber

growth type, and (3) R1 resection margin after surgery [56]. Contraindications to PDT include porphyria, recent use of photosensitizing agents, severe cytopenia, and presence of severe hepatic or renal dysfunction [62].

Clinical Outcomes of PDT

To date, clinical trials of PDT in biliary tract cancer are lacking because these cancers are rare diseases and have heterogeneous biological behaviors according to the location of the tumors. In most controlled and uncontrolled clinical studies, the PDT not only delays bile duct obstruction but also improves survival [57, 63–65]. Most clinical studies about PDT were aimed at delaying bile duct obstruction rather than reducing the tumor. PDT with biliary stenting was superior to stenting alone in patients with unresectable hilar cholangiocarcinoma, regarding the improvement of cholestasis and overall survival in the past two prospective randomized studies [66, 67]. However, recent prospective comparative study between PDT plus stenting and stenting alone in patients with locally advanced or metastatic biliary tract cancer showed that PDT plus stenting was associated with worse clinical outcome than stenting alone. Overall survival (6.2 vs. 9.8 months, HR 1.56, 95% CI 1.00–2.43, $p = 0.048$) and progression-free survival (3.4 vs. 4.3 months, HR 1.43, 95% CI 0.93–2.18, $p = 0.10$) were worse in patients receiving PDT compared with stent alone. However, more patients received subsequent palliative chemotherapy in stenting alone group than in PDT plus stenting group in this study (52% vs. 28%), and it may affect the worse outcome of PDT [68].

Recent prospectively randomized controlled study reported that PDT showed increase survival in patients with malignant biliary obstruction with the combination of systemic chemotherapeutic agents. In this study, the PDT plus S-1 showed promising efficacy in terms of 1-year survival rate (76% vs. 32%, $p = 0.003$), overall survival (median 17 months [95% CI: 12.6–21.4] vs. 8 months [95% CI: 6–10], $p = 0.005$), and progression-free survival (median 10 months [95% CI: 4.1–16] vs. 2 months [95% CI: 0.4–3.5], $p = 0.009$) compared with the PDT alone [69]. Another retrospective study comparing PDT with systemic chemotherapy to PDT alone in patients with advanced hilar cholangiocarcinoma also reported that the median survival was longer in PDT with systemic chemotherapy group than in PDT alone group (538 days [95% CI 475–601] vs. 334 days [95% CI 253–416], $p = 0.05$) [70]. Further larger multicenter clinical trial comparing PDT plus systemic chemotherapy with systemic chemotherapy alone may be warranted.

Regarding the clinical factors associated with better outcome of PDT, higher serum albumin and lower initial bilirubin level, earlier PDT after initial diagnosis, and multiple sessions of PDT were associated with a better overall survival [56]. The main adverse event of PDT is cholangitis which results from the necrosis associated with PDT. Therefore, administration of prophylactic antibiotics is recommended before PDT [71]. Another main adverse event is cutaneous photosensitivity which occurs in approximately 30% of photosensitizer recipients with 5–7% severe sunburn, and avoidance of exposure to sunlight is most important for prevention [62]. Serious phototoxicity may need oral corticosteroid treatment [71].

Radiofrequency Ablation (RFA)

Basics of RFA

RFA has been used for the ablation of small hepatocellular carcinoma and endoscopic treatment of Barrett esophagus or early esophageal cancer [72, 73]. RFA was recently adopted for the endoscopic palliation therapy for malignant biliary obstruction with the development of endobiliary RFA devices.

RFA is physically based on radiofrequency current and a high-frequency alternating current which causes vibration of local ions, thereby producing controlled frictional heat to destroy the target tissue. It is transmitted between an active electrode and a reference electrode, establishing lines of electrical field that generates ionic oscillation, which produces thermal heat around the tip of the electrode. Consequently, the endobiliary RFA delivers high quantity of thermal energy into the target tissue, which may induce coagulation necrosis and prolong the duration of stent patency [74]. The delivery of energy is directly proportional to the amplitude of oscillation, and the amount of coagulation necrosis will be dependent on the temperature and time. However, there is no consensus on the optimal frequency and interval of endobiliary RFA therapy [75]. To deliver thermal energy into the target tissue, selective bile duct cannulation with ERCP and the placement of RFA probe in the stricture site have to be preceded. Sometimes the RFA catheter can be inserted through percutaneous access.

One of the drawbacks of RFA is the "heat-sink effect" that may proceed in treating lesions adjacent to large vasculature. The inflow of cold blood at body temperature may interfere the heating of the tumor closest to the vessels [76].

Two kinds of endobiliary RFA probe have been introduced: Habib EndoHPB (Emcision, UK) and ELRA (Taewoong Medical, Korea). Habib EndoHPB consists of an 8 Fr catheter with a 180 cm working length that can be deployed through endoscope working channel of at least 3.2 mm in diameter. It can be used with a range of commonly available generators such as RITA 1500X RF generator (Angiodynamics, NY) or ERBE electrosurgical generators (Surgical Technology Group, UK) [77]. ELRA consists of a 7 Fr catheter with an 18 mm length of probe, and it has multiple bipolar electrodes which provide linear ablation, and therefore there is no need for ground pads. The VIVA (Taewoong Medical, Korea) combo generator is versatile, and the setting includes power (range 0–200 W), temperature (range 5 °C–95 °C), and time (range 10–600 s). Unlike EndoHPB, ELRA probe can control the temperature, which may result in potentially safe ablation, causing least damage to blood vessels and prevents tissue charring [78]. For this issue, further comparative study for these two probes may be required.

Indication of RFA

Most patients with cholangiocarcinoma have unresectable disease and require palliation of cholestasis with biliary stenting. RFA has been used before the placement of biliary stents or as a treatment of metal stent occlusion [71]. Theoretically, RFA might destroy the tumor tissue and improve malignant stricture, therefore, preventing stent ingrowth or overgrowth and extend stent patency. However, a concern remains about RFA for occluded metal stent that RFA energy may result in damage to the metal stent itself which might affect stent function, properties such as removability, and patency afterward [79]. Because of the friability of endobiliary RFA device and potential risk of thermal injury to nearby tissue, distal bile duct lesion may be preferred than hilar lesion for RFA.

Clinical Outcomes of RFA

Clinical evidence about RFA for the treatment of malignant biliary obstruction remains limited; however, RFA was effective in achieving local tumor control and prolongation of stent patency. First, feasibility study of endobiliary RFA was reported in 2011 [80]. Other clinical studies have shown the feasibility and safety of RFA with the improvement of stricture diameter or improved survival after RFA [78, 81–85]. Recently, first randomized comparative clinical trial was reported and showed that RFA with plastic stenting leads to longer survival than plastic stenting alone in patients with unresectable extrahepatic cholangiocarcinoma (mean 13.2 ± 0.6 vs. 8.3 ± 0.5 months, $p < 0.001$) [75]. The mean stent patency period was also significantly longer in RFA with plastic stenting group than in plastic stenting alone group (6.8 vs. 3.4 months, $p = 0.02$) [75].

Antibiotic prophylaxis is recommended to prevent post-procedural cholangitis and cholangiosepsis [86]. The incidence of adverse events-related RFA ranges from 5.6% to 27.1%, and additional RFA might not increase the post-procedural morbidity than conventional ERCP and stent placement. Most adverse events of RFA are known to be associated with ERCP and biliary stenting except few complications that are solely related to RFA [77]. Rare adverse events of RFA include hemobilia, cholecystitis, gallbladder empyema, and pancreatitis [71]. Given the potential risk of thermal injury to adjacent structures during RFA, accurate pre-interventional imaging assessment of the tumor surroundings is mandatory, especially for proximal biliary strictures [81]. There was one case of liver infarction caused by thermal injury of a segmental liver artery [77]. In addition, two cases of bile duct perforation after percutaneous RFA for malignant biliary obstruction have been reported [87].

Because RFA acts only on local tumors, this treatment alone may not achieve complete tumor destruction [75]. Therefore, the combination with systemic chemotherapy would be beneficial, and further prospective randomized clinical trials are mandatory to clarify the efficacy and safety of the combination of RFA and systemic chemotherapy in treating malignant biliary obstruction.

References

1. Boulay BR, Parepally M. Managing malignant biliary obstruction in pancreas cancer: choosing the appropriate strategy. World J Gastroenterol. 2014;20(28):9345–53.
2. Shah JN, Muthusamy VR. Endoscopic palliation of pancreaticobiliary malignancies. Gastrointest Endosc Clin N Am. 2005;15(3):513–31, ix.
3. Itoi T, Sofuni A, Itokawa F, Tonozuka R, Ishii K. Current status and issues regarding biliary stenting in unresectable biliary obstruction. Dig Endosc. 2013;25(Suppl 2):63–70.
4. Dumonceau JM, Tringali A, Papanikolaou IS, Blero D, Mangiavillano B, Schmidt A, et al. Endoscopic biliary stenting: indications, choice of stents, and results: European Society of Gastrointestinal Endoscopy (ESGE) Clinical guideline – updated October 2017. Endoscopy. 2018;50(9):910–30.
5. Dhir V, Itoi T, Khashab MA, Park DH, Yuen Bun Teoh A, Attam R, et al. Multicenter comparative evaluation of endoscopic placement of expandable metal stents for malignant distal common bile duct obstruction by ERCP or EUS-guided approach. Gastrointest Endosc. 2015;81(4):913–23.
6. Paik WH, Lee TH, Park DH, Choi JH, Kim SO, Jang S, et al. EUS-guided biliary drainage versus ERCP for the primary palliation of malignant biliary obstruction: a multicenter randomized clinical trial. Am J Gastroenterol. 2018;113(7):987–97.
7. Sawas T, Al Halabi S, Parsi MA, Vargo JJ. Self-expandable metal stents versus plastic stents for malignant biliary obstruction: a meta-analysis. Gastrointest Endosc. 2015;82(2):256–67.e7.
8. W-d H, X-w C, W-z W, Zhu Q-h, X-r C. Metal versus plastic stents for malignant biliary obstruction: an update meta-analysis. Clin Res Hepatol Gastroenterol. 2013;37(5):496–500.
9. Tempero MA, Malafa MP, Al-Hawary M, Asbun H, Bain A, Behrman SW, et al. Pancreatic adenocarcinoma, version 2.2017, NCCN clinical practice

guidelines in oncology. J Natl Compr Cancer Netw. 2017;15(8):1028–61.
10. Almadi MA, Barkun A, Martel M. Plastic vs. self-expandable metal stents for palliation in malignant biliary obstruction: a series of meta-analyses. Am J Gastroenterol. 2017;112(2):260–73.
11. Almadi MA, Barkun JS, Barkun AN. Stenting in malignant biliary obstruction. Gastrointest Endosc Clin N Am. 2015;25(4):691–711.
12. Saleem A, Leggett CL, Murad MH, Baron TH. Meta-analysis of randomized trials comparing the patency of covered and uncovered self-expandable metal stents for palliation of distal malignant bile duct obstruction. Gastrointest Endosc. 2011;74(2):321–7.e1-3.
13. Almadi MA, Barkun AN, Martel M. No benefit of covered vs uncovered self-expandable metal stents in patients with malignant distal biliary obstruction: a meta-analysis. Clin Gastroenterol Hepatol. 2013;11(1):27–37.e1.
14. Rerknimitr R, Angsuwatcharakon P, Ratanachu-ek T, Khor CJ, Ponnudurai R, Moon JH, et al. Asia-Pacific consensus recommendations for endoscopic and interventional management of hilar cholangiocarcinoma. J Gastroenterol Hepatol. 2013;28(4):593–607.
15. Wagner HJ, Knyrim K, Vakil N, Klose KJ. Plastic endoprostheses versus metal stents in the palliative treatment of malignant hilar biliary obstruction. A prospective and randomized trial. Endoscopy. 1993;25(3):213–8.
16. Mukai T, Yasuda I, Nakashima M, Doi S, Iwashita T, Iwata K, et al. Metallic stents are more efficacious than plastic stents in unresectable malignant hilar biliary strictures: a randomized controlled trial. J Hepatobiliary Pancreat Sci. 2013;20(2):214–22.
17. Perdue DG, Freeman ML, DiSario JA, Nelson DB, Fennerty MB, Lee JG, et al. Plastic versus self-expanding metallic stents for malignant hilar biliary obstruction: a prospective multicenter observational cohort study. J Clin Gastroenterol. 2008;42(9):1040–6.
18. Sung JY, Leung JW, Shaffer EA, Lam K, Costerton JW. Bacterial biofilm, brown pigment stone and blockage of biliary stents. J Gastroenterol Hepatol. 1993;8(1):28–34.
19. Isayama H, Nakai Y, Kogure H, Yamamoto N, Koike K. Biliary self-expandable metallic stent for unresectable malignant distal biliary obstruction: which is better: covered or uncovered? Dig Endosc. 2013;25(Suppl 2):71–4.
20. Schmidt A, Riecken B, Rische S, Klinger C, Jakobs R, Bechtler M, et al. Wing-shaped plastic stents vs. self-expandable metal stents for palliative drainage of malignant distal biliary obstruction: a randomized multicenter study. Endoscopy. 2015;47(5):430–6.
21. Simmons DT, Petersen BT, Gostout CJ, Levy MJ, Topazian MD, Baron TH. Risk of pancreatitis following endoscopically placed large-bore plastic biliary stents with and without biliary sphincterotomy for management of postoperative bile leaks. Surg Endosc. 2008;22(6):1459–63.
22. Okano N, Igarashi Y, Kishimoto Y, Mimura T, Ito K. Necessity for endoscopic sphincterotomy for biliary stenting in cases of malignant biliary obstruction. Dig Endosc. 2013;25(Suppl 2):122–5.
23. Cui PJ, Yao J, Zhao YJ, Han HZ, Yang J. Biliary stenting with or without sphincterotomy for malignant biliary obstruction: a meta-analysis. World J Gastroenterol. 2014;20(38):14033–9.
24. Hayashi T, Kawakami H, Osanai M, Ishiwatari H, Naruse H, Hisai H, et al. No benefit of endoscopic sphincterotomy before biliary placement of self-expandable metal stents for unresectable pancreatic cancer. Clin Gastroenterol Hepatol. 2015;13(6):1151–8.e2.
25. Tarnasky PR, Cunningham JT, Hawes RH, Hoffman BJ, Uflacker R, Vujic I, et al. Transpapillary stenting of proximal biliary strictures: does biliary sphincterotomy reduce the risk of postprocedure pancreatitis? Gastrointest Endosc. 1997;45(1):46–51.
26. Zhou H, Li L, Zhu F, Luo SZ, Cai XB, Wan XJ. Endoscopic sphincterotomy associated cholangitis in patients receiving proximal biliary self-expanding metal stents. Hepatobiliary Pancreat Dis Int. 2012;11(6):643–9.
27. Pedersen FM, Lassen AT, Schaffalitzky de Muckadell OB. Randomized trial of stent placed above and across the sphincter of Oddi in malignant bile duct obstruction. Gastrointest Endosc. 1998;48(6):574–9.
28. Okamoto T, Fujioka S, Yanagisawa S, Yanaga K, Kakutani H, Tajiri H, et al. Placement of a metallic stent across the main duodenal papilla may predispose to cholangitis. Gastrointest Endosc. 2006;63(6):792–6.
29. Inoue T, Ishii N, Kobayashi Y, Kitano R, Sakamoto K, Ohashi T, et al. Simultaneous versus sequential side-by-side bilateral metal stent placement for malignant hilar biliary obstructions. Dig Dis Sci. 2017;62(9):2542–9.
30. Fukasawa M, Takano S, Shindo H, Takahashi E, Sato T, Enomoto N. Endoscopic biliary stenting for unresectable malignant hilar obstruction. Clin J Gastroenterol. 2017;10(6):485–90.
31. Hong W, Chen S, Zhu Q, Chen H, Pan J, Huang Q. Bilateral stenting methods for hilar biliary obstructions. Clinics (Sao Paulo, Brazil). 2014;69(9):647–52.
32. Adler DG, Baron TH. Endoscopic palliation of malignant gastric outlet obstruction using self-expanding metal stents: experience in 36 patients. Am J Gastroenterol. 2002;97(1):72–8.
33. Mutignani M, Tringali A, Shah SG, Perri V, Familiari P, Iacopini F, et al. Combined endoscopic stent insertion in malignant biliary and duodenal obstruction. Endoscopy. 2007;39(5):440–7.
34. Baron TH. Management of simultaneous biliary and duodenal obstruction: the endoscopic perspective. Gut Liver. 2010;4(Suppl 1):S50–6.
35. Maetani I, Nambu T, Omuta S, Ukita T, Shigoka H. Treating bilio-duodenal obstruction: combining new endoscopic technique with 6 Fr stent introducer. World J Gastroenterol. 2010;16(22):2828–31.

36. Moon JH, Choi HJ. Endoscopic double-metallic stenting for malignant biliary and duodenal obstructions. J Hepatobiliary Pancreat Sci. 2011;18(5):658–63.
37. Nakai Y, Hamada T, Isayama H, Itoi T, Koike K. Endoscopic management of combined malignant biliary and gastric outlet obstruction. Dig Endosc. 2017;29(1):16–25.
38. Novacek G, Potzi R, Kornek G, Hafner M, Schofl R, Gangl A, et al. Endoscopic placement of a biliary expandable metal stent through the mesh wall of a duodenal stent. Endoscopy. 2003;35(11):982–3.
39. Khashab MA, Valeshabad AK, Leung W, Camilo J, Fukami N, Shieh F, et al. Multicenter experience with performance of ERCP in patients with an indwelling duodenal stent. Endoscopy. 2014;46(3):252–5.
40. Staub J, Siddiqui A, Taylor LJ, Loren D, Kowalski T, Adler DG. ERCP performed through previously placed duodenal stents: a multicenter retrospective study of outcomes and adverse events. Gastrointest Endosc. 2018;87(6):1499–504.
41. Giovannini M, Moutardier V, Pesenti C, Bories E, Lelong B, Delpero JR. Endoscopic ultrasound-guided bilioduodenal anastomosis: a new technique for biliary drainage. Endoscopy. 2001;33(10):898–900.
42. Paik WH, Park DH. Endoscopic ultrasound-guided biliary access, with focus on technique and practical tips. Clin Endosc. 2017;50(2):104–11.
43. Lee TH, Choi JH, Park do H, Song TJ, Kim DU, Paik WH, et al. Similar efficacies of endoscopic ultrasound-guided transmural and percutaneous drainage for malignant distal biliary obstruction. Clin Gastroenterol Hepatol. 2016;14(7):1011–9.e3.
44. Ogura T, Higuchi K. Technical tips for endoscopic ultrasound-guided hepaticogastrostomy. World J Gastroenterol. 2016;22(15):3945–51.
45. Imai H, Kitano M, Omoto S, Kadosaka K, Kamata K, Miyata T, et al. EUS-guided gallbladder drainage for rescue treatment of malignant distal biliary obstruction after unsuccessful ERCP. Gastrointest Endosc. 2016;84(1):147–51.
46. Ogura T, Sano T, Onda S, Imoto A, Masuda D, Yamamoto K, et al. Endoscopic ultrasound-guided biliary drainage for right hepatic bile duct obstruction: novel technical tips. Endoscopy. 2015;47(1):72–5.
47. Park SJ, Choi JH, Park DH, Choi JH, Lee SS, Seo DW, et al. Expanding indication: EUS-guided hepaticoduodenostomy for isolated right intrahepatic duct obstruction (with video). Gastrointest Endosc. 2013;78(2):374–80.
48. Dellon ES, Hawk JS, Grimm IS, Shaheen NJ. The use of carbon dioxide for insufflation during GI endoscopy: a systematic review. Gastrointest Endosc. 2009;69(4):843–9.
49. Park DH, Jang JW, Lee SS, Seo DW, Lee SK, Kim MH. EUS-guided biliary drainage with transluminal stenting after failed ERCP: predictors of adverse events and long-term results. Gastrointest Endosc. 2011;74(6):1276–84.
50. Park DH, Lee TH, Paik WH, Choi JH, Song TJ, Lee SS, et al. Feasibility and safety of a novel dedicated device for one-step EUS-guided biliary drainage: a randomized trial. J Gastroenterol Hepatol. 2015;30(10):1461–6.
51. Oh D, Park DH, Song TJ, Lee SS, Seo DW, Lee SK, et al. Optimal biliary access point and learning curve for endoscopic ultrasound-guided hepaticogastrostomy with transmural stenting. Ther Adv Gastroenterol. 2017;10(1):42–53.
52. Ogura T, Masuda D, Takeuchi T, Fukunishi S, Higuchi K. Liver impaction technique to prevent shearing of the guidewire during endoscopic ultrasound-guided hepaticogastrostomy. Endoscopy. 2015;47(S 01):E583–e4.
53. Paik WH, Park DH, Choi JH, Choi JH, Lee SS, Seo DW, et al. Simplified fistula dilation technique and modified stent deployment maneuver for EUS-guided hepaticogastrostomy. World J Gastroenterol. 2014;20(17):5051–9.
54. Choi JH, Kim HW, Lee JC, Paik KH, Seong NJ, Yoon CJ, et al. Percutaneous transhepatic versus EUS-guided gallbladder drainage for malignant cystic duct obstruction. Gastrointest Endosc. 2017;85(2): 357–64.
55. Ogura T, Chiba Y, Masuda D, Kitano M, Sano T, Saori O, et al. Comparison of the clinical impact of endoscopic ultrasound-guided choledochoduodenostomy and hepaticogastrostomy for bile duct obstruction with duodenal obstruction. Endoscopy. 2016;48(2):156–63.
56. Lee TY, Cheon YK, Shim CS. Current status of photodynamic therapy for bile duct cancer. Clin Endosc. 2013;46(1):38–44.
57. Kahaleh M, Mishra R, Shami VM, Northup PG, Berg CL, Bashlor P, et al. Unresectable cholangiocarcinoma: comparison of survival in biliary stenting alone versus stenting with photodynamic therapy. Clin Gastroenterol Hepatol. 2008;6(3):290–7.
58. Bauerfeind P, Ortner M. Radiofrequency ablation for cholangiocarcinoma: it works, but how? Endoscopy. 2018;50(8):741–2.
59. Shim CS, Cheon YK, Cha SW, Bhandari S, Moon JH, Cho YD, et al. Prospective study of the effectiveness of percutaneous transhepatic photodynamic therapy for advanced bile duct cancer and the role of intraductal ultrasonography in response assessment. Endoscopy. 2005;37(5):425–33.
60. Blechacz B, Komuta M, Roskams T, Gores GJ. Clinical diagnosis and staging of cholangiocarcinoma. Nat Rev Gastroenterol Hepatol. 2011;8(9):512–22.
61. Ortner MA. Photodynamic therapy for cholangiocarcinoma: overview and new developments. Curr Opin Gastroenterol. 2009;25(5):472–6.
62. Tomizawa Y, Tian J. Photodynamic therapy for unresectable cholangiocarcinoma. Dig Dis Sci. 2012;57(2):274–83.
63. Cheon YK, Lee TY, Lee SM, Yoon JY, Shim CS. Longterm outcome of photodynamic therapy compared with biliary stenting alone in patients with advanced hilar cholangiocarcinoma. HPB (Oxford). 2012;14(3):185–93.
64. Dumoulin FL, Gerhardt T, Fuchs S, Scheurlen C, Neubrand M, Layer G, et al. Phase II study of pho-

todynamic therapy and metal stent as palliative treatment for nonresectable hilar cholangiocarcinoma. Gastrointest Endosc. 2003;57(7):860–7.
65. Witzigmann H, Berr F, Ringel U, Caca K, Uhlmann D, Schoppmeyer K, et al. Surgical and palliative management and outcome in 184 patients with hilar cholangiocarcinoma: palliative photodynamic therapy plus stenting is comparable to r1/r2 resection. Ann Surg. 2006;244(2):230–9.
66. Ortner ME, Caca K, Berr F, Liebetruth J, Mansmann U, Huster D, et al. Successful photodynamic therapy for nonresectable cholangiocarcinoma: a randomized prospective study. Gastroenterology. 2003;125(5):1355–63.
67. Zoepf T, Jakobs R, Arnold JC, Apel D, Riemann JF. Palliation of nonresectable bile duct cancer: improved survival after photodynamic therapy. Am J Gastroenterol. 2005;100(11):2426–30.
68. Pereira SP, Jitlal M, Duggan M, Lawrie E, Beare S, O'Donoghue P, et al. PHOTOSTENT-02: porfimer sodium photodynamic therapy plus stenting versus stenting alone in patients with locally advanced or metastatic biliary tract cancer. ESMO Open. 2018;3(5):e000379.
69. Park DH, Lee SS, Park SE, Lee JL, Choi JH, Choi HJ, et al. Randomised phase II trial of photodynamic therapy plus oral fluoropyrimidine, S-1, versus photodynamic therapy alone for unresectable hilar cholangiocarcinoma. Eur J Cancer. 2014;50(7):1259–68.
70. Hong MJ, Cheon YK, Lee EJ, Lee TY, Shim CS. Long-term outcome of photodynamic therapy with systemic chemotherapy compared to photodynamic therapy alone in patients with advanced hilar cholangiocarcinoma. Gut Liver. 2014;8(3):318–23.
71. Smith I, Kahaleh M. Biliary tumor ablation with photodynamic therapy and radiofrequency ablation. Gastrointest Endosc Clin N Am. 2015;25(4):793–804.
72. Feng Q, Chi Y, Liu Y, Zhang L, Liu Q. Efficacy and safety of percutaneous radiofrequency ablation versus surgical resection for small hepatocellular carcinoma: a meta-analysis of 23 studies. J Cancer Res Clin Oncol. 2015;141(1):1–9.
73. Orman ES, Li N, Shaheen NJ. Efficacy and durability of radiofrequency ablation for Barrett's esophagus: systematic review and meta-analysis. Clin Gastroenterol Hepatol. 2013;11(10):1245–55.
74. Wadsworth CA, Westaby D, Khan SA. Endoscopic radiofrequency ablation for cholangiocarcinoma. Curr Opin Gastroenterol. 2013;29(3):305–11.
75. Yang J, Wang J, Zhou H, Zhou Y, Wang Y, Jin H, et al. Efficacy and safety of endoscopic radiofrequency ablation for unresectable extrahepatic cholangiocarcinoma: a randomized trial. Endoscopy. 2018;50(8):751–60.
76. Roque J, Ho SH, Reddy N, Goh KL. Endoscopic ablation therapy for biliopancreatic malignancies. Clin Endosc. 2015;48(1):15–9.
77. Rustagi T, Jamidar PA. Intraductal radiofrequency ablation for management of malignant biliary obstruction. Dig Dis Sci. 2014;59(11):2635–41.
78. Nayar MK, Oppong KW, Bekkali NLH, Leeds JS. Novel temperature-controlled RFA probe for treatment of blocked metal biliary stents in patients with pancreaticobiliary cancers: initial experience. Endosc Int Open. 2018;6(5):E513–e7.
79. Rustagi T, Jamidar PA. Endoscopic treatment of malignant biliary strictures. Curr Gastroenterol Rep. 2015;17(1):426.
80. Steel AW, Postgate AJ, Khorsandi S, Nicholls J, Jiao L, Vlavianos P, et al. Endoscopically applied radiofrequency ablation appears to be safe in the treatment of malignant biliary obstruction. Gastrointest Endosc. 2011;73(1):149–53.
81. Dolak W, Schreiber F, Schwaighofer H, Gschwantler M, Plieschnegger W, Ziachehabi A, et al. Endoscopic radiofrequency ablation for malignant biliary obstruction: a nationwide retrospective study of 84 consecutive applications. Surg Endosc. 2014;28(3):854–60.
82. Kallis Y, Phillips N, Steel A, Kaltsidis H, Vlavianos P, Habib N, et al. Analysis of endoscopic radiofrequency ablation of biliary malignant strictures in pancreatic cancer suggests potential survival benefit. Dig Dis Sci. 2015;60(11):3449–55.
83. Sharaiha RZ, Natov N, Glockenberg KS, Widmer J, Gaidhane M, Kahaleh M. Comparison of metal stenting with radiofrequency ablation versus stenting alone for treating malignant biliary strictures: is there an added benefit? Dig Dis Sci. 2014;59(12):3099–102.
84. Sharaiha RZ, Sethi A, Weaver KR, Gonda TA, Shah RJ, Fukami N, et al. Impact of radiofrequency ablation on malignant biliary strictures: results of a collaborative registry. Dig Dis Sci. 2015;60(7):2164–9.
85. Dutta AK, Basavaraju U, Sales L, Leeds JS. Radiofrequency ablation for management of malignant biliary obstruction: a single-center experience and review of the literature. Expert Rev Gastroenterol Hepatol. 2017;11(8):779–84.
86. Alis H, Sengoz C, Gonenc M, Kalayci MU, Kocatas A. Endobiliary radiofrequency ablation for malignant biliary obstruction. Hepatobiliary Pancreat Dis Int. 2013;12(4):423–7.
87. Zhou C, Wei B, Gao K, Zhai R. Biliary tract perforation following percutaneous endobiliary radiofrequency ablation: a report of two cases. Oncol Lett. 2016;11(6):3813–6.
88. Yang Z, Wu Q, Wang F, Ye X, Qi X, Fan D. A systematic review and meta-analysis of randomized trials and prospective studies comparing covered and bare self-expandable metal stents for the treatment of malignant obstruction in the digestive tract. Int J Med Sci. 2013;10(7):825–35.
89. Chen MY, Lin JW, Zhu HP, Zhang B, Jiang GY, Yan PJ, et al. Covered stents versus uncovered stents for unresectable malignant biliary strictures: a meta-analysis. Biomed Res Int. 2016;2016:6408067.
90. Li J, Li T, Sun P, Yu Q, Wang K, Chang W, et al. Covered versus uncovered self-expandable metal stents for managing malignant distal biliary obstruction: a meta-analysis. PLoS One. 2016;11(2):e0149066.

9 Differentiation of Indeterminate Biliary Stricture

Hong Jin Yoon, Sung Ill Jang, and Dong Ki Lee

Introduction

Biliary strictures can be caused by benign and malignant diseases, each of which requires a different treatment approach. The causes of most biliary strictures are malignant (70–80%), but 20–30% are benign. Although differential diagnosis of biliary strictures is difficult, accurate early diagnosis of malignant tumors is important because it influences the likelihood of resection and the overall outcome. If early malignancy is diagnosed correctly, then timely surgery can be performed, and/or the appropriate chemotherapy regimen can be selected. Conversely, exclusion of malignant causes can reduce the frequency of unnecessary surgery. Diagnosis of the causes of indeterminate biliary stricture requires multiple approaches, as many are malignant [1].

Biliary cancer is the most common malignancy in the biliary system and accounts for about 3% of those in the gastrointestinal tract [2]. Biliary cancer is usually diagnosed at an advanced stage when the prognosis is poor. The incidence and mortality of biliary cancer are increasing worldwide [3, 4]. Biliary cancer is classified as intrahepatic or extrahepatic, and cancer of the bile duct is categorized as mass-forming, biliary invasion, or intra-biliary (Fig. 9.1). Patients diagnosed early who undergo surgical resection have an excellent 5-year survival rate [5]. Abdominal ultrasound (US), computed tomography (CT), and magnetic resonance imaging (MRI) are effective for diagnosing bile-duct enlargement, but their ability to assess the cause of biliary obstruction is limited in the absence of a mass. In fact, despite clinical, endoscopic, and hematological tests, it is often difficult to differentiate biliary obstruction of benign and malignant causes [6–8].

About 13–24% of patients with suspected hilar cholangiocarcinoma were in fact shown to have had a benign condition after surgery [6, 7]. Therefore, accurate preoperative diagnosis is important to avoid unnecessary surgery. Patients suspected of having cholangiocarcinoma should be confirmed pathologically before attempting radical curative resection. Although surgical resection of distal cholangiocarcinoma requires pancreaticoduodenectomy (Whipple resection), partial hepatectomy is often used to treat perihilar tumors [9], but has a morbidity rate of 37–64% and a mortality rate of 8–10% [10, 11]. Discriminating benign strictures from malignancies is particularly difficult in patients with primary sclerosing cholangitis (PSC), and caution is required in such cases because it affects the decision to perform transplantation.

H. J. Yoon · S. I. Jang · D. K. Lee (✉)
Department of Internal Medicine, Gangnam Severance Hospital, Yonsei University College of Medicine, Seoul, South Korea
e-mail: aerojsi@yuhs.ac; dklee@yuhs.ac

D. K. Lee (ed.), *Advanced ERCP for Complicated and Refractory Biliary and Pancreatic Diseases*,
https://doi.org/10.1007/978-981-13-0608-2_9

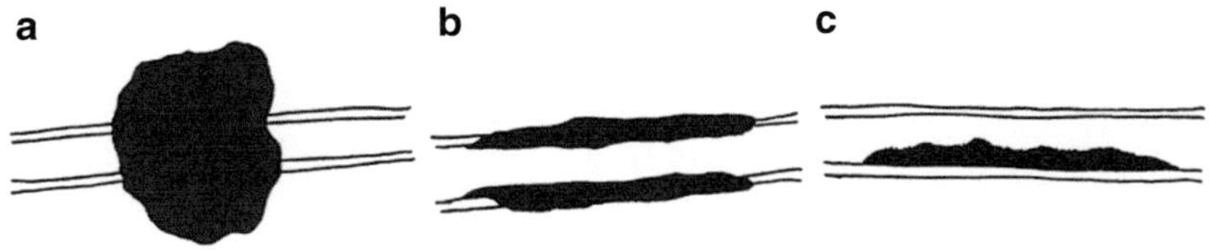

Fig. 9.1 Morphologic classification of intrahepatic and extrahepatic cholangiocarcinoma. Tubule represents the bile duct. Drawings of mass-forming (**a**), periductal-infiltrating (**b**), and intraductal growing (**c**) cholangiocarcinomas. (Adopted for reference [97])

Definition

The definition of indeterminate biliary stricture varies from study to study. We define some cases of clinically indeterminate malignancies based on the patient's history and imaging findings prior to tissue sampling. Most cases are diagnosed as stricture when a previous endoscopic retrograde cholangiopancreatogram (ERCP) using brushing cytology or intraductal biopsy did not provide a diagnosis despite strong clinical suspicion of malignancy [12].

Indeterminate biliary stricture is defined as the absence of other causes (such as stone disease or bile duct injury), at least one of which is detected by an imaging modality, and the result of ERCP-based sampling is negative [13].

Etiology

Bile-duct obstruction with jaundice should always be considered possibly malignant unless a benign cause has been established. Potential causes of benign strictures include cholelithiasis, Mirrizi's syndrome, stricture after liver transplantation or cholecystectomy, chronic pancreatitis, clonorchiasis, PSC, autoimmune pancreatitis, autoimmune cholangitis, and ischemia after liver transplantation (Table 9.1). A malignant biliary stricture is most commonly caused by cancer of the pancreas or bile duct, but can also be due to hepatocellular carcinoma, invasion of the biliary tract by pancreatic cancer, biliary obstruction by gallbladder carcinoma, metastatic carcinoma, or malignant lymph nodes. If the mass is unclear on CT or MRI, it can often be identified by endoscopic ultrasound (EUS) [14, 15]. The possibility of a malignant cause of obstruction of the hilar or upper biliary tract must be considered [16].

Evaluation of Patients with Biliary Strictures

Clinical approaches to indeterminate strictures include medical history-taking and physical examination. In patients with obstructive jaundice, strictures of the bile duct should be regarded

Table 9.1 Biliary strictures: etiology

Benign biliary stricture	Malignant biliary stricture
Stones	Bile duct cancer (cholangiocarcinoma)
Bile duct stone	Pancreatic cancer
Mirizzi's syndrome	Gallbladder cancer
Stenosis of sphincter of Oddi	Ampulla of Vater malignancy
Inflammatory causes	Hepatocellular carcinoma
Primary sclerosing cholangitis	Lymph node metastasis (breast, colon, stomach, lymphoma)
IgG4-associated cholangitis	
Recurrent pancreatitis	
Radiation	
Infection (recurrent cholangitis)	
Parasite (clonorchiasis)	
Surgical injury	
Ischemia (post liver transplantatoin)	
Cholecystectomy, liver transplantation	
Gastric, duodenal, pancreatic, and hepatic surgery	
Idiopathic	

as malignant if no benign cause is identified. The importance of jaundice-free biliary stricture is less certain.

Patients usually present with symptoms such as jaundice, abdominal discomfort, and weight loss, and biliary cancer may be suspected based on the findings of abdominal US, EUS, abdominal CT, or MRI. There are several characteristic differences between benign and malignant strictures (Table 9.2), but these differences are not always present. Therefore, histologic confirmation by abdominal US-guided biopsy, abdominal CT-guided biopsy, ERCP, percutaneous transhepatic biliary drainage (PTBD) biopsy, or brushing cytology is needed before initiation of treatment. A mass visible on abdominal US or CT, which is usually a liver or metastatic mass, can be biopsied using CT (Fig. 9.2a). If these imaging features are absent or the mass cannot be visualized, ERCP or PTBD may be used to perform biopsy and cytology examination (Fig. 9.2b).

Table 9.2 Differences between benign and malignant biliary strictures

	Benign biliary stricture	Malignant biliary stricture
Age	Any age, usually younger	Usually age >50 years
Loss of weight, appetite	Less common	Significant loss
Jaundice	Deep jaundice unusual	Deep jaundice usual
Features of cholangitis	More common	Less common
Presence of lump in abdomen	Not a feature	Favors malignancy
Radiology MRCP/ERCP	Smooth stricture, no mass	Eccentric, irregular stricture, abrupt cutoff, presence of mass
Ca19-9	Normal except in cholangitis	High
Cholangioscopy features	Smooth mucosa, no mass or tumor vessel	Tumor vessels present, nodules, mass
Cytology, biopsy	Not suggestive	Suggestive

Serum Biomarkers

In patients with biliary obstruction, liver function can be tested by assaying the bilirubin level. Patients with high jaundice scores are more likely to have a malignancy than those with normal scores [14].

There are no serum or bile markers specific for bile-duct cancer. The biomarkers of biliary tract malignancies used in the clinic are the serum level of carbohydrate antigen (CA) 19-9 and carcinoembryonic antigen (CEA). The serum CA 19-9 level is elevated in benign diseases such as cholestasis, cholangitis, cirrhosis, pneumonia, and gastric cancer. The sensitivity and specificity values of the serum CA 19-9 level diagnosis of cholangiocarcinoma in patients with PSC are 79% and 98%, respectively, using a cutoff value of 129 U/mL [17]. Sensitivity in patients without PSC is 40–70%, and specificity is 50–80%; these values vary according to the cutoff value used [18–20]. The serum CEA level is elevated in patients with cancer of the digestive system and in those with lung, breast, ovarian, or thyroid cancer [21]. An elevated serum CEA level in patients with cholangiocarcinoma has a sensitivity of 33–68% and specificity of 79–95% [22, 23]. Other markers include the serum mucin 5 AC (MUA5AC) and matrix metalloproteinase (MMP)-7 levels. The serum MUA5AC level in epithelial cancer showed high level in bile duct cancer. A cutoff value of 14 ng/mL was associated with lymph node metastasis [24]. The sensitivity and specificity values of the serum MMP-7 level are 53–76% and 47–92%, respectively, varying depending on the cutoff value used [25]. The clinical utility of the other biomarkers reported requires further study [26].

Radiological Examinations

Abdominal US is typically used in patients with suspected biliary diseases. It is easy to perform and does not involve exposure to radioactivity, but is highly dependent on the skill of the examiner. Abdominal US also shows the rapid expansion and closure of the intrahepatic bile duct in

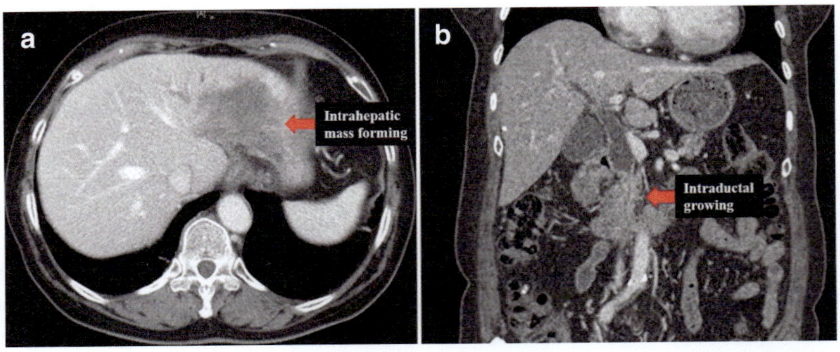

Fig. 9.2 Cholangiocellular adenocarcinoma by computed tomography (CT). (**a**) CT scan showing an irregularly shaped mass (mass-forming intrahepatic cholangiocarcinoma). (**b**) CT scan showing asymmetric thickening of the bile-duct wall and an intraluminal mass representing intraductal-growing extrahepatic cholangiocarcinoma

patients with biliary stricture. However, the peripheral portion of the common bile duct (CBD) cannot be adequately evaluated due to interference by intestinal gas [27]; also, its diagnostic yield for biliary ductal mass is very low [28]. Abdominal CT is helpful in planning diagnostic evaluation and treatment [29]. Abdominal CT has higher sensitivity for diagnosis of bile duct masses compared to US and is particularly useful for hepatic lesions [30]. The sensitivity of CT is 75–80%, and the specificity is 60–80%. However, it is less sensitive for diagnosing cancer at an early stage [31, 32]. Another disadvantage of CT is that its sensitivity for detecting local lymph nodes is only 54% and it tends to underestimate the extent of proximal tumors [33, 34]. Multi-detector helical scanners and rapid injection of contrast agents enable accurate determination of the need for surgical excision by assessing the tumor extent, local lymphadenopathy, and vascular involvement.

Magnetic resonance cholangiopancreatography (MRCP) is an accurate and noninvasive method for the detection of biliary obstruction [35]. MRCP provides a high-resolution image of the entire bile duct without injection of contrast medium directly into the bile duct (Fig. 9.3). However, the specificity and positive predictive value are low, because it is not possible to distinguish benign and malignant strictures [36]. The accuracy of MRCP for assessing vascular invasion and hepatic parenchymal involvement is 67–73% and 78–80%, respectively [37], and its sensitivity and specificity values for distinguishing benign strictures from malignancies are 90% and 65%, respectively; its diagnostic accuracy is similar to that of ERCP [29, 38]. The accuracy of MRCP for predicting involvement of the bile duct in cholangiocarcinoma is 88–96% [39]. A long (>10 mm), asymmetrical, irregular bile duct on MRCP is suggestive of malignancy; however, these features are not particularly sensitive or specific [40]. Therefore, unless the lesion in the biliary tract is located by abdominal imaging, an endoscopic examination should be performed to determine the cause of a bile duct stricture.

Endoscopic Examinations

ERCP

ERCP enables confirmation of the presence, location, and extent of a biliary stricture and collection of tissue. Brushing through ERCP is the first-line approach for sampling the biliary stricture (Fig. 9.4a, b) because it is widely available and technically easy. The specificity of ERCP for diagnosis of malignancy in the bile duct based on examination of sampled tissue is 95%, but the sensitivity is low [41].

The sensitivity of conventional biliary brushing cytology is 27–56% [42, 43]. The sensitivity of biliary brushing cytology is low for bile-duct cancer of a pluricellular nature with submucosal tumor growth or extrinsic malignancy. The results

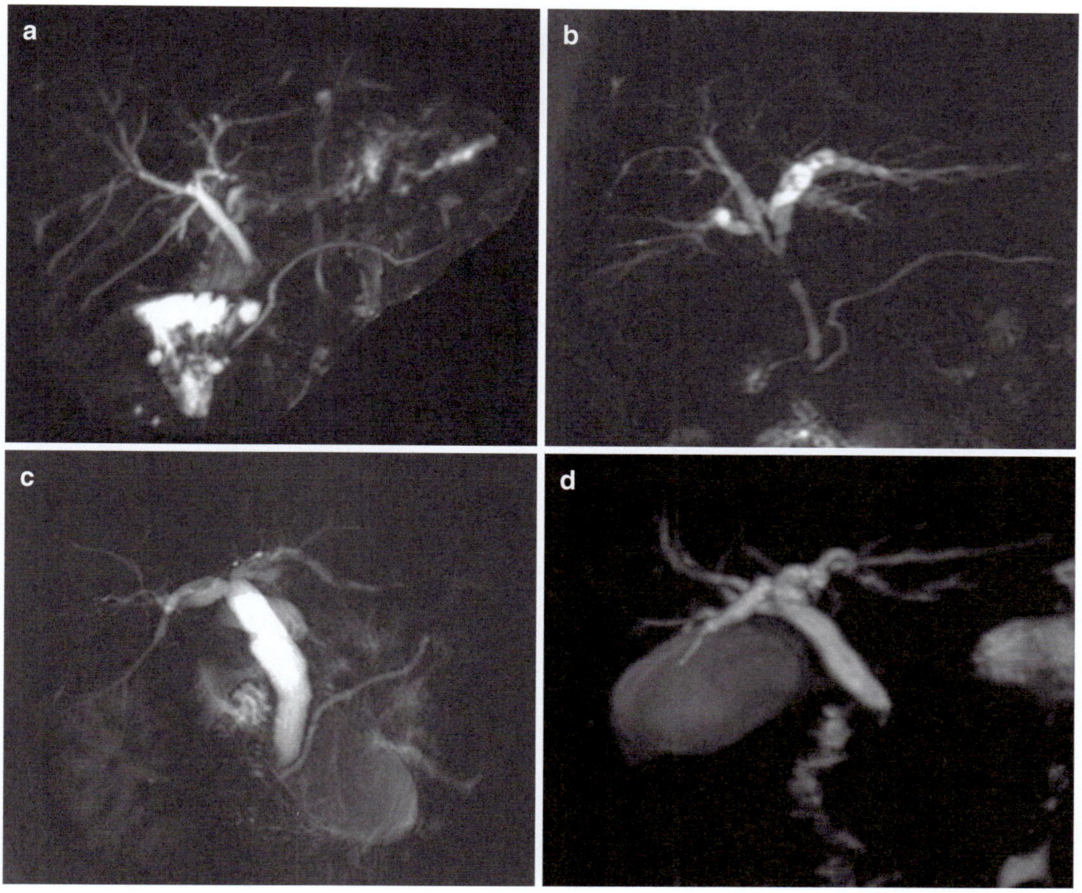

Fig. 9.3 Biliary strictures by magnetic resonance cholangiopancreatography (MRCP). (**a**) Segmental compression of the common bile duct (CBD) by a mass in the head of the pancreas. (**b**) MRCP image showing a high-level stricture and dilatation of the intrahepatic duct caused by intrahepatic cholangiocarcinoma. (**c**) MRCP image showing dilatation of the intrahepatic and extrahepatic duct caused by cholangiocarcinoma in the distal CBD. (**d**) MRCP image of a dilated intrahepatic duct and CBD stricture due to pancreatitis

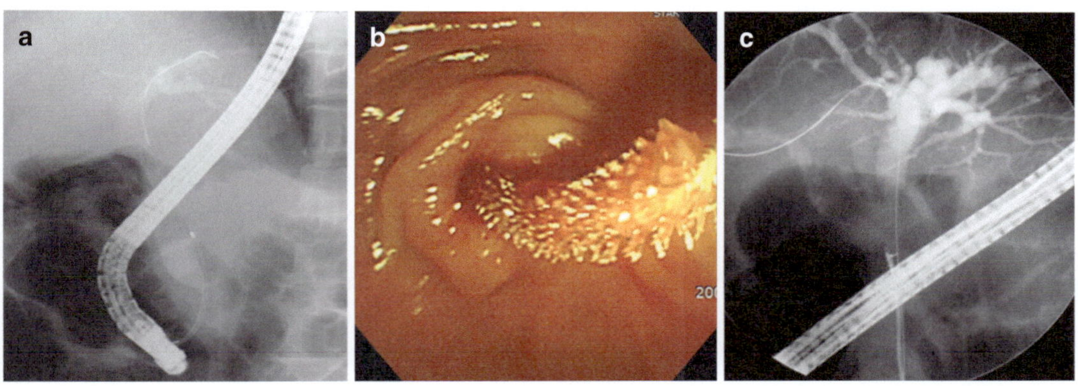

Fig. 9.4 ERCP for determining the cause of biliary strictures. (**a**) ERCP biliary brush cytology of a biliary stricture. (**b**) Brush cytology (endoscopic view). (**c**) Fluoroscopic image obtained during endobiliary forceps biopsy

of cytology for biliary cancer are not satisfactory because of the desmoplastic reaction [44, 45]. A variety of techniques have been used to improve the sensitivity of conventional brush cytology, such as use of a new brush, brushing after biliary stricture extension, and repeated brushing [46, 47]. Several strategies, including endoscopic needle aspiration, immunohistochemical testing, and mutational analysis, have been used to improve the sensitivity [48, 49]. Inadequate biliary cytology specimens are a major cause of nondiagnostic samples; this scenario can be overcome by having pathologists on-site. Real-time evaluation of the cytology sample is possible and reduces the likelihood of improper sampling and sample preparation. Other methods of overcoming inappropriate sampling include cutting the entire brush and having the endoscopy team make and place slides in fixation solution before submitting them to the pathology department.

Endoscopic forceps biopsy by ERCP is routinely performed to sample strictures of the bile duct (Fig. 9.4c). Generally, forceps biopsy has a higher yield than brush cytology but similar sensitivity (36–65%). When using endobiliary forceps, the detection rate is 44–89% for cholangiocarcinoma and 33–71% for pancreatic cancer [50–52]. However, endobiliary biopsy is technically challenging, particularly in stenosis of the proximal bile duct, and may lead to complications such as bleeding and biliary perforation [50, 53].

The combination of biopsy and brushing cytology slightly increases the diagnostic yield to 54–74% compared with either test alone. Repeated testing may increase the diagnostic yield, depending on the location, length, and morphology of the stricture [45, 47].

EUS

EUS is an important method of evaluating indeterminate biliary strictures and enables morphological classification of cholangiocarcinoma (Fig. 9.5). EUS enables visualization of the extrahepatic bile ducts, hilar masses, gallbladder and peri-hilar lymph nodes, and blood vessels. EUS also facilitates real-time confirmation of the digestive tract, surrounding organs, and EUS guided fine-needle aspiration (FNA). The characteristic features of benign strictures on EUS are smooth and concentric narrowing without a significant mass (Fig. 9.6). Several EUS findings can distinguish benign from malignant strictures; however, the accuracy differs markedly depending on the physician. The sensitivity of EUS for diagnosis of pancreatic cancer was 85% and the specificity approached 100% [54]. The role of EUS for diagnosing indeterminate biliary strictures is unclear. The sensitivity for diagnosis of malignancy increased to 86% when the mass was confirmed by EUS [55]. The sensitivity of diagnosis using EUS-FNA was 59% for proximal cholangiocarcinoma and 81% for distal cholangiocarcinoma. This scenario is because proximal lesions are located somewhat farther from the distal end of the endoscope, which hampers collection of tissue, whereas distal lesions are visible by EUS [5, 56]. EUS-FNA is thus not recommended in patients being prepared for liver transplantation because of the potential for tumor seeding [57, 58]. A mass in the bile duct typically appears as a hypoechoic lesion on EUS. However, in the absence of a prominent mass, it may be difficult to differentiate between benign and infiltration-type malignant strictures. The relationships of liver parenchyma, the portal vein system, and hepatic artery masses should be carefully examined to assess the feasibility of tumor removal. EUS can also provide information important for assessing the likelihood of successful resection of cholangiocarcinoma. EUS staging of cancer of the bile duct is based on the tumor, node, and metastasis staging system. Several studies have evaluated the utility of EUS to determine preoperative staging of tumors in the extrahepatic bile duct (Table 9.3) [59–61]. EUS had higher accuracy (88–100%) for predicting portal involvement than US, CT, and angiography (Fig. 9.7a, b) [59–61]. Finally, EUS-FNA can be used to evaluate suspicious local lymph nodes [62].

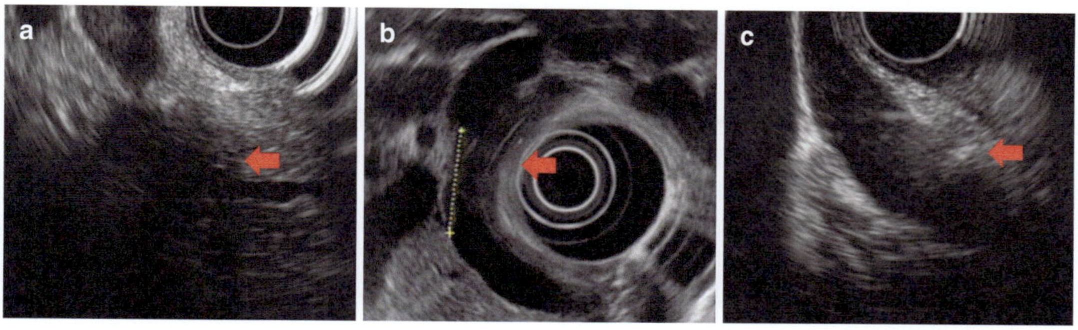

Fig. 9.5 Endoscopic ultrasound (EUS) findings of cholangiocarcinoma according to the morphological classification. EUS demonstrating a hypoechoic mass in the bile duct suggestive of cholangiocarcinoma. (**a**) Mass-forming hypoechoic mass at the intrapancreatic portion shown by EUS (red arrow). (**b**) Periductal infiltrating, CBD wall thickening, irregular mass found by EUS (red arrow). (**c**) Intraductal growing, hypoechoic mass (red arrow)

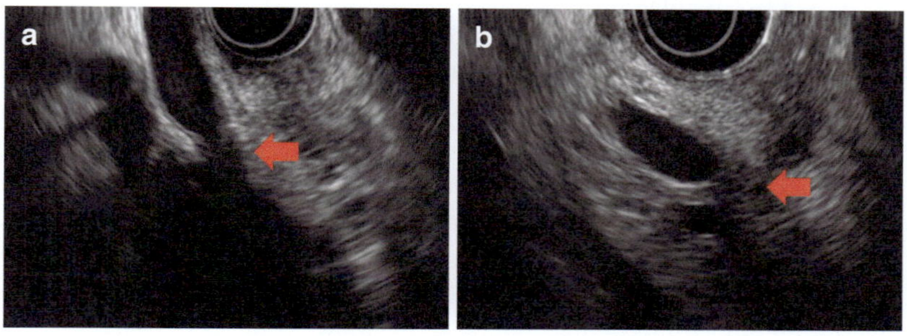

Fig. 9.6 Benign biliary strictures by EUS. Note the smooth, concentric narrowing. (**a**) Distal CBD stricture secondary to autoimmune pancreatitis (red arrow). (**b**) Distal CBD stricture of unknown origin (red arrow)

Table 9.3 Reports on the role of preoperative EUS morphology in staging of cholangiocarcinoma

First author	Publication year	No. patients	Accuracy of tumor staging (%)	Accuracy of node staging (%)	Accuracy of predicting portal vein invasion (%)
Mukai [59]	1992	16	81	81	88
Tio [60]	1993	46	66	64	Not reported
Sugiyama [61]	1997	19	Not reported	Not reported	100

Cholangioscopy

Choledochal examinations are classified into per oral cholangioscopy (POCS) and percutaneous transhepatic cholangioscopy (PTCS). Cholangioscopy allows direct endoscopic observation of the biliary stricture and biopsy as needed. PTCS enables visualization of the inside of the bile duct but requires repeated extension of the tract and puncture of the abdominal wall. The recently introduced single cholangioscopic examination enables tissue biopsy directly in the field of vision, which can overcome the low diagnostic yield of brushing cytology [63]. The device used for this examination, known as SpyGlass (Boston Scientific, Natick, MA), is a small (10 Fr) endoscope that can be inserted into the bile duct through the working channel, allowing direct observation inside the bile duct and histological examination of the lesion. Directed biopsy can be achieved using biopsy forceps. The overall sensitivity, specificity, positive predictive value, and negative predictive value of POCS for malignant and benign biliary strictures were 78%, 82%, 80%, and 80%, respectively. In comparison, the sensitivity and specificity of ERCP alone were 51% and 54%, respectively [64]. The sensitivity of POCS was 84% for malignant tumors of the endoluminal bile ducts and 66% for noninvasive malignant tumors. The incidence of serious adverse events related to diagnostic POCS was 7.5%. The sensitivity of visual inspection using POCS was 95%, and the specificity was 79%, in 36 patients with indeterminate biliary strictures. The sensitivity and specificity values of cholangioscopic biopsy were both 82% [65]. These results suggest the utility of POCS in patients with indeterminate biliary strictures. Gaining a visual impression of malignant tumors is an essential part of cholangioscopy. The presence of abnormal tumor vessels due to neovascularization in biliary strictures suggests biliary malignancy. These irregular, swollen blood vessels are caused by angiogenesis of the stenotic region due to tumor growth. Their presence is 100% specific for malignancy [66]. However, interobserver variability and reproducibility with respect to such observations are unknown. Intraductal nodules and masses can be seen during cholangioscopy and are indicative of malignancy [67]. There is good agreement between the detection of these features by biliary endoscopy and the histopathologic results, but they are present in only a subset of patients with cholangiocarcinoma. Endoscopic sphincterotomy of narrow strictures by POCS is not possible because the scope cannot enter the upper portion of the bile duct. Finally, disposable equipment has the disadvantage of high cost.

Intraductal US

Intraductal ultrasound (IDUS) involves a small, high-frequency ultrasonic probe that provides high-resolution images of the ductal and periductal tissue (Fig. 9.8). Its sensitivity and specificity values were 80% and 90%, respectively, for assessing biliary strictures without visible masses [68, 69]. IDUS with ERCP has a higher diagnostic yield for biliary strictures than ERCP or MRCP alone [70]. The IDUS features suggestive of malignant tumors include eccentric wall thickening with an irregular surface, hypoechoic mass, heterogenicity of the internal echo pattern, papillary surface, destruction of the normal three-layer structure of the bile duct by US, presence of lymph nodes, and vascular invasion [71]. EUS is preferred when the biliary stent is inserted first, but IDUS is more effective than EUS prior to biliary stenting and for hepatic strictures [56]. The disadvantage of IDUS is that the scan range of the mini-probe is only about 25–30 mm, which limits evaluation of metastasis to the surrounding lymph nodes; also, the transducer is expensive and easily damaged.

Chromoendoscopy, Autofluorescence, and Narrow-Band Imaging

Several techniques have been used during cholangioscopy to characterize biliary strictures. In chromoendoscopy, stains are applied to the mucosal surface; for example, methylene blue enables normal mucosa to be distinguished from malignant lesions and ischemic strictures. Narrow-band imaging of the biliary tract enhances the vascular pattern on the mucosal surface, enabling evaluation of the extent of the tumor. Bile ductography with autofluorescence had poor specificity and a high positivity rate [72].

Confocal Laser Endomicroscopy

Probe-based confocal laser endomicroscopy (pCLE) generates an optical biopsy in an instantaneous and minimally invasive manner. This technique is associated with standard histology and enables discrimination of malignant tumors, inflammation, and normal mucosa. In a recent multicenter study, CLE showed significantly greater accuracy for diagnosing biliary strictures than standard ERCP (90% vs. 73%) [73]. In the Miami classification of the pCLE findings of biliary strictures, a thick white band (>20 μm), thick black band (>40 μm), dark lump, epithelial structure, and contrast leakage distinguished biliary strictures with malignant and benign causes (Table 9.4) [74, 75].

The recently proposed Paris classification is based on vascular congestion, dark lines, increased interglandular space, and thickened

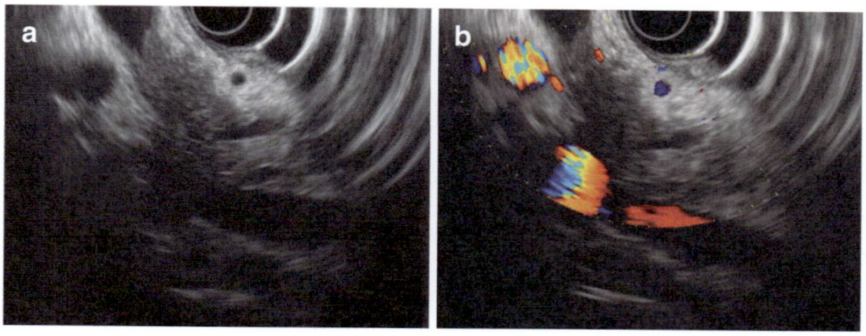

Fig. 9.7 EUS revealing a mass in the middle of the CBD. (**a**) The mass abuts the portal vein. (**b**) Verification of the portal vein on a Doppler view

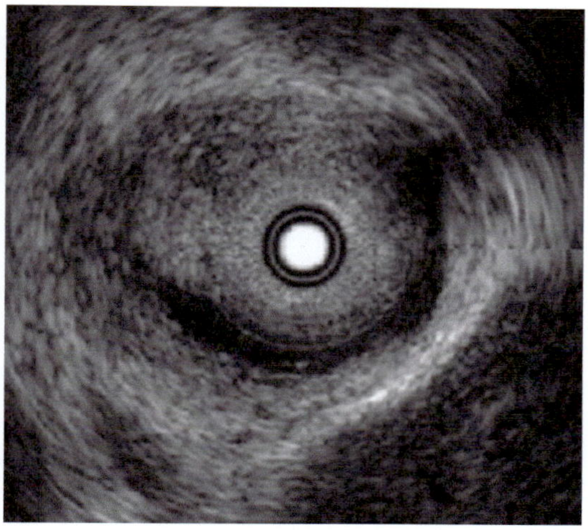

Fig. 9.8 Intraductal ultrasound showing a mass in the bile duct

reticular structures (Table 9.4) [74, 76, 77]. pCLE enabled visualization of 95% of the tumors of 15 patients with PSC and definite strictures, for a sensitivity of 100% and specificity of 61% [78].

Table 9.4 The Miami and Paris classifications of biliary strictures by probe-based confocal endomicroscopy [74–77]

Type of stricture	Miami	Paris
Benign	Thin, dark-branching bands (<20 μm)	Thin, dark-branching bands (<20 μm)
	Thin white bands	Thin white bands
	Light grey background	Light gray background
	Vessels <20 μm	Vessels <20 μm
Inflammatory stricture		Vascular congestion
		Thickened reticular structure
		Increased inter-glandular space
		Multiple white bands
		Dark granular pattern
Malignant stricture	Thick, dark bands (>40 μm)	Thick, dark bands (>40 μm)
	Thick, white bands (>20 μm)	Thick, white bands (>20 μm)
	Villi, glands	Villi, glands
	Fluorescein leak	Fluorescein leak
	Dark clumps	Dark clumps

Development of Diagnostic Methods

Fluorescence In Situ Hybridization

Fluorescence in situ hybridization (FISH) is a cytogenetic technique that uses fluorescent DNA probes to detect chromosomal polysomy under fluorescence microscopy. Cholangiocarcinoma is usually accompanied by chromosomal abnormalities. The sensitivity and specificity values of FISH for diagnosis of malignant disease in the bile duct are 84% and 97%, respectively [79]. FISH may be easier to interpret and more objective than conventional cytology. FISH is particularly useful for the diagnosis of indeterminate biliary strictures because it can detect chromosomal anomalies in fewer cells than conventional cytology [53].

However, in patients with PSC, the abovementioned chromosomal abnormalities can be present in the absence of malignant tumors. In a recent meta-analysis of patients with PSC, FISH had a sensitivity of 68% and specificity of 70% for detecting cancer of the bile duct [80]. FISH increases the sensitivity of brush cytology for indeterminate biliary strictures and so may be useful in groups of patients with high prevalence of malignant biliary strictures.

Immunostaining Methods

p53, Claudin-18, and Maspin

p53 is a tumor suppressor gene, and its product plays a role in DNA repair and apoptosis. P53 alterations are among the most frequent genetic alterations seen in human malignancies, including in neoplasms causing bile-duct strictures [81]. Immunofluorescence staining for P53 in a brushing cytology sample was attempted in 1999; the sensitivity was 43% but has been reported by others to be lower than that of conventional hematoxylin and eosin staining [82]. In a recent study, the sensitivity and specificity values of immunofluorescence staining for P53 were 85% and 100%, respectively. However, p53 was not detected in 28.9% of biliary cancer cells, due to insufficient cell count or cell deformation [83].

Claudin-18 is detected in gastrointestinal and lung tissues and is overexpressed in adenocarcinomas of the pancreas or the bile duct. Mammary serine protease inhibitor, also known as maspin, is a member of the serine protease inhibitor suppressor family and is a tumor suppressor in mammary carcinoma. Moreover, maspin is overexpressed in carcinomas of the pancreas and bile duct. Immunofluorescence staining for claudin-18, maspin, and p53 had sensitivity and specificity values of 100% and 94.7%, respectively [84, 85]. However, these values were obtained using tissue obtained during surgery or by biopsy. Immunofluorescence staining for claudin-18 and maspin had a sensitivity of 97% [85] and that for maspin and p53 had a positive predictive value of 88% [86]. However, maspin is not specific for biliary cancer, and its findings can differ from clinical results. Efforts to identify immunological markers specific for biliary cancer continue.

Methionyl-tRNA Synthetase

Aminoacyl-tRNA synthetases (ARSs) catalyze the coupling of amino acids to their cognate transfer RNAs (tRNAs) [87]. Aminoacyl-tRNA synthetases (ARSs) catalyze the coupling of amino acids to their cognate transfer RNAs (tRNAs) [88]. Because MRS plays an important role in the growth of tumors, it is expected to be highly expressed in cancer of the bile duct; indeed, its utility for differential diagnosis of biliary cancer is currently under investigation. MRS is reportedly overexpressed in malignant fibrous histiocytoma, sarcoma, malignant glioma, glioblastoma, and non-small cell lung cancer, in which it is associated with a poor prognosis [88–92]. The MRS immunostaining signal intensity is higher in malignant biliary strictures than in the normal bile duct (Fig. 9.9). The sensitivity, specificity, positive predictive value, and accuracy of MRS immunostaining for malignant biliary stricture were 98.1%, 96.1%, 98.1%, and 97.5%, respectively, suggesting superior diagnostic performance to conventional cytology (unpublished data). Further studies of these novel diagnostic methods are needed, and their association with the prognosis should be confirmed.

Real-Time Reverse Transcription Polymerase Chain Reaction Assays

The mRNAs of human aspartyl beta-hydroxylase (HAAH) and homeobox (Hox) B7 are molecular markers of cancer of the bile duct. Reverse transcriptase-polymerase chain reaction assays of these molecular markers in brushing cytology specimens improved the sensitivity by 82% [93]. However, these are preliminary results, and discrimination of benign strictures is limited.

Msx2, a member of the Hox gene family, is expressed in the premigratory cranial neural

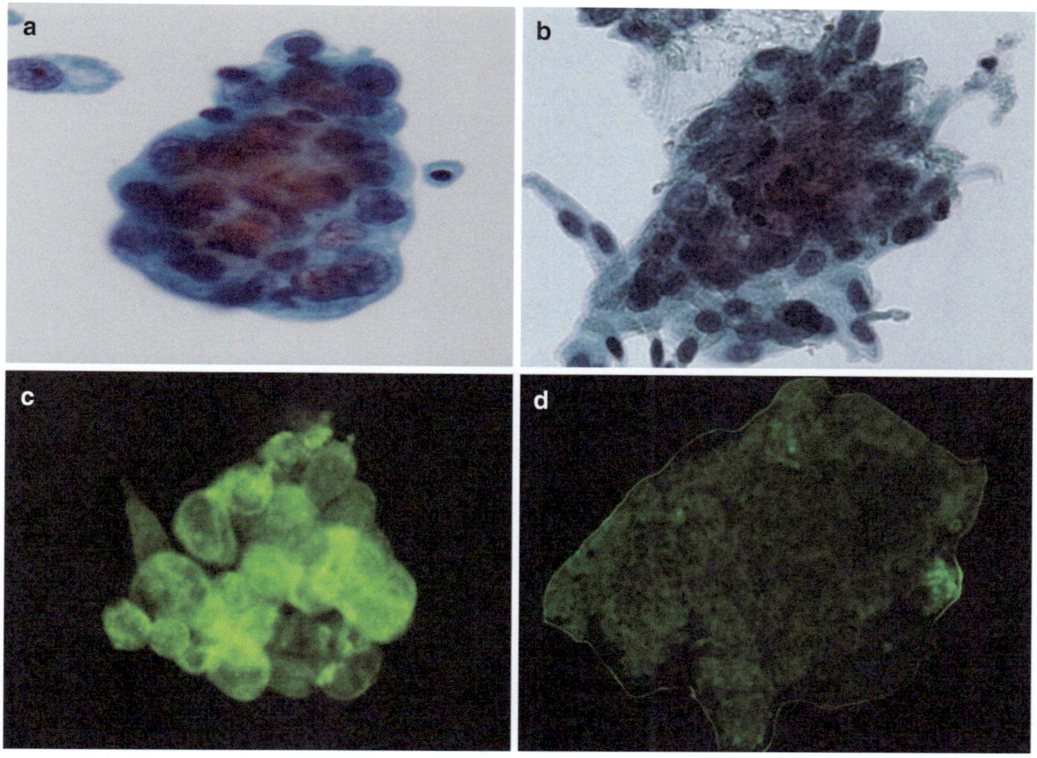

Fig. 9.9 Immunostaining for methionyl-tRNA synthetase (MRS). (**a**) Conventional Papanicolaou staining of a brushing cytology specimen from the distal CBD obtained during ERCP reported as suspicious for malignancy. (**b**) Conventional cytology specimen diagnosed as negative for malignancy; final diagnosis, negative. (**c**) Representative positive immunostaining pattern of MRS in a CBD cancer specimen. (**d**) Representative negative immunostaining pattern of MRS in a benign biliary stricture specimen

crest, tooth, and retina. Msx2 is frequently expressed in carcinoma cells of epithelial origin but not in normal tissues. Msx2 is expressed in pancreatic carcinoma cell lines and tissues but not in benign cultured cells or normal human pancreatic tissues. The sensitivity of MSX2 mRNA for biliary cancer was 72.3%, and the specificity was 58.3% [94]. The sensitivity was improved, but the technique provides additional information rather than a definitive diagnosis.

Among the 13 genes expressed in carcinomas of the bile duct, the degree of methylation of 4 (CDO1, CNRIP1, SEPT9, VIM) was 45–77% [95]. The sensitivity of a biomarker panel comprising these four genes was 85%, and the specificity was 98%, suggesting promise for detection of cancer of the bile duct.

Conclusion

Determining the causes of biliary strictures is problematic. Failure to properly diagnose malignant biliary strictures may delay treatment or lead to missed treatment opportunities. By contrast, if a benign biliary stricture is mistaken for a malignant biliary stricture, unnecessary surgery may be performed. Therefore, accurate diagnosis of biliary strictures is clinically important, and a multifaceted approach should be applied. Several techniques have good ability to determine the cause of biliary strictures, albeit that they vary in sensitivity and specificity (Table 9.5). The advantages and disadvantages of the various endoscopic, hematologic, and imaging techniques have been established (Table 9.6), but further study of novel diagnostic methods, such as MRS immunostaining, is needed.

Table 9.5 Sensitivity and specificity of diagnostic methods for malignant biliary strictures [96]

	Sensitivity (%)	Specificity (%)
ERCP/PTCS	41–77	53–100
Brushing cytology	21–71	83–100
Forceps biopsies	30–84	100
Peroral cholangioscopy/SpyGlass	50–100	87–100
Endoscopic ultrasound	52–94	84–100
FISH/flow cytometry	43–70	82–97
IDUS	83–88	83–92
Confocal laser endomicroscopy	83–98	33–88

Table 9.6 CT, MRCP, ERCP, and IDUS for the diagnosis of malignant biliary strictures

	CT	MRCP	ERCP	EUS (+FNA)	IDUS
Advantage	Assess nodal and vascular involvement, distant metastasis	Assess the level and morphology of strictures High-quality cholangiogram without contrast	Identifying the biliary stricture, determine its location and extent Tissue sampling	Cytological diagnosis	Evaluating biliary stricture without a mass
Disadvantage	Radiation Contrast allergy	Motion artifact Longer imaging process High cost	Invasive	Needle tract tumor seeding	Fragile

References

1. Tummala P, Munigala S, Eloubeidi MA, Agarwal B. Patients with obstructive jaundice and biliary stricture +/− mass lesion on imaging: prevalence of malignancy and potential role of EUS-FNA. J Clin Gastroenterol. 2013;47(6):532–7.
2. Charbel H, Al-Kawas FH. Cholangiocarcinoma: epidemiology, risk factors, pathogenesis, and diagnosis. Curr Gastroenterol Rep. 2011;13(2):182–7.
3. Patel T. Increasing incidence and mortality of primary intrahepatic cholangiocarcinoma in the United States. Hepatology. 2001;33(6):1353–7.
4. Mouzas IA, Dimoulios P, Vlachonikolis IG, Skordilis P, Zoras O, Kouroumalis E. Increasing incidence of cholangiocarcinoma in Crete 1992–2000. Anticancer Res. 2002;22(6B):3637–41.
5. Khashab MA, Fockens P, Al-Haddad MA. Utility of EUS in patients with indeterminate biliary strictures and suspected extrahepatic cholangiocarcinoma (with videos). Gastrointest Endosc. 2012;76(5):1024–33.
6. Gerhards MF, Vos P, van Gulik TM, Rauws EA, Bosma A, Gouma DJ. Incidence of benign lesions in patients resected for suspicious hilar obstruction. Br J Surg. 2001;88(1):48–51.
7. Clayton RA, Clarke DL, Currie EJ, Madhavan KK, Parks RW, Garden OJ. Incidence of benign pathology in patients undergoing hepatic resection for suspected malignancy. Surgeon. 2003;1(1):32–8.
8. Wakai T, Shirai Y, Sakata J, Maruyama T, Ohashi T, Korira PV, et al. Clinicopathological features of benign biliary strictures masquerading as biliary malignancy. Am Surg. 2012;78(12):1388–91.
9. Varadarajulu S, Eloubeidi MA. The role of endoscopic ultrasonography in the evaluation of pancreatico-biliary cancer. Surg Clin. 2010;90(2):251–63.
10. Ortner MAE, Liebetruth J, Schreiber S, Hanft M, Wruck U, Fusco V, et al. Photodynamic therapy of nonresectable cholangiocarcinoma. Gastroenterology. 1998;114(3):536–42.
11. Neuhaus P, Jonas S, Bechstein WO, Lohmann R, Radke C, Kling N, et al. Extended resections for hilar cholangiocarcinoma. Ann Surg. 1999;230(6):808.
12. Korrapati P, Ciolino J, Wani S, Shah J, Watson R, Muthusamy VR, et al. The efficacy of peroral cholangioscopy for difficult bile duct stones and indeterminate strictures: a systematic review and meta-analysis. Endosc Int Open. 2016;4(3):E263.
13. Wani S, Shah RJ. Endoscopic retrograde cholangiopancreatography biliary tissue sampling. Tech Gastrointest Endosc. 2012;14(3):164–71.
14. Marrelli D, Caruso S, Pedrazzani C, Neri A, Fernandes E, Marini M, et al. CA19-9 serum levels in obstructive jaundice: clinical value in benign and malignant conditions. Am J Surg. 2009;198(3):333–9.
15. Navaneethan U, Hasan MK, Lourdusamy V, Njei B, Varadarajulu S, Hawes RH. Single-operator cholangioscopy and targeted biopsies in the diagnosis of indeterminate biliary strictures: a systematic review. Gastrointest Endosc. 2015;82(4):608–14.e2.

16. Singh A, Gelrud A, Agarwal B. Biliary strictures: diagnostic considerations and approach. Gastroenterol Rep. 2015;3(1):22–31.
17. Levy C, Lymp J, Angulo P, Gores GJ, Larusso N, Lindor KD. The value of serum CA 19-9 in predicting cholangiocarcinomas in patients with primary sclerosing cholangitis. Dig Dis Sci. 2005;50(9):1734–40.
18. Patel AH, Harnois DM, Klee GG, LaRusso NF, Gores GJ. The utility of CA 19-9 in the diagnoses of cholangiocarcinoma in patients without primary sclerosing cholangitis. Am J Gastroenterol. 2000;95(1):204–7.
19. Khan .SA, Davidson BR, Goldin RD, Heaton N, Karani J, Pereira SP, et al. Guidelines for the diagnosis and treatment of cholangiocarcinoma: an update. Gut. 2012;61(12):1657–69.
20. Li Y, Zhang N. Clinical significance of serum tumour M2-PK and CA19-9 detection in the diagnosis of cholangiocarcinoma. Dig Liver Dis. 2009;41(8):605–8.
21. Qin XL, Wang ZR, Shi JS, Lu M, Wang L, He QR. Utility of serum CA19-9 in diagnosis of cholangiocarcinoma: in comparison with CEA. World J Gastroenterol. 2004;10(3):427–32.
22. Nehls O, Gregor M, Klump B. Serum and bile markers for cholangiocarcinoma. Semin Liver Dis. 2004;24(2):139–54.
23. Ramage JK, Donaghy A, Farrant JM, Iorns R, Williams R. Serum tumor markers for the diagnosis of cholangiocarcinoma in primary sclerosing cholangitis. Gastroenterology. 1995;108(3):865–9.
24. Ruzzenente A, Iacono C, Conci S, Bertuzzo F, Salvagno G, Ruzzenente O, et al. A novel serum marker for biliary tract cancer: diagnostic and prognostic values of quantitative evaluation of serum mucin 5AC (MUC5AC). Surgery. 2014;155(4):633–9.
25. Leelawat K, Narong S, Wannaprasert J, Ratanashu-Ek T. Prospective study of MMP7 serum levels in the diagnosis of cholangiocarcinoma. World J Gastroenterol: WJG. 2010;16(37):4697.
26. Zeng X, Tao H. Diagnostic and prognostic serum marker of cholangiocarcinoma. Oncol Lett. 2015;9(1):3–8.
27. Songür Y, Temuçin G, Sahin B. Endoscopic ultrasonography in the evaluation of dilated common bile duct. J Clin Gastroenterol. 2001;33(4):302–5.
28. Esnaola NF, Meyer JE, Karachristos A, Maranki JL, Camp ER, Denlinger CS. Evaluation and management of intrahepatic and extrahepatic cholangiocarcinoma. Cancer. 2016;122(9):1349–69.
29. Rosch T, Meining A, Fruhmorgen S, Zillinger C, Schusdziarra V, Hellerhoff K, et al. A prospective comparison of the diagnostic accuracy of ERCP, MRCP, CT, and EUS in biliary strictures. Gastrointest Endosc. 2002;55(7):870–6.
30. Nesbit GM, Johnson CD, James EM, MacCarty RL, Nagorney DM, Bender CE. Cholangiocarcinoma: diagnosis and evaluation of resectability by CT and sonography as procedures complementary to cholangiography. AJR Am J Roentgenol. 1988;151(5):933–8.
31. Sugiyama M, Atomi Y, Kuroda A, Muto T. Bile duct carcinoma without jaundice: clues to early diagnosis. Hepato-Gastroenterology. 1997;44(17):1477–83.
32. Xu A-M, Cheng H-Y, Jiang W-B, Chen D, Jia Y-C, Wu M-C. Multi-slice three-dimensional spiral CT cholangiography: a new technique for diagnosis of biliary diseases. HBPD Int. 2002;1(4):595–603.
33. Vilgrain V. Staging cholangiocarcinoma by imaging studies. HPB. 2008;10(2):106–9.
34. Lee HY, Kim SH, Lee JM, Kim S-W, Jang J-Y, Han JK, et al. Preoperative assessment of resectability of hepatic hilar cholangiocarcinoma: combined CT and cholangiography with revised criteria. Radiology. 2006;239(1):113–21.
35. Taylor AC, Little AF, Hennessy OF, Banting SW, Smith PJ, Desmond PV. Prospective assessment of magnetic resonance cholangiopancreatography for noninvasive imaging of the biliary tree. Gastrointest Endosc. 2002;55(1):17–22.
36. Rösch T, Meining A, Frühmorgen S, Zillinger C, Schusdziarra V, Hellerhoff K, et al. A prospective comparison of the diagnostic accuracy of ERCP, MRCP, CT, and EUS in biliary strictures. Gastrointest Endosc. 2002;55(7):870–6.
37. Vanderveen KA, Hussain HK. Magnetic resonance imaging of cholangiocarcinoma. Cancer Imaging. 2004;4(2):104.
38. Lopera JE, Soto JA, Munera F. Malignant hilar and perihilar biliary obstruction: use of MR cholangiography to define the extent of biliary ductal involvement and plan percutaneous interventions. Radiology. 2001;220(1):90–6.
39. Suthar M, Purohit S, Bhargav V, Goyal P. Role of MRCP in differentiation of benign and malignant causes of biliary obstruction. J Clin Diagn Res. 2015;9(11):Tc08–12.
40. Park M-S, Kim TK, Kim KW, Park SW, Lee JK, Kim J-S, et al. Differentiation of extrahepatic bile duct cholangiocarcinoma from benign stricture: findings at MRCP versus ERCP. Radiology. 2004;233(1):234–40.
41. Navaneethan U, Njei B, Lourdusamy V, Konjeti R, Vargo JJ, Parsi MA. Comparative effectiveness of biliary brush cytology and intraductal biopsy for detection of malignant biliary strictures: a systematic review and meta-analysis. Gastrointest Endosc. 2015;81(1):168–76.
42. Schoefl R, Haefner M, Wrba F, Pfeffel F, Stain C, Poetzi R, et al. Forceps biopsy and brush cytology during endoscopic retrograde cholangiopancreatography for the diagnosis of biliary stenoses. Scand J Gastroenterol. 1997;32(4):363–8.
43. Ponchon T, Gagnon P, Berger F, Labadie M, Liaras A, Chavaillon A, et al. Value of endobiliary brush cytology and biopsies for the diagnosis of malignant bile duct stenosis: results of a prospective study. Gastrointest Endosc. 1995;42(6):565–72.
44. Jo YG, Lee TH, Cho HD, Park SH, Park JM, Cho YS, et al. Diagnostic accuracy of brush cytology with direct

smear and cell-block techniques according to preparation order and tumor characteristics in biliary strictures. Korean J Gastroenterol. 2014;63(4):223–30.
45. Glasbrenner B, Ardan M, Boeck W, Preclik G, Moller P, Adler G. Prospective evaluation of brush cytology of biliary strictures during endoscopic retrograde cholangiopancreatography. Endoscopy. 1999;31(9):712–7.
46. Fogel EL, McHenry L, Watkins JL, Chappo J, Cramer H, Schmidt S, et al. Effectiveness of a new long cytology brush in the evaluation of malignant biliary obstruction: a prospective study. Gastrointest Endosc. 2006;63(1):71–7.
47. De Bellis M, Fogel EL, Sherman S, Watkins JL, Chappo J, Younger C, et al. Influence of stricture dilation and repeat brushing on the cancer detection rate of brush cytology in the evaluation of malignant biliary obstruction. Gastrointest Endosc. 2003;58(2):176–82.
48. Howell D, Beveridge R, Bosco J, Jones M. Endoscopic needle aspiration biopsy at ERCP in the diagnosis of biliary strictures. Gastrointest Endosc. 1992;38(5):531–5.
49. Fritcher EGB, Kipp BR, Halling KC, Oberg TN, Bryant SC, Tarrell RF, et al. A multivariable model using advanced cytologic methods for the evaluation of indeterminate pancreatobiliary strictures. Gastroenterology. 2009;136(7):2180–6.
50. De Bellis M, Sherman S, Fogel EL, Cramer H, Chappo J, McHenry L, et al. Tissue sampling at ERCP in suspected malignant biliary strictures (part 2). Gastrointest Endosc. 2002;56(5):720–30.
51. Mansfield J, Griffin S, Wadehra V, Matthewson K. A prospective evaluation of cytology from biliary strictures. Gut. 1997;40(5):671–7.
52. Higashizawa T, Tamada K, Tomiyama T, Wada S, Ohashi A, Satoh Y, et al. Biliary guidewire facilitates bile duct biopsy and endoscopic drainage. J Gastroenterol Hepatol. 2002;17(3):332–6.
53. Victor DW, Sherman S, Karakan T, Khashab MA. Current endoscopic approach to indeterminate biliary strictures. World J Gastroenterol. 2012;18(43):6197–205.
54. Harewood GC, Wiersema MJ. Endosonography-guided fine needle aspiration biopsy in the evaluation of pancreatic masses. Am J Gastroenterol. 2002;97(6):1386–91.
55. Eloubeidi MA, Chen VK, Jhala NC, Eltoum IE, Jhala D, Chhieng DC, et al. Endoscopic ultrasound-guided fine needle aspiration biopsy of suspected cholangiocarcinoma. Clin Gastroenterol Hepatol. 2004;2(3):209–13.
56. Mohamadnejad M, DeWitt JM, Sherman S, LeBlanc JK, Pitt HA, House MG, et al. Role of EUS for preoperative evaluation of cholangiocarcinoma: a large single-center experience. Gastrointest Endosc. 2011;73(1):71–8.
57. Heimbach JK, Sanchez W, Rosen CB, Gores GJ. Trans-peritoneal fine needle aspiration biopsy of hilar cholangiocarcinoma is associated with disease dissemination. HPB. 2011;13(5):356–60.
58. El Chafic AH, Dewitt J, Leblanc JK, El H II, Cote G, House MG, et al. Impact of preoperative endoscopic ultrasound-guided fine needle aspiration on postoperative recurrence and survival in cholangiocarcinoma patients. Endoscopy. 2013;45(11):883–9.
59. Mukai H, Nakajima M, Yasuda K, Mizuno S, Kawai K. Evaluation of endoscopic ultrasonography in the pre-operative staging of carcinoma of the ampulla of Vater and common bile duct. Gastrointest Endosc. 1992;38(6):676–83.
60. Tio T, Reeders J, Sie L, Wijers O, Maas J, Colin E, et al. Endosonography in the clinical staging of Klatskin tumor. Endoscopy. 1993;25(01):81–5.
61. Sugiyama M, Hagi H, Atomi Y, Saito M. Diagnosis of portal venous invasion by pancreatobiliary carcinoma: value of endoscopic ultrasonography. Abdom Imaging. 1997;22(4):434–8.
62. Blechacz B, Komuta M, Roskams T, Gores GJ. Clinical diagnosis and staging of cholangiocarcinoma. Nat Rev Gastroenterol Hepatol. 2011;8(9):512.
63. Chen YK, Pleskow DK. SpyGlass single-operator peroral cholangiopancreatoscopy system for the diagnosis and therapy of bile-duct disorders: a clinical feasibility study (with video). Gastrointest Endosc. 2007;65(6):832–41.
64. Chen YK, Parsi MA, Binmoeller KF, Hawes RH, Pleskow DK, Slivka A, et al. Single-operator cholangioscopy in patients requiring evaluation of bile duct disease or therapy of biliary stones (with videos). Gastrointest Endosc. 2011;74(4):805–14.
65. Ramchandani M, Reddy DN, Gupta R, Lakhtakia S, Tandan M, Darisetty S, et al. Role of single-operator peroral cholangioscopy in the diagnosis of indeterminate biliary lesions: a single-center, prospective study. Gastrointest Endosc. 2011;74(3):511–9.
66. Kim H-J, Kim M-H, Lee S-K, Yoo K-S, Seo D-W, Min Y-I. Tumor vessel: a valuable cholangioscopic clue of malignant biliary stricture. Gastrointest Endosc. 2000;52(5):635–8.
67. Parsi MA. Peroral cholangioscopy in the new millennium. World J Gastroenterol: WJG. 2011;17:1):1.
68. Vazquez-Sequeiros E, Baron TH, Clain JE, Gostout CJ, Norton ID, Petersen BT, et al. Evaluation of indeterminate bile duct strictures by intraductal US. Gastrointest Endosc. 2002;56(3):372–9.
69. Stavropoulos S, Larghi A, Verna E, Battezzati P, Stevens P. Intraductal ultrasound for the evaluation of patients with biliary strictures and no abdominal mass on computed tomography. Endoscopy. 2005;37(8):715–21.
70. Domagk D, Wessling J, Reimer P, Hertel L, Poremba C, Senninger N, et al. Endoscopic retrograde cholangiopancreatography, intraductal ultrasonography, and magnetic resonance cholangiopancreatography in bile duct strictures: a prospective comparison of imaging diagnostics with histopathological correlation. Am J Gastroenterol. 2004;99(9):1684–9.
71. Tamada K, Ueno N, Tomiyama T, Oohashi A, Wada S, Nishizono T, et al. Characterization of biliary strictures using intraductal ultrasonography: comparison with

percutaneous cholangioscopic biopsy. Gastrointest Endosc. 1998;47(5):341–9.
72. Itoi T, Neuhaus H, Chen YK. Diagnostic value of image-enhanced video cholangiopancreatoscopy. Gastrointest Endosc Clin. 2009;19(4):557–66.
73. Meining A, Chen YK, Pleskow D, Stevens P, Shah RJ, Chuttani R, et al. Direct visualization of indeterminate pancreaticobiliary strictures with probe-based confocal laser endomicroscopy: a multicenter experience. Gastrointest Endosc. 2011;74(5):961–8.
74. Meining A, Shah RJ, Slivka A, Pleskow D, Chuttani R, Stevens PD, et al. Classification of probe-based confocal laser endomicroscopy findings in pancreaticobiliary strictures. Endoscopy. 2012;44(3):251–7.
75. Slivka A, Gan I, Jamidar P, Costamagna G, Cesaro P, Giovannini M, et al. Validation of the diagnostic accuracy of probe-based confocal laser endomicroscopy for the characterization of indeterminate biliary strictures: results of a prospective multicenter international study. Gastrointest Endosc. 2015;81(2):282–90.
76. Caillol F, Filoche B, Gaidhane M, Kahaleh M. Refined probe-based confocal laser endomicroscopy classification for biliary strictures: the Paris Classification. Dig Dis Sci. 2013;58(6):1784–9.
77. Kahaleh M, Giovannini M, Jamidar P, Gan SI, Cesaro P, Caillol F, et al. Probe-based confocal laser endomicroscopy for indeterminate biliary strictures: refinement of the image interpretation classification. Gastroenterol Res Pract. 2015;2015:675210.
78. Heif M, Yen RD, Shah RJ. ERCP with probe-based confocal laser endomicroscopy for the evaluation of dominant biliary stenoses in primary sclerosing cholangitis patients. Dig Dis Sci. 2013;58(7):2068–74.
79. Kipp BR, Stadheim LM, Halling SA, Pochron NL, Harmsen S, Nagorney DM, et al. A comparison of routine cytology and fluorescence in situ hybridization for the detection of malignant bile duct strictures. Am J Gastroenterol. 2004;99(9):1675–81.
80. Navaneethan U, Njei B, Venkatesh PG, Vargo JJ, Parsi MA. Fluorescence in situ hybridization for diagnosis of cholangiocarcinoma in primary sclerosing cholangitis: a systematic review and meta-analysis. Gastrointest Endosc. 2014;79(6):943–50. e3.
81. Tascilar M, Sturm PD, Caspers E, Smit M, Polak MM, Huibregtse K, et al. Diagnostic p53 immunostaining of endobiliary brush cytology: preoperative cytology compared with the surgical specimen. Cancer. 1999;87(5):306–11.
82. Stewart C, Burke G. Value of p53 immunostaining in pancreatico-biliary brush cytology specimens. Diagn Cytopathol. 2000;23(5):308–13.
83. Yeo M, Kim K, Lee Y, Lee BS, Choi S. The usefulness of adding p53 immunocytochemistry to bile drainage cytology for the diagnosis of malignant biliary strictures. Diagn Cytopathol. 2017;45(7):592–7.
84. Keira Y, Takasawa A, Murata M, Nojima M, Takasawa K, Ogino J, et al. An immunohistochemical marker panel including claudin-18, maspin, and p53 improves diagnostic accuracy of bile duct neoplasms in surgical and presurgical biopsy specimens. Virchows Arch. 2015;466(3):265–77.
85. Tokumitsu T, Sato Y, Yamashita A, Moriguchi-Goto S, Kondo K, Nanashima A, et al. Immunocytochemistry for Claudin-18 and Maspin in biliary brushing cytology increases the accuracy of diagnosing pancreatobiliary malignancies. Cytopathology. 2017;28(2):116–21.
86. Kanzawa M, Sanuki T, Onodera M, Fujikura K, Itoh T, Zen Y. Double immunostaining for maspin and p53 on cell blocks increases the diagnostic value of biliary brushing cytology. Pathol Int. 2017;67(2):91–8.
87. Kim S, You S, Hwang D. Aminoacyl-tRNA synthetases and tumorigenesis: more than housekeeping. Nat Rev Cancer. 2011;11(10):708–18.
88. Kwon NH, Kang T, Lee JY, Kim HH, Kim HR, Hong J, et al. Dual role of methionyl-tRNA synthetase in the regulation of translation and tumor suppressor activity of aminoacyl-tRNA synthetase-interacting multifunctional protein-3. Proc Natl Acad Sci U S A. 2011;108(49):19635–40.
89. Palmer JL, Masui S, Pritchard S, Kalousek DK, Sorensen PH. Cytogenetic and molecular genetic analysis of a pediatric pleomorphic sarcoma reveals similarities to adult malignant fibrous histiocytoma. Cancer Genet Cytogenet. 1997;95(2):141–7.
90. Reifenberger G, Ichimura K, Reifenberger J, Elkahloun AG, Meltzer PS, Collins VP. Refined mapping of 12q13-q15 amplicons in human malignant gliomas suggests CDK4/SAS and MDM2 as independent amplification targets. Cancer Res. 1996;56(22):5141–5.
91. Kim EY, Jung JY, Kim A, Kim K, Chang YS. Methionyl-tRNA synthetase overexpression is associated with poor clinical outcomes in non-small cell lung cancer. BMC Cancer. 2017;17(1):467.
92. Nilbert M, Rydholm A, Mitelman F, Meltzer PS, Mandahl N. Characterization of the 12q13-15 amplicon in soft tissue tumors. Cancer Genet Cytogenet. 1995;83(1):32–6.
93. Feldmann G, Nattermann J, Nischalke H, Gorschlüter M, Kuntzen T, Ahlenstiel G, et al. Detection of human aspartyl (asparaginyl) beta-hydroxylase and homeobox B7 mRNA in brush cytology specimens from patients with bile duct cancer. Endoscopy. 2006;38(06):604–9.
94. Ito H, Satoh K, Hamada S, Hirota M, Kanno A, Ishida K, et al. The evaluation of MSX2 mRNA expression level in biliary brush cytological specimens. Anticancer Res. 2011;31(3):1011–7.
95. Andresen K, Boberg KM, Vedeld HM, Honne H, Jebsen P, Hektoen M, et al. Four DNA methylation biomarkers in biliary brush samples accurately identify the presence of cholangiocarcinoma. Hepatology. 2015;61(5):1651–9.
96. Voigtlander T, Lankisch TO. Endoscopic diagnosis of cholangiocarcinoma: From endoscopic retrograde cholangiography to bile proteomics. Best Pract Res Clin Gastroenterol. 2015;29(2):267–75.
97. Lim JH. Cholangiocarcinoma: morphologic classification according to growth pattern and imaging findings. AJR Am J Roentgenol. 2003;181(3):819–27.

Characteristics of Benign Pancreatic Duct Stricture

10

Resheed Alkhiari and Michel Kahaleh

Introduction

Benign pancreatic duct stricture (PDS) is a common pancreatic condition that results from a previous or existing injury to the main pancreatic duct. The most common etiology for PDS includes chronic pancreatitis, trauma, previous pancreatic surgery, pancreatic pseudocyst, IgG4 disease, and benign neoplasm (Table 10.1). It may participate in the events of recurrent acute pancreatitis, chronic abdominal pain, and local pancreatic complication [1–4].

PDS can be classified into single or multiple and dominant or nondominant. Dominant stricture has been defined by upstream dilatation of the main pancreatic duct to 6 mm or more in diameter, occlusion of contrast outflow alongside a 6-Fr size catheter placed upstream from the stricture or provocation of symptoms, mainly abdominal pain during continuous infusion of 1 l saline at the upstream area using a nasopancreatic catheter for 12–24 h [5–8].

The first step when PDS is found is to identify the nature of the stricture and to rule out underlying malignancy. History and physical examination could be a guide to the etiology, as well as a history of alcohol abuse and previous pancreatitis.

R. Alkhiari
Qassim Unviersity, Buraydah, Saudi Arabia

M. Kahaleh (✉)
Robert Wood Johnson University Hospital,
Rutgers Robert Wood Johnson Johnson University,
New Brunswick, NJ, USA

All pancreatic strictures should be taken seriously to rule out underlying malignancy. Younger age <50, history of pancreatitis, absence of jaundice, normal bile duct, strictures in the body or tail of the pancreas, irregular duct and multiple strictures, and presence of main pancreatic stones may suggest benign process (Table 10.2) [4].

Workup

Roles of different modalities to characterize benign PDS.

Computed Tomography (CT) Scan

This scan has an important role in evaluation of PDS (Fig. 10.1), which is usually seen in dilation in the pancreatic duct during the venous phase after contrast injection. Underlying etiology could be viewed as an obstructive lesion or with chronic pancreatitis features such as atrophic pancreas, ductal dilation, and calcification [8–10].

Magnetic Resonance Imaging (MRI)

Magnetic resonance cholangiopancreatography (MRCP) is a form of MRI that uses T2-weighted sequences to assess the fluid-filled structure without the need for contrast (Fig. 10.2). It has

D. K. Lee (ed.), *Advanced ERCP for Complicated and Refractory Biliary and Pancreatic Diseases*,
https://doi.org/10.1007/978-981-13-0608-2_10

Table 10.1 Benign pancreatic stricture etiology

Causes of benign pancreatic duct stricture
Chronic pancreatitis
Trauma
Previous pancreatic surgery
Pancreatic pseudocyst
IgG4 disease
Benign neoplasm

Table 10.2 Characteristics of benign versus pancreatic duct stricture

Characteristics of benign and malignant pancreatic stricture		
Characteristics	Benign	Malignant
Age	<55	>55
History of pancreatitis	yes	No
Duct morphology	Multiple stricture with irregular duct	Focal stricture with dilated duct upstream
Location	Pancreatic body or tail	Pancreatic head or neck
Pancreatic duct stones	Present	Absent
Pancreatic divisum	May be present	Absent
Bile duct	Normal	May be dilated
Jaundice	Absent	May be present

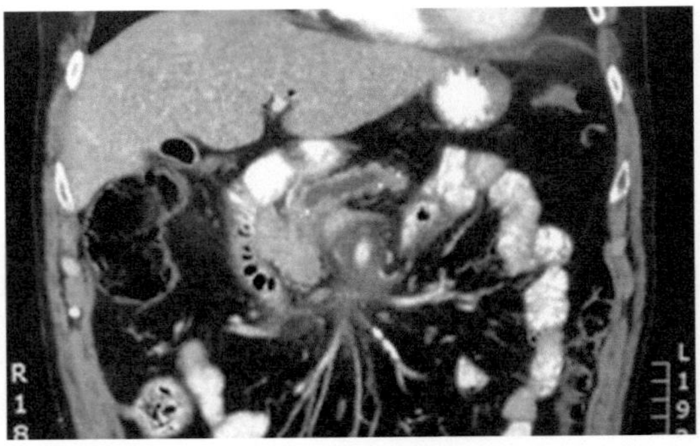

Fig. 10.1 CT showing dilated pancreatic duct with benign pancreatic stricture with stone in patient with chronic pancreatitis

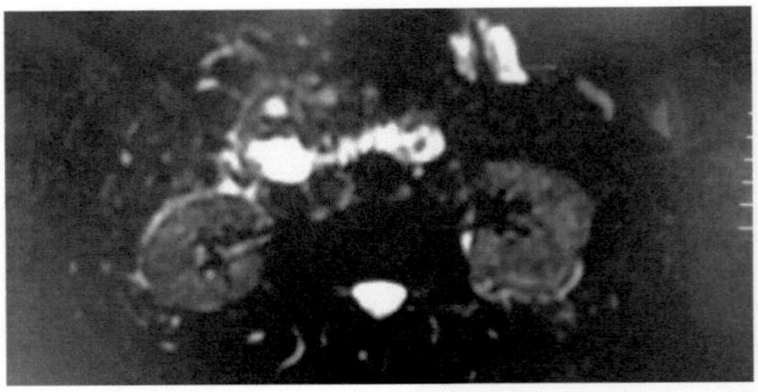

Fig. 10.2 MRCP showing dilated pancreatic duct with multiple stricture in chronic recurrent pancreatitis

the ability to identify the ductal stricture in 70–92% of chronic pancreatitis. In addition to PDS, it also provides invaluable details about the underlying etiology such as intraductal stones, neoplasm, and cysts [11–14].

Endoscopic Retrograde Pancreatography (ERP)

ERP is the main modality to provide diagnostic and therapeutic options to evaluate PDS. Fluoroscopic image and endoscopic view of ERP can characterize pancreatic stricture (Fig. 10.3) and underlying etiology such as pancreatic divisum, ampullary lesions, and chronic pancreatitis.

Pancreatic duct stricture is seen as segmental or focal. Segmental PDS is usually an alternation between dilation and stenosis in fluoroscopy which gives the appearance of a chain of lakes. Focal PDS is usually seen as the dilation of upstream pancreatic duct with focal narrowing. A pancreatic leak, main pancreatic duct stones (as a filling defect) in addition to pancreatic stricture, is favorable for benign pancreatic stricture in chronic pancreatitis [15, 16].

Peroral Pancreatoscopy

POP is a direct way to evaluate pancreatic stricture visually and obtain a biopsy. The physical appearance of benign pancreatic stricture can be better evaluated for scars, calcification, lesions, and ductal erythema (Fig. 10.4) [17, 18].

Echoendosonography (EUS)

EUS is one of the best modalities to characterize PDS and identify underlying etiology. In

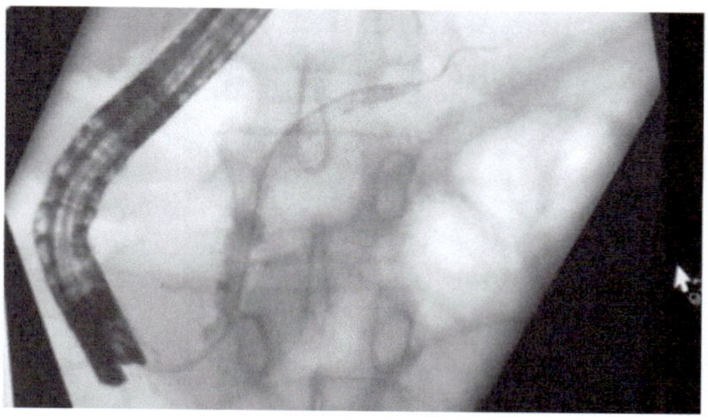

Fig. 10.3 ERP: showing dilated pancreatic duct with pancreatic head stricture in chronic pancreatitis

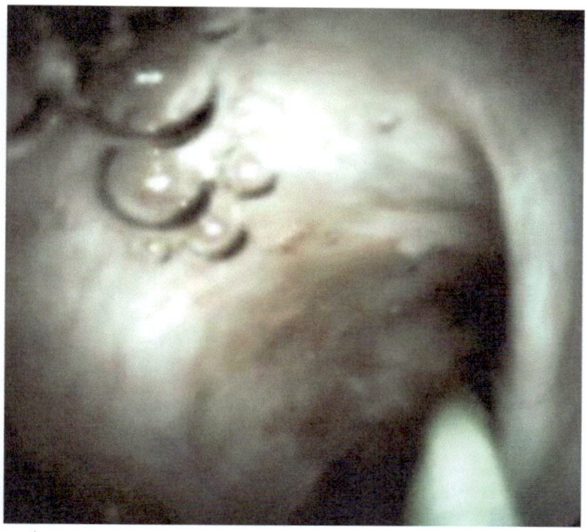

Fig. 10.4 Pancreatoscopy showing a focal narrowing and local erythema

EUS, PDS found in the form of dilated main pancreatic duct with a narrowing point represents the stricture. It also a gold standard for evaluation of pancreatic parenchyma and obtained biopsy to rule out malignancy if needed [19, 20].

Optical Coherence Tomography (OCT)

OCT is one of the new hypermagnification modalities to provide cross-sectional imaging at the structure level. A newer generation was tested and showed dilated hyporeflective structure at the level of benign stricture in the main pancreatic duct [21].

References

1. Steer ML, Waxman I, Freedman S. Chronic pancreatitis. N Engl J Med. 1995;332:1482–90.
2. Witt H, Apte MV, Keim V, et al. Chronic pancreatitis: challenges and advances in pathogenesis, genetics, diagnosis, and therapy. Gastroenterology. 2007;132:1557–73.
3. Sah RP, Chari ST. Autoimmune pancreatitis: an update on classification, diagnosis natural history, and management. Curr Gastroenterol Rep. 2012;14:95–105.
4. Kalady M, Peterson B, Baillie J. Pancreatic duct strictures: identifying risk of malignancy. Ann Surg Oncol. 2004;11(6):581–8.
5. Cohen SA, Siegel JH, Kasmin FE. Treatment of pancreatic strictures. Curr Treat Options Gastroenterol. 2007;10:347–54.
6. Oza VM, Kahaleh M. Endoscopic management of chronic pancreatitis. World J Gastrointest Endosc. 2013;5:19–28.
7. Catalano MF. Endoscopic treatment of pancreatic duct strictures. Tech Gastrointest Endosc. 1999;1:168–74.
8. Remer EM, Baker ME. Imaging of chronic pancreatitis. Radiol Clin N Am. 2002;40:1229–42.
9. Siddiqi AJ, Miller F. Chronic pancreatitis: ultrasound, computed tomography, and magnetic resonance imaging features. Semin Ultrasound CT MR. 2007;28:384–94.
10. Miller FH, Keppke A, Balthazar E. Imaging pancreatitis. In: RMLM G, editor. Textbook of gastrointestinal radiology. 3rd ed. Philadelphia, PA: W.B. Saunders; 2008.
11. oto JA, Barish MA, Yucel EK, et al. Pancreatic duct: MR cholangiopancreatography with a three-dimensional fast spin-echo technique. Radiology. 1995;196:459–64.
12. Matos C, Metens T, Deviere J, et al. Pancreatic duct: morphologic and functional evaluation with dynamic MR pancreatography after secretin stimulation. Radiology. 1997;203:435–41.
13. Sanyal R, Stevens T, Novak E, et al. Secretin-enhanced MRCP: review of technique and application with proposal for quantification of exocrine function. AJR Am J Roentgenol. 2012;198:124–32.
14. Hansen TM, Nilsson M, Gram M, Frøkjær JB. Morphological and functional evaluation of chronic pancreatitis with magnetic resonance imaging. World J Gastroenterol. 2013;19(42):7241–6.
15. Dumonceau JM, Delhaye M, Tringali A, et al. Endoscopic treatment of chronic pancreatitis: European Society of Gastrointestinal Endoscopy (ESGE) clinical guideline. Endoscopy. 2012;44:784–800.
16. Cohen SA, Siegel JH, Kasmin FE. Treatment of pancreatic strictures. Curr Treat Options Gastroenterol. 2007 Oct;10(5):347–54.
17. Ringold DA, Shah RJ. Peroral pancreatoscopy in the diagnosis and management of intraductal papillary

mucinous neoplasia and indeterminate pancreatic duct pathology. Gastrointest Endosc Clin N Am. 2009;19(4):601–13.
18. Kodama T, Koshitani T, Sato H, et al. Electronic pancreatoscopy for the diagnosis of pancreatic diseases. Am J Gastroenterol. 2002;97(3):617–22.
19. Stevens T. Update on the role of endoscopic ultrasound in chronic pancreatitis. Curr Gastroenterol Rep. 2011;13:117–22.
20. Varadarajulu S, Tamhane A, Eloubeidi MA. Yield of EUS-guided FNA of pancreatic masses in the presence or the absence of chronic pancreatitis. Gastrointest Endosc. 2005;62:728–36; quiz 751, 753.
21. Tyberg A, Xu MM, Gaidhane M, Kahaleh M. Second generation optical coherence tomography: Preliminary experience in pancreatic and biliary strictures. Dig Liver Dis. 2018;50:1214–7.

11 Management of Benign Pancreatic Strictures

Resheed Alkhiari and Michel Kahaleh

Introduction

Treatment of a pancreatic stricture depends on the underlying etiology and ongoing symptoms. The first step when pancreatic stricture is found is to rule out underlying malignancy. After this, any therapeutic option depends on the patient's symptoms and the presence of local complication. An asymptomatic patient may not need an intervention if malignant stricture has been excluded. The management of benign pancreatic stricture requires a multidisciplinary approach which includes medical, endoscopic, and surgical therapy [1–5].

Medical Therapy

Medical therapy provides the first line of modality which is mainly used in patients with chronic pancreatitis to prevent further injury to the pancreas. These measures include alcohol and smoking cessation, a low-fat diet, and small frequent meals with pancreatic enzyme therapy if they have exocrine dysfuntion [1, 2].

Endoscopic Therapy

Over the last few decades, a huge advancement in endoscopic technology has put endotherapy first as the mainstay therapy in pancreatic stricture due to its feasibility and safety with lower rates of morbidity and mortality compared with surgery [1, 4].

Endoscopic Retrograde Pancreatography (ERP)

ERP has a major role in diagnosis and provides therapy especially in the presence of chronic recurrent pancreatitis with features of pancreatic duct stricture with obstruction (Fig. 11.1). These actions mainly include pancreatic sphincterotomy, dilation, and stenting in addition to using diagnostic modalities such as brushing and pancreatoscopy with biopsy. The technical success rate of ERP with pancreatic stenting in patients with chronic pancreatitis ranges from 85% to 98% (Fig. 11.2).

Pancreatic sphincterotomy (PS) is an endoscopic therapy that has shown symptomatic relief when the stricture of the duct is located at the ampulla and is used as well prior to stent placement. It can be done using a sphincterotome to pull up at the direction of the pancreatic duct or by using needle knife sphincterotomy. The success rate is as high as 98% with minimal adverse

R. Alkhiari
Qassim Unviersity, Buraydah, Saudi Arabia

M. Kahaleh (✉)
Robert Wood Johnson University Hospital,
Rutgers Robert Wood Johnson Johnson University,
New Brunswick, NJ, USA

D. K. Lee (ed.), *Advanced ERCP for Complicated and Refractory Biliary and Pancreatic Diseases*,
https://doi.org/10.1007/978-981-13-0608-2_11

events which can reaches up to 4%. The first technique may have a higher risk for post-sphincterotomy pancreatitis compared to needle knife sphincterotomy (Fig. 11.3) [6–8].

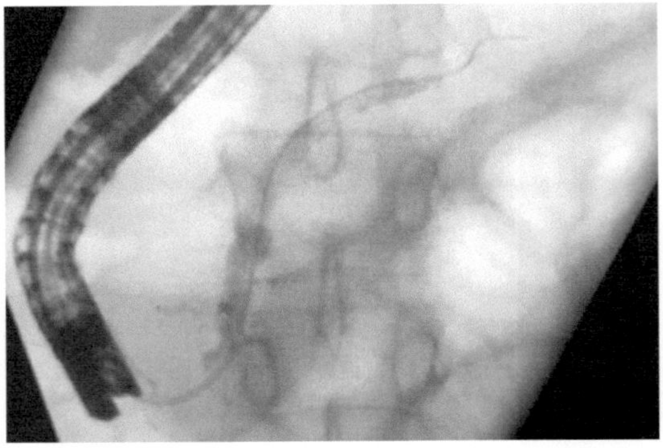

Fig. 11.1 Pancreatogram showing a distal pancreatic stricture with proximal dilation

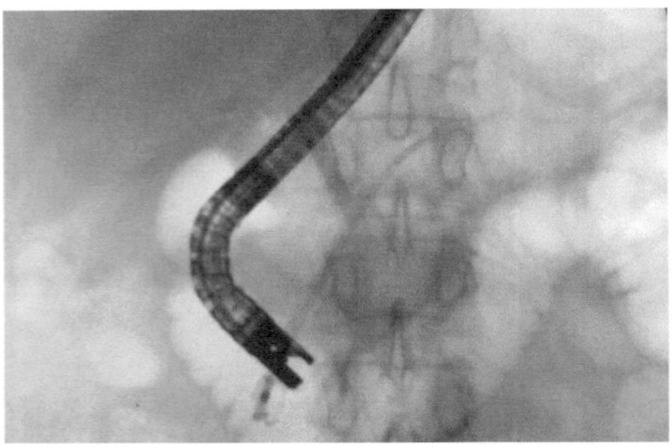

Fig. 11.2 Pancreatogram after placement of two 7 Fr pancreatic stents to treat a distal pancreatic stricture

Biliary sphincterotomy is selective in the management of pancreatic stricture and is considered in the presence of cholangitis, jaundice, and a dilated bile duct of >12 mm with elevated alkaline phosphatase more than twice of the upper limit of normal (Fig. 11.4) [8].

Main pancreatic stenting for benign pancreatic stricture is considered to be a cornerstone in the management. The success rate has been reported between 70% and 94% after single stent placement for pain relief. Stenting therapy is ideal for the focal segment stricture in the head, the genu, or the body. Pancreatic tail stricture could be stented but is less likely to participate in pancreatic duct hypertension (Fig. 11.5) [9, 10].

Prior to the stent placement, dilation is usually performed using dilating catheter, a wire-guided balloon dilator, or a Soehendra stent retriever as a rescue option when the first two were not successful. These dilators achieve dilation up to 4–6 mm which is needed to place a large bore plastic pancreatic stent, 7–10 Fr. Following the stent placement, attention should be placed on any local complications that could occur with stent placement such as pancreatitis, infection, migration, stent occlusion, and perforation. Stent exchange is required between 2 and 6 months, depending on the recurrence of symptoms, to achieve resolution of the stricture. The timeline for the resolution of the stricture varies depending on the severity of the stricture and that may be required 8 to 15 months or longer after stenting. Upsizing the stent should be evaluated at each session to achieve a favorable outcome [9, 10].

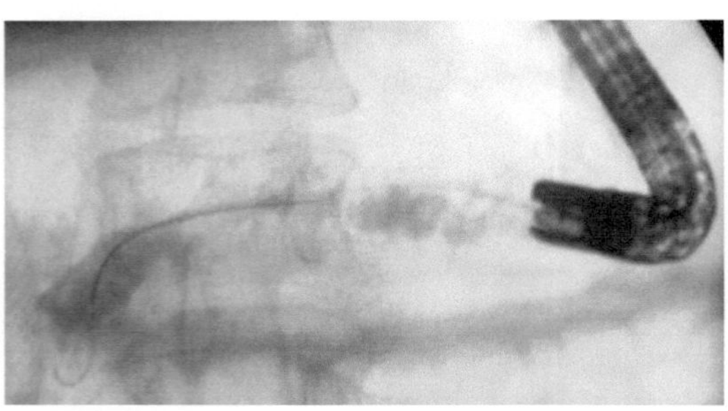

Fig. 11.3 EUS-guided access of a dilated pancreatic duct in an antegrade fashion

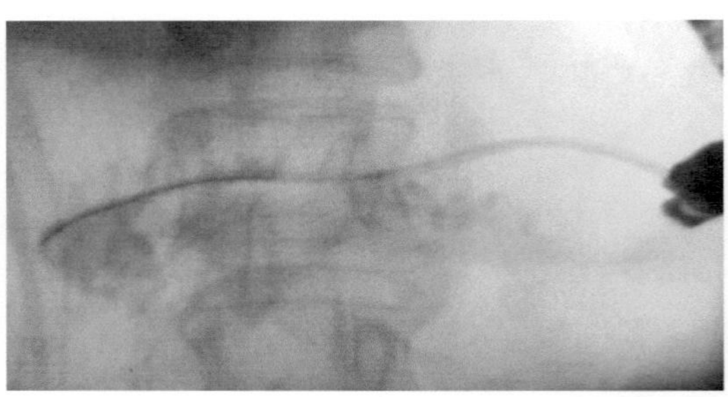

Fig. 11.4 EUS-guided placement of a 7 Fr double pigtail in an antegrade fashion

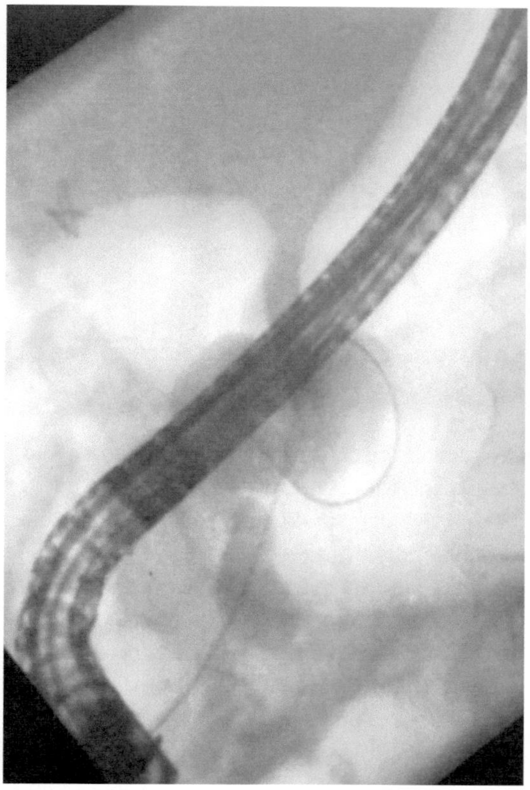

Fig. 11.5 Pancreatogram showing pancreatic stricture following pancreaticojejunostomy

Plastic Pancreatic Stents

Plastic pancreatic stents are mainly polyethylene and come with a single pigtail tailored to shape the pancreatic duct. They are usually good for 2–3 months before occlusion depending on the pancreatic condition. They have different sizes ranging from 5 to 10 Fr; however, the smaller diameter stent has been associated with recurrence of symptoms compared with a larger size (i.e., the 10 Fr). The choice of stent is highly affected by the degree of the stricture, location, and the diameter of the main pancreatic duct. In general, ESGE has recommended placing a 10 Fr for dominant stricture with frequent exchange for one year, regardless of the patient's symptoms. The insertion of multiple pancreatic stents side by side is a feasible option especially when the stricture persists for more than one year.

The overall efficacy of pancreatic stent placement for dominant strictures has a technical success in 72%–100% with resolution of pancreatic pain in 75%–94% of cases. The long-term outcomes have been reported as 52%–74%. The results of these studies are summarized in Table 11.1 [18, 19].

Table 11.1 Data on using plastic stents for benign pancreatic stricture

Author	Patinet's number	Technical success (%)	Immidtae clinical reponse (%)	Long term clinical response	Duration of the follow up (months)
Cremer et al. (1991) [11]	75	98.6	94	52	37
Rösch et al. (2002) [12]	478	72	N/A	63	52
Vitale et al. (2004) [13]	89	100	83	63	43
Fleftherladis et al. (2005) [14]	100	100	100	70	69
Cosamagna et al. (2006) [15]	13	100	100	84	38
Weber et al. (2007) [16]	17	89	89	83	24
Sauer et al. (2009) [17]	163	NA	NA	56	36

The decision to terminate pancreatic stenting can be considered when adequate contrast drainage from the pancreatic duct within 1–2 min following contrast injection at the upstream location from the stricture. The passage of 6 Fr catheter through the stricture with no resistance is another indicator to terminate stenting. The relapse rate following stents removal has been reported in up to one third of the patients and management of the relapse including restenting but should be discussed at the level of a multidisciplinary team considering the underlying etiology, the patient's comorbidities, and preferences [13, 20–22].

The predictors for successful endostenting therapy include alcohol and smoking cessation, location of the PDS in the head, shorter duration of symptoms with fewer attachments prior to endoscopic therapy, and the clearance of pancreatic duct stones if present (Table 11.2).

Fully Covered Metal Stent

Temporary placement of FCSEMS has been reported to be safe and achieved a resolution of main pancreatic stricture in most of the patients. The use of metal stents has been limited to refractory pancreatic stricture. Migration and de novo stricture have been seen in 31% and 16%, respectively [24, 25].

A recent study for the use of FCSEMS with long-term follow up has shown feasibility with resolution of the symptoms at 3 years follow-up in up to 90% of the patients. However, migration, despite the small number of patients, was up to 47% which was higher than previously reported. The use of uncovered SEMSs has been limited and is not recommended [1, 2].

Endosonography-Guided Access and Drainage of the MPD

Despite the current success with endoscopic retrograde pancreatography with stent placement for the management of benign pancreatic stricture, technical failure may occur mainly due to failed cannulation of the pancreatic duct or the inability to pass the stricture. These cases remain challenging to endoscopists. EUS-guided pancreatic duct drainage (EUS-PD) is another endoscopic solution that offers a minimally invasive alternative therapeutic option. EUS-PD has been evaluated and has shown to be a reasonable technical and clinical success. In one review of 222 patients, the technical success was achieved in 70%–80% using a rendezvous technique or intergrade with clinical success ranging between 70% and 90% which was defined as a resolution of symptoms [31–37].

Table 11.2 Data on using fully covered self-expandable metal stents for benign pancreatic stricture

Author	Number of patients	Technical success (%)	Clinical response (%)	Duration of the stent placement (months)	Duration of the follow up (months)
Park et al. (2008) [23]	13	100	100	2	5
Sauer et al. (2008) [24]	6	100	66	3	8
Moon et al. (2010) [25]	32	100	100	5	20
Akbar et al. (2012) [26]	9	100	90	NA	18
Giacino et al. (2012) [27]	10	100	90	NA	19.8
Landi et al. (2016) [28]	15	100	54	6	18.5
Ogura et al. (2016) [29]	13	100	92	5.7	8.6
Matsubara et al. (2016) [30]	10	100	70	3	35

Complications have been reported in up to 40% of patients, which includes pain, bleeding, hematoma, perforation, and severe pancreatitis [35–37].

EUS-PD is indicated in symptomatic patients who have failed conventional ERP. Due to the complexity of the procedure, it is recommended that this procedure be performed at a tertiary center with expertise in therapeutic EUS.

Pancreatic Duct Strictures Following Pancreatoduodenectomy

Patients with main pancreatic duct stricture following pancreatoenteric anastomosis is common up to 30% following pancreaticogastrostomy and up to 10% following pancreaticojejunostomy. Patients may present with recurrent abdominal pain, dilated pancreatic duct, and acute or recurrent pancreatitis. Endoscopy role remains is the first line for decompression and stenting [38–40].

Surgery

For patients that do not respond to endoscopic therapy, surgery remains an option which could provide adequate outcomes in terms of pain control, quality of life, and symptom control in a selected group of patients. Surgical management includes partial tail resection, Whipple, Berger, and Frey procedures [41]. Finally, the last decade has seen the rise of islet cell transplant in patients with preserved endocrine function [42].

References

1. Dumonceau JM, Delhaye M, Tringali A, et al. Endoscopic treatment of chronic pancreatitis: European Society of Gastrointestinal Endoscopy (ESGE) clinical guideline. Endoscopy. 2012;44:784–800.
2. Dominguez-Munoz JE, Drewes AM, Lindkvist B, et al. Recommendations from the United European Gastroenterology evidence-based guidelines for the diagnosis and therapy of chronic pancreatitis. Pancreatology. 2018;18(8):847–54.
3. Cahen DL, Gouma DJ, Nio Y, Rauws EA, Boermeester MA, Busch OR, Stoker J, Laméris JS, Dijkgraaf MG, Huibregtse K, Bruno MJ. Endoscopic versus surgical drainage of the pancreatic duct in chronic pancreatitis. N Engl J Med. 2007;356:676–84. https://doi.org/10.1056/NEJMoa060610. [PMID: 17301298].
4. Dawod E, Kahaleh M. Management of benign and malignant pancreatic duct strictures. Clin Endosc. 2018;51:156–60.
5. Tandan M, et al. Endoscopic therapy in chronic pancreatitis. World J Gastroenterol. 2013;19(37):6156–64.
6. Ell C, Rabenstein T, Schneider HT, Ruppert T, Nicklas M, Bulling D. Safety and efficacy of pancreatic sphincterotomy in chronic pancreatitis. Gastrointest Endosc. 1998;48:244–9.
7. Varadarajulu S, Wilcox CM. Randomized trial comparing needle-knife and pull-sphincterotome techniques for pancreatic sphincterotomy in high-risk patients. Gastrointest Endosc. 2006;64:716–22.
8. Kim MH, Myung SJ, Kim YS, et al. Routine biliary sphincterotomy may not be indispensable for endoscopic pancreatic sphincterotomy. Endoscopy. 1998;30:697–701.
9. Cohen SA, Siegel JH, Kasmin FE. Treatment of pancreatic strictures. Curr Treat Options Gastroenterol. 2007;10:347–54.
10. Oza VM, Kahaleh M. Endoscopic management of chronic pancreatitis. World J Gastrointest Endosc. 2013;5:19–28.
11. Cremer M, Devière J, Delhaye M, Baize M, Vandermeeren A. Stenting in severe chronic pancreatitis: results of medium-term follow-up in seventy-six patients. Endoscopy. 1991;23:171–6.
12. Rösch T, Daniel S, Scholz M, et al. Endoscopic treatment of chronic pancreatitis: a multicenter study of 1000 patients with long-term follow-up. Endoscopy. 2002;34:765–71.
13. Vitale GC, Cothron K, Vitale EA, et al. Role of pancreatic duct stenting in the treatment of chronic pancreatitis. Surg Endosc. 2004;18:1431–4.
14. Eleftherladis N, Dinu F, Delhaye M, et al. Long-term outcome after pancreatic stenting in severe chronic pancreatitis. Endoscopy. 2005;37:223–30.
15. Costamagna G, Bulajic M, Tringali A, et al. Multiple stenting of refractory pancreatic duct strictures in severe chronic pancreatitis: long-term results. Endoscopy. 2006;38:254–9.
16. Weber A, Schneider J, Neu B, et al. Endoscopic stent therapy for patients with chronic pancreatitis: results from a prospective follow-up study. Pancreas. 2007;34:287–94.
17. Sauer BG, Gurka MJ, Ellen K, et al. Effect of pancreatic duct stent diameter on hospitalization in chronic pancreatitis: does size matter? Pancreas. 2009;38:728–31.
18. Nguyen-Tang T, Dumonceau J-M. Endoscopic treatment in chronic pancreatitis, timing, duration and type of intervention. Best Pract Res Clin Gastroenterol. 2010;24:281–98.

19. Ponchon T, Bory RM, Hedelius F, et al. Endoscopic stenting for pain relief in chronic pancreatitis: results of a standardized protocol. Gastrointest Endosc. 1995;42:452–6.
20. Smits ME, Badiga SM, Rauws EA, et al. Long-term results of pancreatic stents in chronic pancreatitis. Gastrointest Endosc. 1995;42:461–467 61.
21. Morgan DE, Smith JK, Hawkins K, et al. Endoscopic stent therapy in advanced chronic pancreatitis: relationships between ductal changes, clinical response, and stent patency. Am J Gastroenterol. 2003;98:821–6.
22. Costamagna G, Bulajic M, Tringali A, et al. Multiple stenting of refractory pancreatic duct strictures in severe chronic pancreatitis: long-term results. Endoscopy. 2006;38:254–9.
23. Park DH, Kim MH, Moon SH, Lee SS, Seo DW, Lee SK. Feasibility and safety of placement of a newly designed, fully covered self-expandable metal stent for refractory benign pancreatic ductal strictures: a pilot study (with video). Gastrointest Endosc. 2008;68:1182–9.
24. Sauer B, Talreja J, Ellen K, et al. Temporary placement of a fully covered self-expandable metal stent in the pancreatic duct for management of symptomatic refractory chronic pancreatitis: preliminary data (with videos). Gastrointest Endosc. 2008;68:1173–8.
25. Moon S-H, Kim M-H, Park DH, et al. Modified fully covered self-expand- able metal stents with antimigration features for benign pancreatic- duct strictures in advanced chronic pancreatitis, with a focus on the safety profile and reducing migration. Gastrointest Endosc. 2010;72:86–91.
26. Akbar A, Baron TH. Covered self-expanding metal stent use in the pancreatic duct: a case series. Endoscopy. 2012;44:869–73.
27. Giacino C, Grandval P, Laugier R. Fully covered self-expanding metal stents for refractory pancreatic duct strictures in chronic pancreatitis. Endoscopy. 2012;44:874–7.
28. Landi R, Tringali A, Bove V, et al. Fully covered self-expandable metal stents to dilate pancreatic duct strictures due to chronic pancreatitis: a pilot study. Gastrointest Endosc. 2016;83(5 Suppl):AB251–2.
29. Ogura T, Onda S, Takagi W, et al. Placement of a 6 mm, fully covered metal stent for main pancreatic head duct stricture due to chronic pancreatitis: a pilot study (with video). Therap Adv Gastroenterol. 2016;9:722–8.
30. Matsubara S, Sasahira N, Isayama H, et al. Prospective pilot study of fully covered self-expandable metal stents for refractory benign pancreatic duct strictures: long-term outcomes. Endosc Int Open. 2016;4:E1215–22.
31. Chapman C, Waxman I, SiddiquiI U. The basics of when and how to perform EUS-guided pancreatic duct interventions. Clin Endosc. 2016;49:161–7.
32. Mallery S, Matlock J, Freeman ML. EUS-guided rendezvous drainage of obstructed biliary and pancreatic ducts: report of 6 cases. Gastrointest Endosc. 2004;59:100–7.
33. Will U, Fueldner F, Thieme A-K, et al. Transgastric pancreatography and EUS-guided drainage of the pancreatic duct. J Hepato-Biliary-Pancreat Surg. 2007;14:377–82.
34. Tessier G, Bories E, Arvanitakis M, et al. EUS-guided pancreatogastrostomy and pancreatobulbostomy for the treatment of pain in patients with pancreatic ductal dilatation inaccessible for transpapillary endoscopic therapy. Gastrointest Endosc. 2007;65:233–41.
35. François E, Kahaleh M, Giovannini M, Matos C, Devière J. EUS-guided pancreaticogastrostomy. Gastrointest Endosc. 2002;56:128–33.
36. Brauer BC, Chen YK, Fukami N, Shah RJ. Single-operator EUS-guided cholangiopancreatography for di cult pancreaticobiliary access (with video). Gastrointest Endosc. 2009;70:471–9.
37. Tyberg A, Sharaiha RZ, Kedia P, et al. EUS-guided pancreatic drainage for pancreatic strictures a er failed ERCP: a multicenter international collaborative study. Gastrointest Endosc. 2017;85:164–9.
38. Takano S, Ito Y, Oishi H, et al. A retrospective analysis of 88 patients with pancreaticogastrostomy after pancreaticoduodenectomy. Hepato-gastroenterology. 2000;47:1454–7.
39. Kikuyama M, Itoi T, Ota Y, et al. Therapeutic endoscopy for stenotic pancreatodigestive tract anastomosis after pancreatoduodenectomy (with videos). Gastrointest Endosc. 2011;73:376–82.
40. Kurihara T, Itoi T, Sofuni A, Itokawa F, Moriyasu F. Endoscopic ultrasonography-guided pancreatic duct drainage after failed endoscopic retro grade cholangiopancreatography in patients with malignant and benign pancreatic duct obstructions. Dig Endosc. 2013;25(Suppl 2):109–16.
41. Bellon E, Roswora MD, Melling N, Grotelueschen R, Grupp K, Reeh M, Ghadban T, Izbicki JR, Bachmann K. Duodenum-preserving pancreatic head resection: a retrospective analysis of the Hamburg modification. Surgery. 2019;165:938–45.
42. McEachron KR, Bellin MD. Total pancreatectomy and islet autotransplantation for chronic and recurrent acute pancreatitis. Curr Opin Gastroenterol. 2018;34:367–73.

Functional Biliary Stents

12

Jin-Seok Park, Seok Jeong, and Don Haeng Lee

Introduction

Since the last decade, stents have been used as a safe and effective alternative to surgery or repetitive endoscopic procedures to improve the quality of life for patients with malignant biliary obstruction. Indications for the use of stenting have gradually expanded to include a variety of malignant strictures, external compressions of the biliary tract, and selected cases of benign stricture that are resistant to repeated balloon dilation or surgical bougienage [5–7]. However, a significant number of patients still require re-intervention for stent malfunctions, including obstruction, migration, and other related complications [8]. Therefore, studies are ongoing to enhance the functions of stents, strengthen their merits, and reduce their drawbacks. In recent years, considerable advances have been made in the design of these stents, and several types of high-quality devices have been developed. Moreover, various functional stents are being developed to serve a diverse range of purposes, including anti-migratory stents, drug-eluting stents, radioactive stents, and easily removable or shape-modifying stents, and bioabsorbable stent. In this review, we describe an update on the most recent technologies.

J.-S. Park · S. Jeong · D. H. Lee (✉)
Department of Internal Medicine, Inha University School of Medicine, Incheon, South Korea
e-mail: ldh@inha.ac.kr

Anti-migratory Stents

Since the self-expandable metal stent (SEMS) has an especially long patency compared with those of plastic stent, it is widely recognized to be an effective standard biliary endoprosthesis [9–11]. Full-covered SEMS (FCSEMS) have also been developed to prevent tumor ingrowth through the stent mesh and to prolong the stent patency. Although FCSEMSs show longer patency than uncovered SEMS, they associated with significantly higher rate of stent migration [12, 13]. With this regard, several newly designed stents aimed at preventing FCSEMS migration have been developed. An anchoring component, such as anchoring fin, flared ends, and anchoring flaps, is typical of these recent designs. Among studies on stent with anchoring fin to prevent stent migration, Mahajan et al. reported a study on FCSEMS covered with Gore-Tex expanded polytetrafluoroethylene (Viabil; Conmed, Utica, NY, USA) [14]. This stent has serrated anchoring pin protruding from a section of the stent, contributing to potent anti-migratory effect. The FCSEMS with anchoring fin show high biliary stricture resolution rate (83%) and significantly stifling its migration. However, stent removal was difficult, and biliary mucosal ulcer and hemorrhage after the stent removal were found on cholangioscopic examination. A flared end is a commonly used technique to prevent migration, which has an expanded shape at both ends that

D. K. Lee (ed.), *Advanced ERCP for Complicated and Refractory Biliary and Pancreatic Diseases*,
https://doi.org/10.1007/978-981-13-0608-2_12

prevents migration while allowing for easier removal. In a small size study, the flared end FCSEMS (Niti-S; Taewoong Medical, Goyang, Korea) showed superior efficacy and a lower migration rate than conventional FCSEMS [15] (Fig. 12.1).

A study using the anchoring-flap fully covered metal stent (M.I. Tech; Seoul, South Korea) which has four anti-migrating flaps at the proximal end that prevent distal migration by Park et al. [16] reported excellent results for the prevention of migration (0% for 6 month). In this study, the investigators also compared the anti-migration effect of the anchoring flap and flared end and found that none of the 22 patients in the anchoring flap group had stent migration, compared with 33% of patients (7 of 21, 1 proximal and 6 distal) in the flared end group ($P = 0.004$). They thus concluded that the anchoring flap is superior to the flared end with regard to stent migration.

Drug-Eluting Stent (DES)

Biliary metal stenting is an effective means of relieving obstruction and is the preferred method of palliating patients with malignancy [17]. Malignant obstructions in particular cause high stent obstruction rate, despite the relatively short lifespan of patients with biliary tract cancers [18, 19]. Stent failure is associated with recurrent morbidity and often necessitates repeat endoscopy with stent retrieval and replacement [10]. These procedures carry an increased risk for procedural complication such as pancreatitis and can result in additional hospital admissions. Stent failure can be stratified into four primary etiologies: internal stent failure from biliary clogging, external failure caused by tumor ingrowth or overgrowth of excessive epithelial or malignant cells, and stent migration, and stent migration [20]. In this literature, the use of stent drug elution as prophylaxis agent to internal and external failure of stent will be addressed.

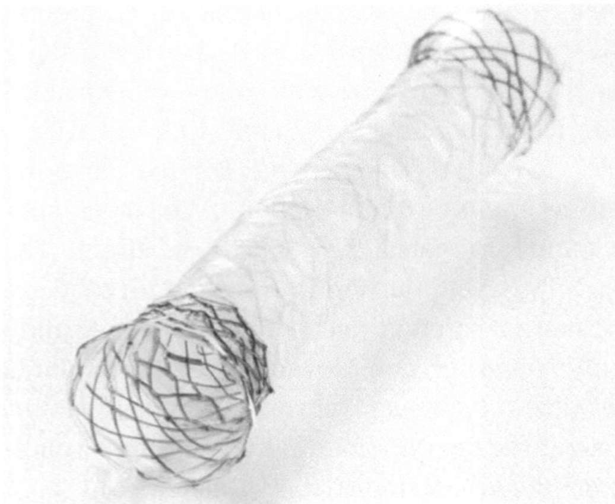

Fig. 12.1 Fully covered self-expandable metal stent attached with antimigratory flare ends. (Adapted from http://www.stent.net, with permission from Taewoong [66])

Drug-Eluting Stent for Internal Stent Failure

Internal stent failure results from the accumulation of obstructing material in the stent lumen. It is a complex process involving microbial colonization and biofilm generation. After stent placement across the papilla, reflux of intestinal content and bacteria into biliary system is allowed, and biliary stents are quickly colonized by a diverse polymicrobial community [21]. Aerobic and anaerobic bacteria are readily isolated from occluded biliary stents with Enterococcus, *Escherichia coli*, and Klebsiella being the most common aerobic bacteria isolated from biliary sludge, while Clostridium being the most common anaerobe isolated. Anaerobic bacteria may be the first to attach and may play a crucial role on biofilm initiation [21–24]. Therefore, drug to inhibit bacterial growth including antibiotics can theoretically improve internal failure rates by decreasing bacterial colonization and biofilm formation. Regarding this concept, systemic antibiotics were tried to decrease bacterial colonization. Since 1989, numerous studies were conducted to identify systemic antibiotic treatments which could decrease internal stent failure rates [25, 26]. However, multiple studies and meta-analysis have failed to show a direct benefit from any systemic treatment in decreasing internal failure rates [25–27].

Along with a lack of benefit when given systemically, the locally antibiotics eluting biliary metal stent was studied. However, local eluting antibiotics have also failed to show any benefit. Weickert et al. analyzed the effect of antibiotic elution on internal failure by incubating stents in human bile [28]. Their experiment examined the combined effect of stents combined with hydrophobin and ampicillin/sulbactam, and hydrophobin and levofloxacin showed that neither antibiotic reduced the amount of biofilm generation compared with hydrophobin alone. In 2012, Gwon et al. developed a cefoxitime-eluting stent and for testing in a canine model. Upon both gross inspection and analysis with electron microscopy, they found no effect from cefotaxime in preventing biofilm development [29]. The reasons behind the lack of local antibiotic efficacy may be the selection of resistant organisms in the polymicrobial biliary environment, the inability of antibiotics to permeate through biofilms, or local breakdown and inactivation of antibiotics. Therefore, further evaluation would be warrant to use the antibiotics-eluting stent in clinical practices.

Drug-Eluting Stent for External Stent Failure

Biliary metal stent failures frequently occur due to the ingrowth and overgrowth of tumor cells or benign granulation tissue, despite the stent providing clinical improvement [18]. The ingrowth and overgrowth could cause shorten stent occlusion and restricted patency and result in shortened patient survival [30]. Although covered SEMSs are designed to withstand tumor growth, occlusion is inevitable over time in most cases because the polyurethane used is biodegraded in vivo by hydrolysis, oxidation, and continuous contact with biliary tract content [31]. In addition, from analysis of biopsied obstruction tissue, it was found that 44% of the tissue ingrowth was nonmalignant in nature, suggesting epithelial hyperplasia plays a significant role in stent obstruction [32]. Given these limitations, there have been efforts to develop DESs, which are expected to prolong stent patency by adding antihyperplasia or antitumor functions. Paclitaxel is an extremely potent agent that causes the dose-dependent inhibition of proliferation of human epithelial gallbladder cells, fibroblasts, and pancreatic carcinoma cells in vitro [33]. Because of this inhibitory effect, local delivery of paclitaxel using covered metallic biliary stents is now under investigation at many centers. Lee et al. introduced a metallic stent covered with a paclitaxel-incorporated membrane and conducted a study to evaluate the safety of this device in the porcine bile duct [34]. Lee group also reported new generation of metallic stents covered with a paclitaxel-incorporated membrane using a Pluronic® mixture (MSCPM) was compared prospectively with those of covered metal stents (CMSs) in patients with malignant biliary obstructions. Safety with enhanced local drug delivery of MSCPM was demonstrated in a previous animal study. Although compared with a CMS, the MSCPM did not significantly influence time to RBO or survival duration in patients with malignant biliary obstructions, and MSCPM reduced tumor volume and was used safely in humans [35, 36]. The decision to use paclitaxel was based on bench data from Kalinowski et al. [33] which showed that paclitaxel, inhibited human gallbladder cells, human fibroblasts, and pancreatic cells in a dose-dependent fashion. In this study, results were promising, finding acceptable histologic changes. Epithelial denudation, mucin hypersecretion, and epithelial metaplasia were noted in the bile ducts that were in contact with stents containing paclitaxel, and no significant complications including transmural necrosis and perforation occurred. With these results, the investigators concluded that a paclitaxel-incorporated metallic stent can be safely used in the normal bile duct. Another study regarding local delivery into the bile duct compared paclitaxel-eluting SEMS and control stents [37]. Even though mucosal hyperplasia was noted in three of six dogs in the paclitaxel-eluting SEMS group, all experimental animals survived until death without evidence of jaundice. The group concluded that paclitaxel-eluting SEMSs are safe in normal canine biliary tracts and do not exhibit technical difficulties. As regards these positive results in animal studies, several human studies followed, a few of which demonstrated the antitumor effect of paclitaxel-eluting SEMS [38]. However, recent prospective comparative studies using a metallic stent covered with a paclitaxel-incorporated membrane did not show significant differences between paclitaxel-eluting SEMS and conventional FCSEMS when it comes to stent patency or patient survival [35, 39]. Therefore, efforts to improve and demonstrate the effectiveness of DES remain ongoing. One of these efforts entails selecting an adequate antitumor agent depending on the nature of the cancer; in that regard, gemcitabine and 5-fluorouracile (5-FU) have gained attention.

Gemcitabine is the standard chemotherapeutic agent in advanced pancreatic and biliary tract cancer. However, it is hydrophilic and its local delivery is challenging due to the initial burst of the gemcitabine. Prolonged gemcitabine release (over 2 weeks) is also hardly realizable. Therefore, a new design is required to allow longer drug elution throughout a broader contact surface between the stent and tumor that maintains a continuous and slow release of drug. Moon et al. [40] introduced a gemcitabine-eluting stent using pullulan acetate. Pullulan is a natural polysaccharide that can be acetylated to varying degrees to form pullulan acetate, which has a greater drug-loading capacity. When pullulan acetate was layered onto polytetrafluoroethylene and applied as part of a gemcitabine-loaded controlled-release membrane for drug-eluting nonvascular stents, the gemcitabine released lasted for 30 days. In addition, Na et al. [41] reported pullulan acetate-conjugated PDT stent. They designed photosensitizer-embedded self-expanding metal stent (PDT-stent) which allows repeatable photodynamic treatment of cholangiocarcinoma without systemic injection of photosensitizer. Polymeric photosensitizer (pullulan acetate-conjugated pheophorbide A; PPA) was incorporated in self-expanding nonvascular metal stent. Covered SEMS with polymeric photosensitizer functions in palliative treatment for biliary drainage and also has potential as a repeatable and efficient PDT therapy. Chen et al. [42] also reported the prototype of gemcitabine-eluting stent (PDT-chemo stent) in 2014. The stent was made through electrospinning and electrospraying dual processes with an electrical charge to cover the stent with a drug-storing membrane from polymer liquid, and they reported that this stent may provide a new prospect of localized and controlled release treatment for cholangiocarcinoma because drug release on the stent showed regular pattern in drug release study. However, local drug delivery from the DES has a risk of damaging the adjacent normal biliary tract mucosa and causing nontarget organ toxicity and systemic exposure. Various studies are currently still ongoing to determine the type and shape of stent membranes and appropriate drug concentrations to prevent stent-induced adverse events and to allow for longer drug release [42, 43].

Radioactive Stents

As mentioned above, stent dysfunction due to tumor ingrowth or compression is a problem for biliary stenting. External beam radiotherapy has been used to prolong stent patency, however, almost inevitably results in normal tissue toxicity because of the proximity of vital organs [43]. More recently, good results have been reported with the use of a combination of intraluminal ^{192}Ir brachytherapy and stenting. Brachytherapy takes longer to relieve the symptoms of biliary obstruction, while provides longer patency and fewer complications compared with stent placement [44, 45]. The combination of stent insertion and brachytherapy is likely to be a feasible and safe palliative treatment strategy in patients with unresectable cholangiocarcinoma. Therefore, radioactive stents have been developed with the aim of combining the advantages of the immediate relief of biliary obstruction by stent insertion with the longer-term benefits achieved through brachytherapy. Radioactive stents contain attached ^{125}I seeds, a radioactive material. The inside of the stent comprises a conventional metal stent to facilitate insertion. Results from a randomized controlled clinical trial with 12 patients in the radioactive stent (stent loaded with ^{125}I seeds) group versus 12 patients in the conventional stent group showed encouraging results in terms of clinical outcomes and stent patent period. The jaundice and pruritus disappeared, and the performance status was markedly improved in all patients with radioactive stent group. The median and mean overall survivals in the irradiation stent group were significantly higher than those in the control group (7.40 months vs. 2.50 months, 8.03 months vs. 3.36 months, $P = 0.006$) [46]. In addition to this study, almost all studies on radioactive stents in biliary malignant obstruction reported that radioactive stents were relatively safe and easy to apply [47–49]. However, these previous investigations involved too small a sample size to determine safety and feasibility. In addition, seed activity, reference point of prescription dose, and the irradiation dose of target were different in the related studies. Therefore, comparison of clinical efficacy among different studies becomes difficult. The American Association of Physicists in Medicine recommend that, for each type of radioactive stent (i.e., of various lengths, diameters, and activities), the 3D dose distributions should be carefully determined before clinical application [50]. Therefore, large-scale studies are required before clinical application.

Anti-reflux Stent

In inoperable biliary tract cancers, SEMSs provide long-term biliary tract patency and relieve progressive symptoms of biliary obstruction as they have larger lumens than plastic stents as mentioned previously. However, refluxed content through the SEMS can cause various diseases including ascending cholangitis due to duodenobiliary reflux, and also it could cause stent obstruction by inducing biofilm formation or introducing undigested food. As a result, refluxed content leads to lower the quality of life in the patients [51]. Dua et al. [52] first developed a plastic stent with an anti-reflux valve (ARV) (attaching 4-cm windsock-shaped tubular valve), demonstrating longer patency than that of standard plastic stents. This scenario suggests that duodenobiliary reflux may contribute to stent malfunction. Also, anti-reflux valves do not interfere with antegrade flow, because the complication rates of plastic stents with an anti-reflux valve are similar to that of standard plastic stents. Therefore, there is a growing need for, and interest in, stents designed to prevent reflux. Currently, anti-reflux stents are being developed in which an anti-reflux valve is attached, and studies on SEMS with these valves have been conducted in biliary cancer patients [53, 54] (Fig. 12.2). According to retrospective study reported by Hu el al., metal stent with anti-reflux valve (ARV) was effective to prolong the stent patency. The metal stent with ARV was made by adding 2-cm length silicon membrane on the duodenal side of SEMS and evaluating the efficacy of this stent in 22 patients with distal malignant biliary obstruction [53]. In the results, the median duration of stent patency of this stent was 14 months, with cumulative patency rates at 3, 6, and 12 months of 95%, 74%, and 56%, respectively. Furthermore, Lee et al. [54] also demonstrated the superiority of metal stent with newly designed ARV over the conventionally covered SEMS in patients with unresectable distal malignant biliary obstruction. The anti-reflux stent consists of an SEMS partially covered by an e-polytetrafluoroethylene (ePTFE) membrane that extends as a pliable tube beyond the distal end of the stent creating a windsock-type ARV. The length of the valve portion is 20 mm. On the results of this study, overall reflux of barium was significantly lower in the metal stent with ARV group than the covered SEMS group (7.7% vs. 100%, $P < 0.001$). The cumulative duration of stent patency was significantly longer in the metal stent with ARV group than in the covered SEMS group (median ± SD, 407 ± 92 vs. 220 ± 37 days; $P = 0.013$). However, the results of recently published studies evaluating anti-reflux stents were not always positive because the attached valve often malfunctioned depending on its design [55, 56]. Hamada et al. [56] conducted a pilot study for the evaluation of feasibility of metal stents with ARV in 13 patients with unresectable distal malignant biliary obstruction. Although the patency of metal stent with ARV was longer than that of SEMS, stent

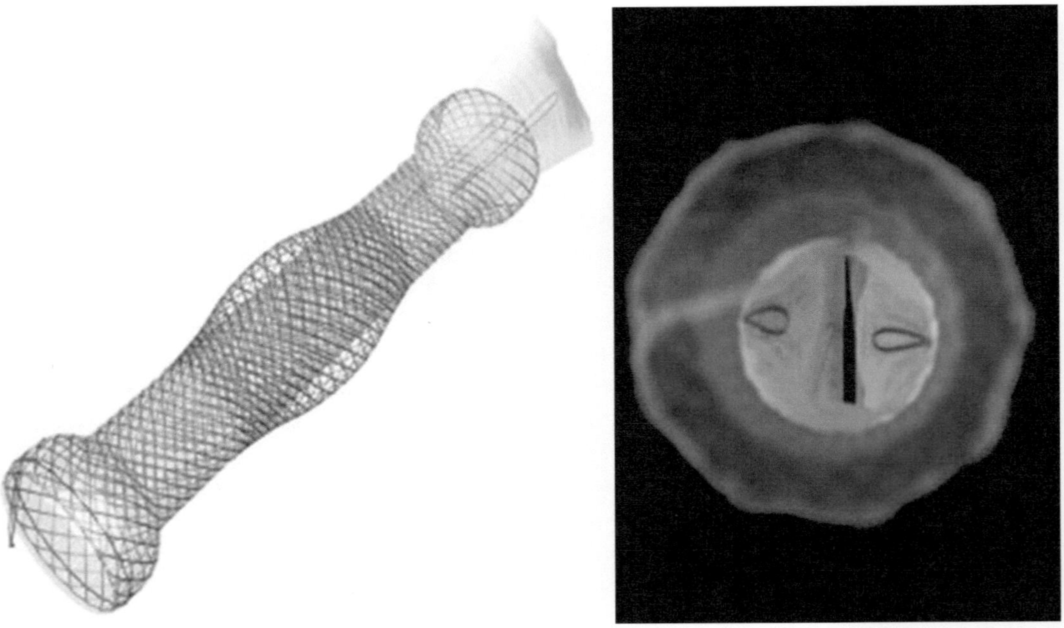

Fig. 12.2 Anti-reflux fully covered self-expandable metal stent. FCSEMS attached with anti-reflux valve at distal end for preventing reflux of contents. (Adapted from http://www.stent.net, with permission from Taewoong [66])

occlusion rate is high (15%), and stent migration frequently occurred (31%). Anti-reflux valves designed to minimize the risk of stent malfunction led to decreased efficacy against reflux; however, those designed for greater resistance is able to be interfered with natural stent patency. Therefore, a more optimal anti-reflux valve design is still required.

Shape-Modified Stent

Modification of stent design is one of the strategies to reduce adverse events of stent and to improve stent function and patency. In a condition of short stricture including anastomotic stenosis after liver transplantation or hilar bile duct stricture, long SEMS may cause tissue necrosis and fibrosis due to pressure injuries to normal biliary tract, and short SEMS may increase the risk of stent migration. To overcome these flaws, several modifications of stent design were studied. One of the interesting shape-modified stents is a dumbbell-type covered SEMS (BONASTENT M-Intraductal, Standard Sci-Tech Inc., Seoul, South Korea) which has narrower waist to prevent stent migration [57]. Both ends of this stent are covered with a silicone membrane to create efficient flare. These stents have a convex margin at both ends to prevent tissue hyperplasia, and the central portion of 12 cm has a cross-wired structure and smaller diameter at the waist, whereas the remainder has a fixed hook and a cross-wired structure. This stent has a long lasso for easier removal of the stent as occasion demands. Moon et al. [57] studied with Dumbbell-type FCSEMS for the treatment of benign biliary strictures. In this study, Dumbbell-type FCSEMS were deployed above the papilla in 21 patients with benign biliary strictures and removed from all of them despite migration in four. None of their patients developed stent-induced ductal change. They concluded dumbbell-type FCSEMS can prevent stent migration and stent-induced ductal change and can be deployed above the papilla.

This shape modification conferred clinical benefit in endoscopic ultrasound-guided procedure also (Fig. 12.3). Because endoscopic ultrasound (EUS) is frequently utilized for stent insertion, modification of the stent shape is also

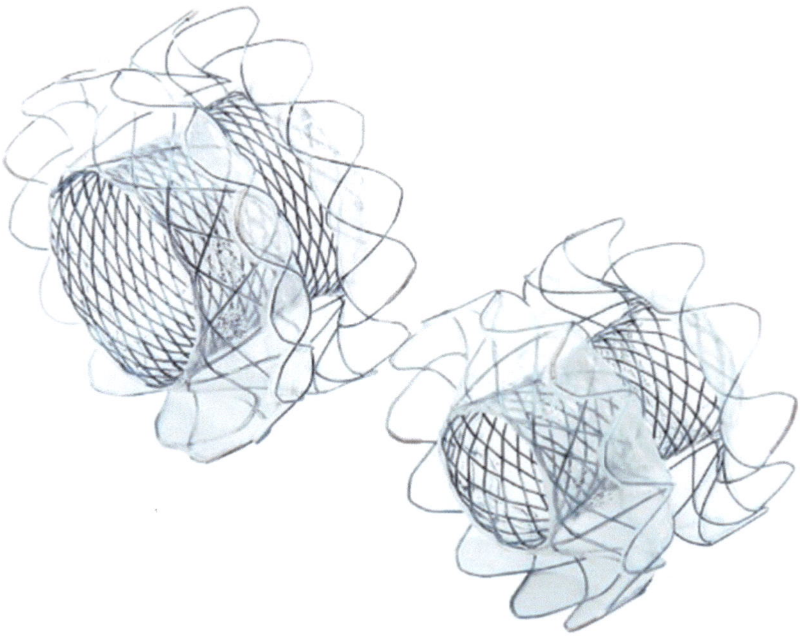

Fig. 12.3 A shape-modifying fully covered self-expandable metal stent for endoscopic ultrasound procedure. (Adapted from http://www.stent.net, with permission from Taewoong [66])

required for a successful procedure. Because conventional SEMS has a high risk of migration and bile leakage during EUS-guided gallbladder drainage, modified SEMS have been developed to avoid these complications by means of a dumbbell-shape modification (AXIOS stent: Xlumena Inc.; Mountain View, CA, USA). In one case study reporting clinical results, AXIOS stents showed high technical success (84.61%) and clinical success (100%) rates with respect to gallbladder drainage, and major complications did not occur [58]. The effort for developing effective shape modification to improve stent is underway still, and these efforts achieve the desired result and provide valuable information for future modifications of biliary stent shapes.

Biodegradable Stents

Biodegradable stent has various advantages compared to conventional plastic stent or SEMS. Biodegradable self-expandable stents have larger lumen than plastic stent that allows improved patency rate and reduced biofilm formation. In addition, since the nature of the degradable stent does not require its removal, this scenario can reduce hyperplastic tissue reaction and adverse event associated with stent removal compared to SEMS. Furthermore, the biodegradable stent can be equipped with antibacterial or antitumor agent the same way as drug-eluting stent [59]. These stents consist of a braided structure of filaments made of absorbable polylactic acid polymers. Currently, stents constructed from biodegradable materials are one of the ideal tools for treating benign strictures. The initial use of biodegradable stents was in the digestive tract, and its first indications were for benign esophageal and colonic stricture [60, 61] (biodegradable). Fry et al. [62] reported a case treated with a biodegradable esophageal stent (AB-esophacoil: Instent; Eden Prairie, MN, USA) for benign esophageal strictures due to a radiation injury. The investigators used a self-expanding coil-shaped biodegradable stent, which was effective in alleviating their patient's symptoms. They concluded that coiled-shaped biodegradable stents might be plausible treatment modalities for treating benign esophageal strictures. The first publications referring to the possible use in the bile duct date back to the mid-2000s. Later, several animal studies confirmed their feasibility and absence of deleterious effects in their utilization or degradation; all these studies allowed these stents to be subsequently used in human beings. Recently, Gimenez et al. [63] reported a case series treated with a biodegradable biliary stent (ELLA-CS, s.r.o., Hradec Kralove, Czech Republic) for the management of hepaticojejunostomy stricture. The stent is made of polydioxanone, that is, a semicrystalline, biodegradable polymer of the polyester family. In this study, 16 biodegradable stents were placed in 13 patients with hepaticojejunostomy strictures secondary to bile duct repair of a biliary surgical injury, and 84.6% of stricture resolution rate was reported with a mean follow-up of 20 months without recurrence. In addition, promising results of biodegradable stent in benign biliary stricture were reported in some animal studies and case reports [64, 65]. However, biodegradable stents remain in the investigative stages; thus, long-term follow-up in many more cases should be required to assess the future efficacy of these types of stents.

Conclusion

The role of stenting in the management of patients with biliary tract obstruction has expanded in recent years. Recent advances in stent technology have improved stent patency and reduced stent-induced complications, resulting in an improved quality of life for the patients. However, biliary stents continue to undergo design changes to address their limitations. Further technical refinements and studies to improve and demonstrate their efficacy are needed.

References

1. Huibregtse K, Cheng J, Coene P, et al. Endoscopic placement of expandable metal stents for biliary strictures-a preliminary report on experience with 33 patients. Endoscopy. 1989;21:280–2.
2. Neuhaus H, Hagenmüller F, Classen M. Self-expanding biliary stents: preliminary clinical experience. Endoscopy. 1989;21:225–8.
3. Irving JD, Adam A, Dick R, et al. Gianturco expandable metallic biliary stents: results of a European clinical trial. Radiology. 1989;172:321–6.
4. Dumonceau J, Tringali A, Blero D, et al. Biliary stenting: indications, choice of stents and results: European Society of Gastrointestinal Endoscopy (ESGE) clinical guideline. Endoscopy. 2012;44:277–98.
5. Varadarajulu S, Banerjee S, Barth B, et al. Enteral stents. Gastrointest Endosc. 2011;74:455–64.
6. Pfau PR, Pleskow DK, Banerjee S, et al. Pancreatic and biliary stents. Gastrointest Endosc. 2013;77:319–27.
7. McLoughlin MT, Byrne MF. Endoscopic stenting—where are we now and where can we go? World J Gastroenterol: WJG. 2008;14:3798.
8. Kim JH. Endoscopic stent placement in the palliation of malignant biliary obstruction. Clin Endosc. 2011;44:76–86.
9. Davids PH, Groen AK, Rauws E, et al. Randomised trial of self-expanding metal stents versus polyethylene stents for distal malignant biliary obstruction. Lancet. 1992;340:1488–92.
10. Knyrim K, Wagner H, Pausch J, et al. A prospective, randomized, controlled trial of metal stents for malignant obstruction of the common bile duct. Endoscopy. 1993;25:207–12.
11. Lammer J, Hausegger KA, Fluckiger F, et al. Common bile duct obstruction due to malignancy: treatment with plastic versus metal stents. Radiology. 1996;201:167–72.
12. Isayama H, Komatsu Y, Tsujino T, et al. A prospective randomised study of "covered" versus "uncovered" diamond stents for the management of distal malignant biliary obstruction. Gut. 2004;53:729–34.
13. Park DH, Kim M, Choi JS, et al. Covered versus uncovered wall stent for malignant extrahepatic biliary obstruction: a cohort comparative analysis. Clin Gastroenterol Hepatol. 2006;4:790–6.
14. Mahajan A, Ho H, Sauer B, et al. Temporary placement of fully covered self-expandable metal stents in benign biliary strictures: midterm evaluation (with video). Gastrointest Endosc. 2009;70:303–9.
15. Tringali A, Familiari P, Mutignani M, et al. S1467: self-expandable, removable, fully covered metal stents to dilate common bile duct strictures secondary to chronic pancreatitis: preliminary results. Gastrointest Endosc. 2010;71:AB169–70.
16. Park DH, Lee SS, Lee TH, et al. Anchoring flap versus flared end, fully covered self-expandable metal stents to prevent migration in patients with benign biliary strictures: a multicenter, prospective, comparative pilot study (with videos). Gastrointest Endosc. 2011;73:64–70.
17. Barkay O, Mosler P, Schmitt CM, et al. Effect of endoscopic stenting of malignant bile duct obstruction on quality of life. J Clin Gastroenterol. 2013;47:526–31.
18. Hausegger KA, Kleinert R, Lammer J, et al. Malignant biliary obstruction: histologic findings after treatment with self-expandable stents. Radiology. 1992;185:461–4.
19. Kim HS, Lee DK, Kim HG, et al. Features of malignant biliary obstruction affecting the patency of metallic stents: a multicenter study. Gastrointest Endosc. 2002;55:359–65.

20. Donelli G, Guaglianone E, Di Rosa R, et al. Plastic biliary stent occlusion: factors involved and possible preventive approaches. Clin Med Res. 2007;5:53–60.
21. Sung J, Leung J, Shaffer E, et al. Ascending infection of the biliary tract after surgical sphincterotomy and biliary stenting. J Gastroenterol Hepatol. 1992;7:240–5.
22. Speer AG, Cotton PB, Rode J, et al. Biliary stent blockage with bacterial biofilm: a light and electron microscopy study. Ann Intern Med. 1988;108:546–53.
23. Leung J, Ling T, Kung J, et al. The role of bacteria in the blockage of biliary stents. Gastrointest Endosc. 1988;34:19–22.
24. Di Rosa R, Basoli A, Donelli G, et al. A microbiological and morphological study of blocked biliary stents. Microb Ecol Health Dis. 1999;11:84–8.
25. Barrioz T, Besson I, de Ledinghen V, et al. Randomised trial of prevention of biliary stent occlusion by ursodeoxycholic acid plus norfloxacin. Lancet. 1994;344:581–2.
26. Coene P, Groen A, Davids P, et al. Bile viscosity in patients with biliary drainage: effect of co-trimoxazole and N-acetylcysteine and role in stent clogging. Scand J Gastroenterol. 1994;29:757–63.
27. Smit J, Out M, Groen A, et al. A placebo-controlled study on the efficacy of aspirin and doxycycline in preventing clogging of biliary endoprostheses. Gastrointest Endosc. 1989;35:485–9.
28. Weickert U, Wiesend F, Subkowski T, et al. Optimizing biliary stent patency by coating with hydrophobin alone or hydrophobin and antibiotics or heparin: an in vitro proof of principle study. Adv Med Sci. 2011;56:138–44.
29. Gwon DI, Lee SS, Kim E. Cefotaxime-eluting covered self-expandable stents in a canine biliary model: scanning electron microscopic study of biofilm formation. Acta Radiol. 2012;53:1127–32.
30. Yang MJ, Kim JH, Yoo BM, et al. Partially covered versus uncovered self-expandable nitinol stents with anti-migration properties for the palliation of malignant distal biliary obstruction: a randomized controlled trial. Scand J Gastroenterol. 2015;50:1490–9.
31. Lee DK. Drug-eluting stent in malignant biliary obstruction. J Hepato-Biliary-Pancreat Surg. 2009;16:628–32.
32. Loew BJ, Howell DA, Sanders MK, et al. Comparative performance of uncoated, self-expanding metal biliary stents of different designs in 2 diameters: final results of an international multicenter, randomized, controlled trial. Gastrointest Endosc. 2009;70:445–53.
33. Kalinowski M, Alfke H, Kleb B, et al. Paclitaxel inhibits proliferation of cell lines responsible for metal stent obstruction: possible topical application in malignant bile duct obstructions. Investig Radiol. 2002;37:399–404.
34. Lee DK, Kim HS, Kim K, et al. The effect on porcine bile duct of a metallic stent covered with a paclitaxel-incorporated membrane. Gastrointest Endosc. 2005;61:296–301.
35. Jang SI, Lee SJ, Jeong S, et al. Efficacy of a multiplex paclitaxel emission stent using a pluronic((R)) mixture membrane versus a covered metal stent in malignant biliary obstruction: a prospective randomized comparative study. Gut Liver. 2017;11:567–73.
36. Jang SI, Lee KT, Choi JS, et al. Efficacy of a paclitaxel-eluting biliary metal stent with sodium caprate in malignant biliary obstruction: a prospective randomized comparative study. Endoscopy. 2019;51(9):843–51.
37. Lee SS, Shin JH, Han JM, et al. Histologic influence of paclitaxel-eluting covered metallic stents in a canine biliary model. Gastrointest Endosc. 2009;69:1140–7.
38. Suk KT, Kim JW, Kim HS, et al. Human application of a metallic stent covered with a paclitaxel-incorporated membrane for malignant biliary obstruction: multicenter pilot study. Gastrointest Endosc. 2007;66:798–803.
39. Jang SI, Kim J, You JW, et al. Efficacy of a metallic stent covered with a paclitaxel-incorporated membrane versus a covered metal stent for malignant biliary obstruction: a prospective comparative study. Dig Dis Sci. 2013;58:865–71.
40. Moon S, Yang S, Na K. An acetylated polysaccharide-PTFE membrane-covered stent for the delivery of gemcitabine for treatment of gastrointestinal cancer and related stenosis. Biomaterials. 2011;32:3603–10.
41. Bae B, Yang S, Jeong S, et al. Polymeric photosensitizer-embedded self-expanding metal stent for repeatable endoscopic photodynamic therapy of cholangiocarcinoma. Biomaterials. 2014;35:8487–95.
42. Chen M, Liang P, Chang K, et al. Prototype of biliary drug-eluting stent with photodynamic and chemotherapy using electrospinning. Biomed Eng Online. 2014;13:118.
43. Válek V, Kysela P, Kala Z, et al. Brachytherapy and percutaneous stenting in the treatment of cholangiocarcinoma: a prospective randomised study. Eur J Radiol. 2007;62:175–9.
44. Jain S, Kataria T, Bisht SS, et al. Malignant obstructive jaundice – brachytherapy as a tool for palliation. J Contemp Brachyther. 2013;5:83–8.
45. Mattiucci GC, Autorino R, D'Agostino GR, et al. Chemoradiation and brachytherapy in extrahepatic bile duct carcinoma. Crit Rev Oncol. 2014;90:58–67.
46. Zhu H, Guo J, Zhu G, et al. A novel biliary stent loaded with 125I seeds in patients with malignant biliary obstruction: Preliminary results versus a conventional biliary stent. J Hepatol. 2012;56:1104–11.
47. Yao LH, Wang JJ, Shang C, et al. In vitro dosimetric study of biliary stent loaded with radioactive (125)I seeds. Chin Med J. 2017;130:1093–9.
48. Guo Y, Liu Y, Lu Z, et al. Obstructive component analysis of radioactive stents and common plastic stents in the bile duct. Eur J Gastroenterol Hepatol. 2014;26:795–802.
49. Liu Y, Liu J, Cai Z, et al. A novel approach for treatment of unresectable extrahepatic bile duct carcinoma: design of radioactive stents and an experimental trial in healthy pigs. Gastrointest Endosc. 2009;69:517–24.

50. Nath R, Amols H, Coffey C, et al. Intravascular brachytherapy physics: report of the AAPM Radiation Therapy Committee Task Group no. 60. Med Phys. 1999;26:119–52.
51. Misra SP, Dwivedi M. Reflux of duodenal contents and cholangitis in patients undergoing self-expanding metal stent placement. Gastrointest Endosc. 2009;70:317–21.
52. Dua KS, Reddy ND, Rao VG, et al. Impact of reducing duodenobiliary reflux on biliary stent patency: an in vitro evaluation and a prospective randomized clinical trial that used a biliary stent with an antireflux valve. Gastrointest Endosc. 2007;65:819–28.
53. Hu B, Wang T, Shi Z, et al. A novel antireflux metal stent for the palliation of biliary malignancies: a pilot feasibility study (with video). Gastrointest Endosc. 2011;73:143–8.
54. Lee YN, Moon JH, Choi HJ, et al. Effectiveness of a newly designed antireflux valve metal stent to reduce duodenobiliary reflux in patients with unresectable distal malignant biliary obstruction: a randomized, controlled pilot study (with videos). Gastrointest Endosc. 2016;83:404–12.
55. Kim DU, Kwon C, Kang DH, et al. New antireflux self-expandable metal stent for malignant lower biliary obstruction: In vitro and in vivo preliminary study. Dig Endosc. 2013;25:60–6.
56. Hamada T, Isayama H, Nakai Y, et al. Novel antireflux covered metal stent for recurrent occlusion of biliary metal stents: a pilot study. Dig Endosc. 2014;26:264–9.
57. Moon JH, Choi HJ, Koo HC, et al. Feasibility of placing a modified fully covered self-expandable metal stent above the papilla to minimize stent-induced bile duct injury in patients with refractory benign biliary strictures (with videos). Gastrointest Endosc. 2012;75:1080–5.
58. de la Serna-Higuera C, Pérez-Miranda M, Gil-Simón P, et al. EUS-guided transenteric gallbladder drainage with a new fistula-forming, lumen-apposing metal stent. Gastrointest Endosc. 2013;77:303–8.
59. Kwon CI, Ko KH, Hahm KB, et al. Functional self-expandable metal stents in biliary obstruction. Clin Endosc. 2013;46:515–21.
60. Boland ED, Coleman BD, Barnes CP, et al. Electrospinning polydioxanone for biomedical applications. Acta Biomater. 2005;1:115–23.
61. Janík V, Horák L, Hnaníček J, et al. Biodegradable polydioxanone stents: a new option for therapy-resistant anastomotic strictures of the colon. Eur Radiol. 2011;21:1956.
62. Fry SW, Fleischer DE. Management of a refractory benign esophageal stricture with a new biodegradable stent. Gastrointest Endosc. 1997;45:179–82.
63. Gimenez ME, Palermo M, Houghton E, et al. Biodegradable biliary stents: a new approach for the management of hepaticojejunostomy strictures following bile duct injury. Prospective study. Arq Bras Cir Dig. 2016;29:112–6.
64. Shi J, Lv Y, Yu L, et al. Interest of a new biodegradable stent coated with paclitaxel on anastomotic wound healing after biliary reconstruction. Eur J Gastroenterol Hepatol. 2013;25:1415–23.
65. Siiki A, Sand J, Laukkarinen J. A systematic review of biodegradable biliary stents: promising biocompatibility without stent removal. Eur J Gastroenterol Hepatol. 2018;30:813–8.
66. TaeWoong Medical. Taewoong Niti-S biliary stent. Goyang: TaeWoong Medical; 2012. http://www.stent.net. Accessed 14 Oct 2018.

MIX
Papier aus verantwortungsvollen Quellen
Paper from responsible sources
FSC® C105338

If you have any concerns about our products,
you can contact us on
ProductSafety@springernature.com

In case Publisher is established outside the EU,
the EU authorized representative is:
Springer Nature Customer Service Center GmbH
Europaplatz 3, 69115 Heidelberg, Germany

Printed by Libri Plureos GmbH
in Hamburg, Germany